Asthma as an Inflammatory Disease

ALLERGIC DISEASE AND THERAPY

Series Editor
David G. Tinkelman
Medical College of Georgia,
Augusta, Georgia, and
Atlanta Allergy Clinic,
Atlanta, Georgia

Volume 1 Histamine and H_2 Antagonists in Inflammation and Immunodeficiency, *edited by Ross E. Rocklin*

Volume 2 Asthma as an Inflammatory Disease, *edited by Paul M. O'Byrne*

Volume 3 Childhood Rhinitis and Sinusitis, *edited by Charles K. Naspitz and David G. Tinkleman*

Additional Volumes in Preparation

Asthma as an Inflammatory Disease

Edited by

Paul M. O'Byrne

Ambrose Cardiorespiratory Unit
McMaster University
Hamilton, Ontario, Canada

MARCEL DEKKER, Inc. New York and Basel

Library of Congress Cataloging-in-Publication Data

Asthma as an inflammatory disease / edited by Paul M. O'Byrne.
p. cm. -- (Allergic disease and therapy : v. 2)
ISBN 0-8247-8220-8 (alk. paper)
1. Asthma. 2. Inflammation. 3. Asthma--Pathophysiology.
I. O'Byrne, Paul M. II. Series.
[DNLM: 1. Asthma. 2. Asthma--therapy. 3. Bronchitis. WF 553
A8522]
RC591.A75 1990
616.2'38-dc20
DNLM/DLC
for Library of Congress 89-25931
CIP

This book is printed on acid-free paper.

MARCEL DEKKER, INC.
270 Madison Avenue, New York, New York 10016

Current printing (last digit):
10 9 8 7 6 5 4 3 2 1

PRINTED IN THE UNITED STATES OF AMERICA

Preface

Descriptions of asthma as a disease entity are present in the earliest medical literature from the cultures of Ancient Greece and Egypt. The word ***asthma*** originates from the Greek word meaning "to breathe." While the first accurate description of an attack of asthma was made by Aretaeus of Cappadocia (81-131 AD), Hippocrates, five centuries before, had recognized that asthma "has its own nature and arises from external causes."

Despite these remarkable insights made 25 centuries ago, identification of the "external causes" that cause asthma and the way these stimuli cause asthma remains very incomplete. More than 100 years ago, Blackley recognized that the inhalation of environmental allergens can mimic the symptoms of asthma. As the majority of patients with asthma are sensitized to one or more environmental allergens, it is possible that inhaled allergens are one very important "external cause." Others that have been clearly described include occupational sensitizing agents, viral respiratory infections, and atmospheric pollutant ozone.

Over the past 5 to 10 years, it has been realized that these inhaled stimuli which cause asthma also cause airway inflammation at the same time. However, the idea that airway inflammation may be important in the pathogenesis of asthma has existed much longer. In his textbook, ***The Principles and Practice of Medicine***, published in 1892, Sir William Osler mentions that others have documented severe airway inflammation in patients dying from asthma (for a more complete description see Chapter 2). What is more recent, however, is the understanding that airway inflammation exists in the airways of all asthmatic subjects, even those with mild, stable disease.

This improved understanding of the importance of airway inflammation in the pathogenesis of asthma has changed the way asthma is currently being treated in many countries. The purpose of this volume is to describe the current understanding of the epidemiology, genetics, pathophysiology, and treatment of asthma, with special reference to the ways in which improved understanding of the pathophysiology of asthma has led to improved treatment of asthma. The authors of these chapters have been asked to keep in mind that this volume will be perused by physicians who manage patients with asthma. For this reason, chapters include information on not only the current understanding of specific inflammatory cells and mediators in causing asthma, but also the pharmacology of the various drugs available, the way these drugs should be used to treat both acute and persisting asthma, and the variation in patterns of treatment throughout the world. This hopefully will mean that this text is useful to all physicians and scientists who are interested in this common and continually perplexing disease.

Paul M. O'Byrne

Contents

Contributors

Luigi Allegra, M.D. Interuniversity Center on Cellular and Molecular Mechanisms of Lung Injury, Universities of Brescia, Ferrara, Milan, Padova, and Parma, Italy

K. F. Chung, M.D. Department of Thoracic Medicine, National Heart and Lung Institute, Brompton Hospital, London, England

Donald W. Cockcroft, M.D., F.R.C.P.(C) Section of Respiratory Medicine, University Hospital, Saskatoon, Saskatchewan, Canada

Francis M. C. Cuss, M.D. Respiratory Clinical Research, Schering-Plough Research, Kenilworth, New Jersey

Jerry Dolovich, M.D. Department of Medicine, McMaster University, Hamilton, Ontario, Canada

Michael Duddridge, M.D., MRCP The Chest Unit, Newcastle General Hospital University of Newcastle Upon Tyne, Newcastle Upon Tyne, England

Leonardo M. Fabbri, M.D. Interuniversity Center on Cellular and Molecular Mechanisms of Lung Injury, Universities of Brescia, Ferrara, Milan, Padova, and Parma, Italy

J. Mark Fitzgerald, M.B., MRCP(I), FRCP(C) Department of Medicine, University of British Columbia, Vancouver, British Columbia, Canada

Frederick E. Hargreave, M.D., FRCP (C) Firestone Regional Chest and Allergy Unit, St. Joseph's Hospital, Hamilton, Ontario, Canada

James C. Hogg, M.D. Department of Pathology and Pulmonary Research Laboratory, University of British Columbia, Vancouver, British Columbia, Canada

Russell J. Hopp, D.O. Department of Internal Medicine, Allergic Disease Center, Creighton University School of Medicine, Omaha, Nebraska

Jean-Luc Malo, M.D. Department of Chest Medicine, Hôpital du Sacré-Coeur, Montreal, Quebec, Canada

Cristina E. Mapp, M.D. Interuniversity Center on Cellular and Molecular Mechanisms of Lung Injury, Universities of Brescia, Ferrara, Milan, Padova, and Parma, Italy

Paul M. O'Byrne, M.D. Department of Medicine, Ambrose Cardiorespiratory Unit, McMaster University, Hamilton, Ontario, Canada

E. H. Ramsdale, M.D. Department of Medicine, St. Joseph's Hospital and McMaster University, Hamilton, Ontario, Canada

Marina Saetta, M.D. Interuniversity Center on Cellular and Molecular Mechanisms of Lung Injury, Universities of Brescia, Ferrara, Milan, Padova, and Parma, Italy

Malcolm R. Sears, M.D. Department of Medicine, University of Otago Medical School, Dunedin, New Zealand

Pierre Tessier, M.D., M.Sc. Department of Chest Medicine, Hôpital du Sacré-Coeur, Montreal, Quebec, Canada

Robert G. Townley, M.D. Department of Internal Medicine and Chief, Allergic Disease Center, Creighton University School of Medicine, Omaha, Nebraska

E. Haydn Walters, M.A., D.M., MRCP Chest Unit, Newcastle General Hospital, University of Newcastle Upon Tyne, Newcastle Upon Tyne, England

Asthma as an Inflammatory Disease

1

Pathology of Asthma

JAMES C. HOGG

University of British Columbia
Vancouver, British Columbia, Canada

INTRODUCTION

The concept that the inflammatory response causes the structural changes in the airways of patients who died of asthma was well established in the last century. The following quotation from Osler (1) discussing the pathologic descriptions of asthma shows the list of theories that were then current concerning the pathogenesis of this condition:

(1) That asthma is due to spasm of the bronchial muscles, a theory which has perhaps the largest number of adherents. The original experiments of C.J.B. Williams upon which this is largely based have not however been confirmed of late years.
(2) That the attack is due to swelling of the bronchial mucus membrane hyperemia (Traube), vasomotor turgescence (Webber), diffuse hyperemic swelling (Clark).
(3) That in many cases it is a special form of inflammation of the smaller bronchioles–bronchiolitis, exudative (Curschmann).

Items 2 and 3 on Osler's list clearly show the importance of the inflammatory response in asthma in that the hyperemia and swelling of the bronchial mucus membrane and the exudative bronchiolitis in the more distal airways are direct manifestations of this response. He also indicated the importance of smooth muscle shortening (i.e., spasm) in producing the airways obstruction that characterizes asthma. In this chapter the general characteristics of an inflammatory process in tissue with a mucosal surface are reviewed and discussed in relation to the structural features of the airways in asthma. Some recent studies showing that muscle shortening, which is well within the normal range, can combine with these inflammatory changes in the airway wall and lumen to produce abnormal airways function are then presented. These data suggest that the importance of the inflammatory response in chronic asthma may be that it thickens the submucosa and mucosa of the airway wall and partially or completely fills the lumen with exudate. These changes then act in series with muscle shortening to narrow airway calibre and produce symptoms.

THE STRUCTURAL FEATURES OF THE INFLAMMATORY RESPONSE

Lord Florey (2) credits Burdon-Sanderson with defining inflammation as the response of living tissue to injury. Following this injury, a rapid series of changes occurs in the small blood vessels which increases both blood volume and blood flow. This vascular congestion is associated with an escape of plasma from the vessels and a later migration of cells from the microvessels into the interstitial space. This increase in tissue fluid enhances lymphatic drainage and the balance between exudation from the vessels and drainage by the lymphatics determines the degree of tissue swelling. This acute exudation of fluid and cells into the tissues is followed by a repair phase where disruptions in the epithelium are replaced, new vessels grow into the inflamed area, and connective tissue accumulates in the interstitial space. When the inflammatory stimulus is chronic, the injured tissue shows the changes produced by both the acute exudative and the chronic repair phase of the response which combine to alter the normal structure of the tissue. In tissue such as the airways that are covered by a mucosal surface, the additional changes of epithelial shedding and excessive mucus secretions are added to these basic structural features (2,3).

Mediators of the Inflammatory Response

The mediators of the various events that characterize the inflammatory response to injury are chemical in nature and are derived from three basic sources. The first major source of mediators is the tissue where peroxidation of the arachidonic acid released from the disrupted membranes of damaged cells is an important source of mediators. Other mediators are generated from intact cells that reside in the tissue, such as the mast cells and nerves. The second source of mediators is the plasma which when activated by coming into contact with a foreign surface, produces mediators via several enzymatic cascades. The third source of mediators is from cells that migrate into the tissue in response to injury. The exact chemical nature and specific function of some mediators is known but it is probable that many important mediators of the inflammatory response remain to be discovered; the following account provides only the briefest overview of this complex subject.

Tissue-Derived Mediators

An important group of mediators of the inflammatory reaction is derived from peroxidation of arachidonic acid which is a major constituent of lipid in cell membranes. Arachidonic acid can be metabolized in two ways. The cyclooxygenase pathway involves two unstable endoperoxide intermediates which are metabolized to stable prostaglandins. The lipoxygenase pathway of arachidonic acid peroxidation, on the other hand, produces a family of compounds known as leukotrienes. Leukotrienes C4, D4, and E4 are now known to be identical with slow-reacting substance of anaphylaxis, which has been thought to be an important mediator of the prolonged smooth muscle contraction seen in asthma.

Histamine is formed by decarboxylation of histidine in the granules of mast cells that are distributed throughout the body and can be found in high concentration around the airways, particularly in the distal parts of the lung. An important group of neuropeptides called tachykinins can be generated from nerve endings following antidromic nerve conduction and contribute to the inflammatory process.

Plasma-Derived Mediators

Hageman factor is activated when plasma comes in contact with a foreign surface during the exudative phase of the inflammatory response. Once activated, Hageman factor acts on plasma proenzymes to convert them to their active form. This results in activation of the complement, coagulation, kinin, and fibrinolytic cascades which generate a host of mediators that help to control the exudation of fluid and cells into the inflammatory site.

Mediators Derived from Cells that Migrate into the Tissue

The cell population that migrates into an acutely inflamed area can also contribute a variety of mediators. This applies not only to neutrophils, but also to other cell types such as platelets, eosinophils, monocytes, and lymphocytes. The neutrophil contributes cationic proteins, acid, and neutral proteases from its granules and the membrane of this cell is also capable of generating a superoxide anion, hydroxyl radical, and hydrogen peroxide, which can in turn, react with halide ions and myeloperoxidase to destroy invading bacteria. Monocytes migrating into the tissue can transform to macrophages which are capable of processing antigen and stimulating the proliferation of both T and B lymphocytes which take an active part in the host response. The lymphocytes are capable of releasing a large number of lymphokines which can influence the changes that occur in the tissue.

RELATIONSHIP BETWEEN MEDIATORS AND THE STRUCTURAL CHANGES OF INFLAMMATION

Although our knowledge of inflammatory mediators is growing rapidly, the precise nature of the structural changes that they produce when they are released in the tissue is not. How the individual mediators act, and more importantly, how they interact with each other in living tissue to produce the observed structural changes is poorly understood. Furthermore, as the inflammatory response of tissue to injury is a fundamental survival mechanism of the host, the basic structural and functional changes can probably be produced by a variety of combinations of mediator release. This means that if one pathway were blocked by a specific antagonist, it is very likely that the structural features of the inflammatory response will be produced by pathways of mediator release that are not blocked. Therefore, whether or not an inflammatory airways disease such as asthma can be cured by specific antagonists directed against single mediators remains open to question.

A general summary of the relationship between mediator release and the structural changes in inflamed tissue is presented in Table 1. Immediately after injury, the actual damage to the epithelium and subepithelial structures that result from the insult are less obvious than those that are subsequently produced by the tissues response to the injury. Although pathologists have been unable to visualize many of the mediators that must be released into the tissue, the introduction of monoclonal antibody techniques and the ability to identify the messenger RNA for specific mediators will no doubt improve the ability to correlate structure with function in the future.

The acute vascular events of the inflammatory response (2-4) include changes in blood volume and flow as well as exudation of fluid and cells from the microvessels. The changes in blood volume are readily visualized as congestion, but changes in blood flow must be measured by experiment. Recently (5) it has become possible to measure both blood volume and flow and calculate the transit times through the blood vessels in tissue. This provides information about blood velocity which shows that circulating cells tend to marginate along the walls of the microvessels as the velocity slows. This margination occurs as a preparatory step prior to adherence of the leukocyte to the endothelium and migration from the vascular space into the tissue. Histology provides a sensitive technique for determining the passage of fluid and cells from the vascular to the interstitial space, but this technique is seldom applied in a quantitative fashion to provide exact information about cell and fluid traffic into the tissue.

TABLE 1 Major Events in an Inflammatory Response to Injury

Tissue injury:

Disrupted epithelium and damaged subepithelial structure

Mediator release:

From damaged cells	From activated plasma
Lipid peroxidation of arachidonic acid	Complement system
From resident tissue cells	Kinin system
Mast cells	Fibrinolytic system
Nerve endings	Coagulation system
	From cells migrating into damaged site
	Neutrophils
	Eosinophils
	Monocytes
	Macrophages
	Lymphocytes

Vascular response:

Increased blood volume leading to congestion of the vascular bed and fluid exudation from microvessels. A lesser increase in blood flow causing a longer transit time (volume/flow = time) and slower blood velocity so that leukocytes can adhere to the endothelium in preparation for migration.

Cellular response:

Migration of inflammatory cells from the vessels into the tissue and lumen of the airways.

Repair:

Stimulation of epithelium leading to replacement of disrupted epithelium, goblet cell metaplasia, squamous cell metaplasia, increased amounts of basement membrane formation

Stimulation of subepithelial connective tissue leading to connective tissue deposition and increased smooth muscle

Stimulation of microvessels leading to revascularization of the inflamed tissue

The repair phase of the inflammatory response begins almost immediately after the injury (2,4), but the histological changes only become apparent at a later time. These changes are seen in the airway tissue where there is an increase in the number of microvessels and deposition of connective tissue including an increase in the amount of smooth muscle. In tissue such as the airways, which are covered by a mucosa, there is also epithelial shedding, regeneration of the shedded epithelial cells leads to a thickened basement membrane and mucus hypersecretion (3).

ASTHMA AS AN INFLAMMATORY AIRWAYS DISEASE

The changes that characterize an inflammatory process in tissue covered by a mucosal surface which are reviewed above, have been repeatedly documented in histological studies of asthmatic airways. As already mentioned, they were well known to Osler (1) at the turn of the century and have been confirmed by postmortem studies (6-15) and in tissue obtained at open lung (16) and bronchial biopsy (17). Figure 1 shows an airway from a patient who died of asthma; exudate of fluid and cells from the bronchial microvasculature into the airway wall and lumen can be clearly seen. This exudate contains plasma proteins as well as many inflammatory cells including eosinophils. The epithelium and subepithelium contain mast cells (8,10) and there is goblet cell metaplasia (10), basement membrane thickening (7,8,11), and smooth muscle hypertrophy and hyperplasia (14). In very recent studies using biopsy and bronchoalveolar lavage (18) to investigate mild asthmatics, epithelial and submucosal changes that are consistent with milder forms of the changes seen at postmortem were reported. This study (18) showed an inverse correlation between airway hyperresponsiveness and lavage epithelial cell count and evidence of deposition of collagen below the epithelial basement membrane, mast cell degranulation, mucosal infiltration with eosinophils, and migration of eosinophils and monocytes from vessels to tissue in the asthmatics. These changes are all highly predictable markers of the inflammatory response and suggest that the severity of the inflammatory process correlates with increased airways responsiveness. They (18) also show that inflammatory changes are present early in the course of asthma suggesting that this condition, like many other important disease processes, has a long preclinical phase.

MECHANISM OF AIRWAY NARROWING

The exact mechanism by which the inflammatory changes that are well documented to be present in airways lead to a reversible reduction in airway calibre is less clearly established. Although most studies favor the hypothesis that excess smooth muscle shortening accounts for airway narrowing in asthma, there is surprisingly little evidence to support this view. Studies that have attempted to correlate in vivo airways responsiveness and the ability of airway strips to generate tension in vitro have been disappointing (19-21). Furthermore, recent studies (22) have shown that airways from asthmatics can close with smooth

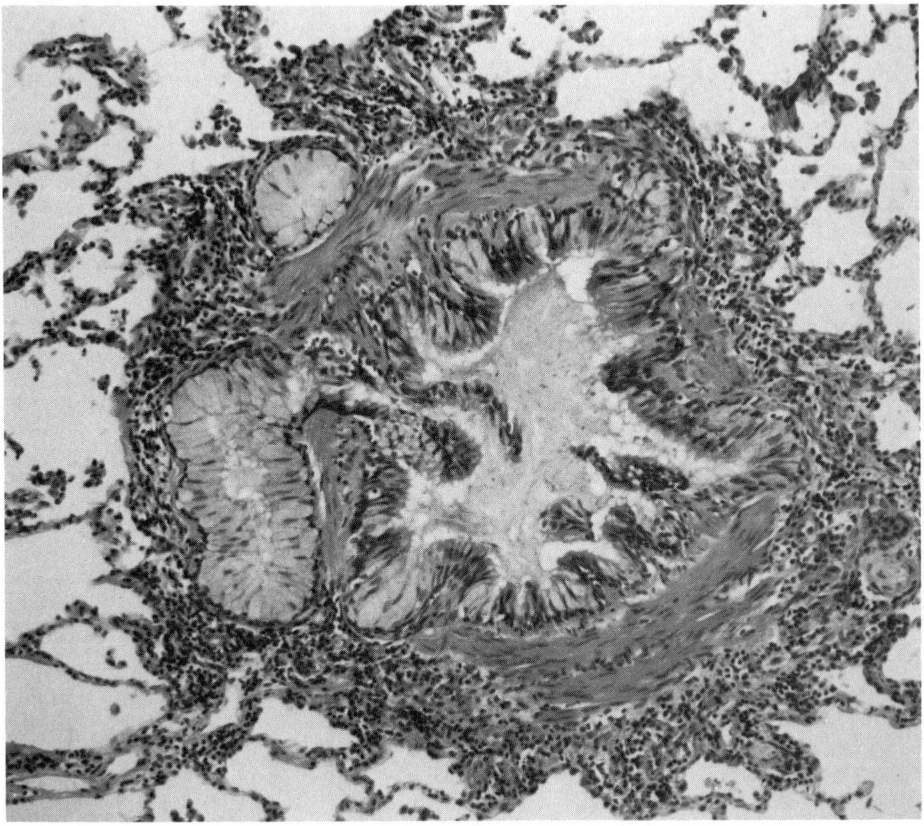

FIGURE 1 A histological section of a bronchiole from a patient who died of asthma showing that the airway wall is thickened and infiltrated by inflammatory cells that are also present in the airways lumen. The epithelium has a large number of goblet cells and the lumen contains an exudate.

muscle shortening that is well within the normal range. This suggests that the airways hyperresponsiveness that characterizes asthma is a property of intact airways and that abnormal airway smooth muscle shortening may not be required to produce the reversible reduction in airway calibre that characterizes asthma.

An alternate hypothesis is that the airway wall thickening associated with the chronic inflammatory process responsible for asthma gives rise to exaggerated changes in airway calibre when the smooth muscle shortens normally (23,24), and a recent analysis of this hypothesis (25) showed that changes in airway wall

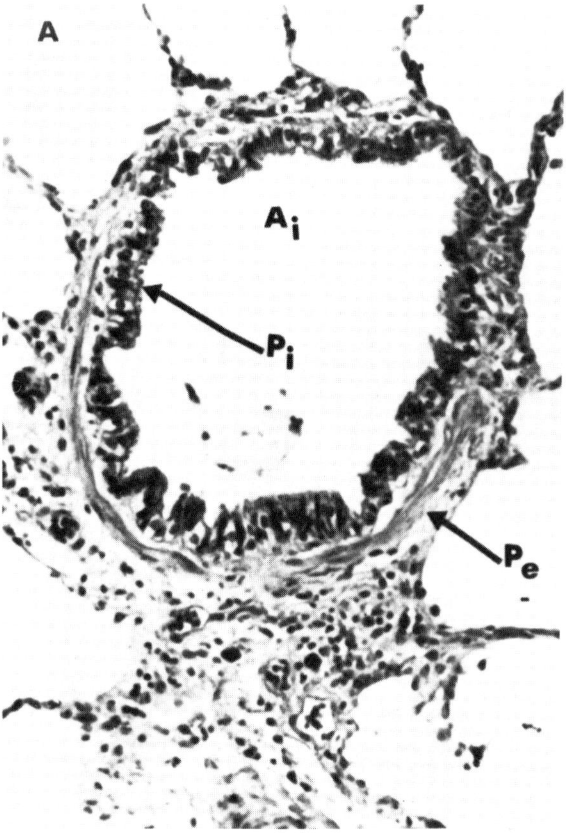

FIGURE 2 The internal perimeter Pi and area of the lumen Ai from an airway represented on two surfaces after the lung had been sliced in half. Half of the lung was incubated in theophylline (A) and the other half in carbachol (B). Note that muscle contraction reduces Ai and folds Pi. (From Ref. 22; photograph courtesy of Dr. Carol Bosken.)

thickness that have little effect on baseline airways resistance can markedly increase airway responsiveness to inhaled agonists as the smooth muscle shortens.

Recent studies from our laboratory have shown that the internal perimeter and wall area of airways remains constant at different degrees of airway smooth muscle shortening (26,27). One study (27) was performed on human lungs obtained from patients who had lobar resection for a solitary peripheral lung

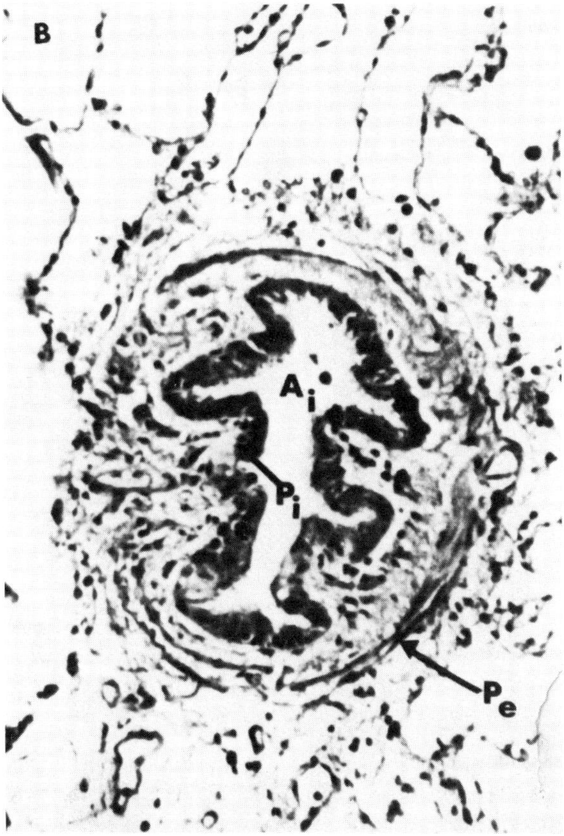

tumor. The resected specimens were inflated with Krebs' solution, bisected in the sagittal plane, and submerged for 30 minutes at room temperature in Krebs' solution containing either supersaturated theophylline or 10^{-3} M carbachol. The Krebs' solution was then replaced with 2.5% buffered glutaraldehyde and the specimens were left in this fixative for 24 hours. After fixation, blocks of tissue containing large and small airways were taken from the apposing cut surface of the specimens to observe the effect of relaxation and contraction on airways from a similar region of the same lung.

The data show (Fig. 2) that treatment of the resected lungs with carbachol 10^{-3} M produced contraction of both large and small airways and caused the lumen area to decrease and the mucosal surface to fold. It also showed that when the square root of WA was plotted against Pi (Fig. 3), there was a linear

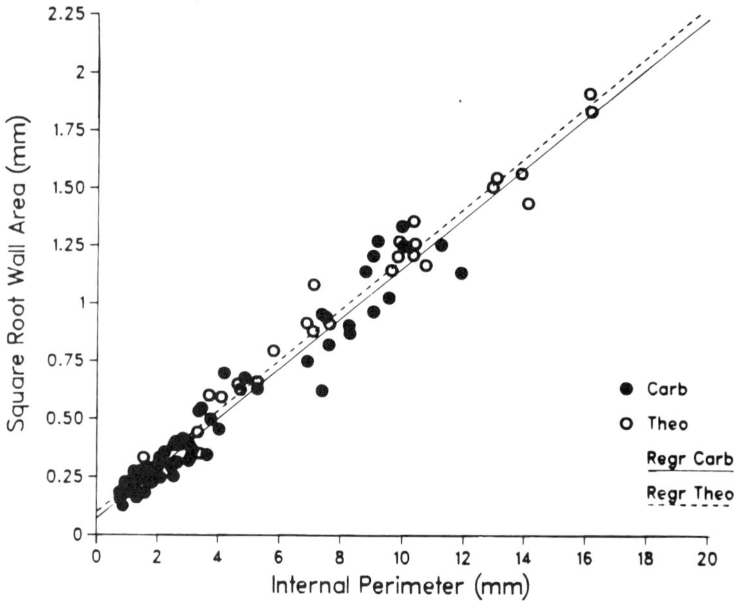

FIGURE 3 Data showing a linear relationship between the square root of wall area and the internal perimeter of airways when they are either contracted with catecholamine or relaxed with theophylline. (From Ref. 27, with permission.)

relationship. In other postmortem studies (22) where 18 human lung specimens from patients with asthma were compared to 23 lung specimens from patients who died suddenly without evidence of chronic or acute lung disease, it was found that the degree of muscle shortening required to produce airway closure was less in the asthmatic subjects. This was because the wall area of airways from asthmatic patients was greater than those of nonasthmatic patients (22) due to an increase in epithelium, submucosa, and muscle. These airways were similar to those in Figure 1 where there was infiltration of inflammatory cells, thickening of the basement membrane, goblet cell metaplasia, and partial occlusion of the lumen with mucus and cellular debris. All of these changes are characteristic of what is known of the pathology of asthma and have been repeatedly demonstrated in structural studies. When the effect of airway wall thickening on airway responsiveness was estimated (Fig. 4) by calculating the increase in airway resistance that occurred as the smooth muscle shortened (22) in a cartilaginous airway > 10 mm in internal perimeter, it showed that smooth muscle shortening of 40% results in approximately a 15-fold increase in resistance in the 'airway' of the nonasthmatic subjects, whereas the same degree of muscle shortening causes approximately a 290-fold increase in resistance in

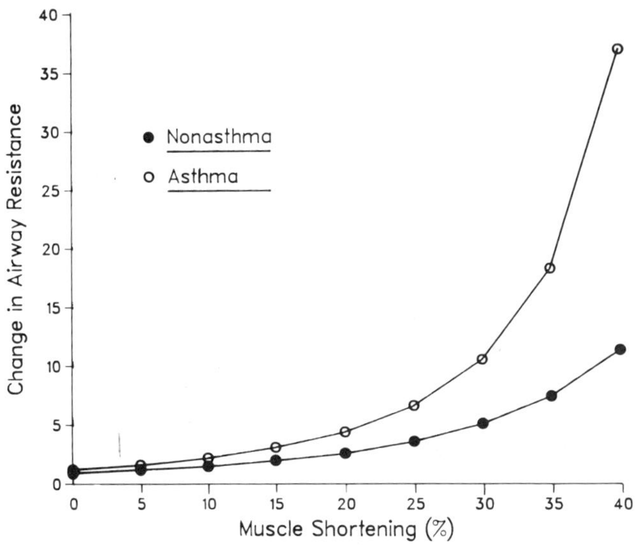

FIGURE 4 Data showing calculated changes in resistance of cartilaginous airways (Pi = 10 mm) using the mean dimensions measured in nonasthmatic and asthmatic subjects. (From Ref. 27, with permission.)

the 'asthmatic airway.' The increase in resistance with 40% smooth muscle shortening for the 'airways' of asthmatic subjects were 256-, 72-, and 37-fold for membranous airways (< 2 mm), membranous airways (> 2 mm), and cartilaginous (> 10 mm) internal perimeter, respectively. Corresponding values for the airways of nonasthmatic subjects were 20-, 13-, and 9-fold increases in the resistance of these airways. This suggests that a thickened airway wall can cause a marked increase in airways resistance with normal smooth muscle shortening by a mechanism that would also account for a rapid reversal of airways resistance if the smooth muscle relaxed. This shows that smooth muscle shortening and relaxation within the normal range can act in series with an airway wall that has been thickened by the inflammatory response to reversibly narrow the airway calibre in a way that would account for the reversible changes in airways resistance that characterizes asthma.

In summary, studies of the structural changes in the airways of asthmatics show changes that are consistent with an inflammatory response. These changes include congestion in the vascular space, exudation of fluid and cells from the vessels into the airway wall and lumen, hypertrophy of the interstitial connective tissue and excess deposition of interstitial matrix and revascularization of the inflamed tissue. Although the increased airways obstruction seen during attacks is often attributed to abnormal smooth muscle shortening, there is little or no evidence that the muscle contracts abnormally (19-21). Therefore, it is reasonable to consider that the major problem of asthmatic airways is the wall thickening that is produced by the chronic inflammatory process. The early studies of Traube, Webber, Clark, and Curschmann quoted by Osler (1) show that these changes were recognized as an important feature of asthma in the last century. More recent studies have confirmed that fluid exudation, cellular infiltration, deposition of connective tissue, hypertrophy of smooth muscle, thickening of the basement membrane, and goblet cell metaplasia of the epithelium are constant features of asthma (6,8-18). These structural changes are fully consistent with an inflammatory process involving tissue with a mucosal surface (2,3), and a recent analysis of this problem (22) suggests that airway walls thickened in this way act in series with smooth muscle shortening to narrow airways calibre. Although therapies designed to relax smooth muscle may be expected to produce a rapid increase in the calibre of the airways narrowed in this way, they are likely to have less lasting value than those designed to reverse the chronic inflammatory process that causes the thickening of the airway wall.

REFERENCES

1. Osler W. *Principles and Practice of Medicine*. Third Edition, 1899.
2. Florey HW. Inflammation. In: *General Pathology*. Lloyd Luke (Medical Books) Ltd., London, 1962; pp. 1-167.
3. Florey HW. Secretion of mucus and inflammation of mucus membranes. In: *General Pathology*. Lloyd Luke (Medical Books) Ltd., London, 1962; pp. 167-197.
4. Taussig MJ. Inflammation. In: *Processes in Pathology and Microbiology*. Blackwell Scientific, Oxford, London, 1984; pp. 3-68.
5. Hogg JC. Neutrophil kinetics and lung injury. Physiol Rev 1987; 67:1249-1295.
6. Huber HL, Koessler KK. The pathology of bronchial asthma. Arch Int Med 1922; 30:689-760.
7. Unger L. Pathology of bronchial asthma. Southern Med J 1945; 38:513-522.
8. Bullen SS. Correlation of clinical and autopsy findings in 176 cases of asthma. J Allergy 1952; 23:193-203.
9. Houston JC, De Vavasquez S, Trounce JR. A clinical and pathological study of fatal cases of status asthmaticus. Thorax 1953; 8:207-213.
10. Dunnill MS. The pathology of asthma with special reference to changes in the bronchial mucosa. J Clin Pathol 1960; 13:27-33.
11. Messer J, Peters GA, Bennett WA. Cause of death and pathological findings in 304 cases of bronchial asthma. Dis Chest 1960; 38:616-624.

12. Richards W, Patrick JR. Death from asthma in children. Am J Dis Child 1965; 110:4–21.
13. Dunnill MS, Massarella GR, Anderson JA. A comparison of the quantitative anatomy of the bronchi in normal subjects, in status asthmaticus, in chronic bronchitis and in emphysema. Thorax 1969; 24:176–9.
14. Heard BE, Hossain S. Hyperplasia of bronchial muscle in asthma. J Pathol 1921; 110:319–331.
15. Takizawa T, Thurlbeck WM. Muscle and mucous gland size in the major bronchi of patients with chronic bronchitis, asthma and asthmatic bronchitis. Am Rev Respir Dis 1971; 104:331–336.
16. Cudz E, Levison H, Cooper DM. Ultrastructure of airways in children with asthma. Histopathology 1978; 2:407–421.
17. Salvato G. Some histological changes in chronic bronchitis and asthma. Thorax 1968; 23:168–172.
18. Beasley R, Roche WR, Roberts JA, Holgate ST. Cellular events in the bronchi in mild asthma and after bronchial provocation. Am Rev Respir Dis 1989; 139:806–817.
19. Vincenc KS, Black JL, Yan K, Armour CL, Donnelly PD, Woolcock AJ. A comparison of in vivo and in vitro responses to histamine in human airway. Am Rev Respir Dis 1983; 128:875–879.
20. Armour CL, Lazar NM, Schellenberg RR, Taylor SM, Chan N, Hogg JC, Pare PD. A comparison of in vivo and in vitro human airway reactivity to histamine. Am Rev Respir Dis 1980; 129:907-910.
21. Cerrina J, Ladurie ML, Labat C, Raffestin B, Bayol A, Brink C. Comparison of human bronchial smooth muscle responses to histamine in vivo with histamine and isoproteronol in vitro. Am Rev Respir Dis 1986; 134:51–61.
22. James AL, Pare PD, Hogg JC. Mechanisms of airway narrowing in asthma. Am Rev Respir Dis 1989; 139:242–6.
23. Freedman BJ. The functional geometry of the bronchi. Bull Physiopathol Resp 1972; 8:545–551.
24. Benson MK. Bronchial hyperreactivity. Br J Dis Chest 1975; 69:227–239.
25. Moreno RH, Hogg JB, Pare PD. Mechanisms of airway narrowing. Am Rev Respir Dis 1986; 133:1171–1180.
26. James AL, Pare PD, Moreno RH, Hogg JC. Quantitative measurement of smooth muscle shortening in the isolated pig trachea. J Appl Physiol 1987; 63:1360–1365.
27. James AL, Hogg JC, Dunn LA, Pare PD. The use of internal perimeter to compare airway size and calculate smooth muscle shortening. Am Rev Respir Dis 1988; 138:136–9.

2

Epidemiology of Asthma

MALCOLM R. SEARS

University of Otago Medical School
Dunedin, New Zealand

Epidemiology may be defined as a science that deals with the incidence, distribution, and control of disease in a population; the sum of the factors controlling the presence or absence of a disease; and the interrelationship of a disease with its environment (1). Unlike epidemiology, asthma cannot yet be precisely defined (2,3), and therein lies a considerable part of the difficulty in summarizing its epidemiology. The literature reporting the incidence, prevalence, and distribution of the condition known as "asthma" and factors influencing its development, expression, and control is growing rapidly. Despite this, the fundamental nature of asthma remains obscure; whether or not asthma is one disease with many inciting and provocative factors modifying its expression, or a syndrome with multiple etiologies and therefore outcomes, continues to be debated.

RECOGNITION OF ASTHMA

Scadding defined asthma as

> a disease characterized by wide variations over short periods of time in resistance to flow in intrapulmonary airways (4).

Increasingly, asthma is referred to as "variable airflow obstruction." Its recognition depends primarily on interpretation of a variable cluster of symptoms; wheeze, cough, chest tightness, and dyspnea. That such symptoms are due to asthma may be firmly established by documentation of variable or reversible airflow obstruction accompanying symptoms (5). Airway hyperresponsiveness to nonallergic stimuli usually accompanies asthma symptoms (6). However, airway hyperresponsiveness is very occasionally absent in some subjects with asthma, and has been present in some children and adults without significant respiratory symptoms (7-10). Hence the presence or absence of airway hyperresponsiveness is less useful as a diagnostic tool for studying the epidemiology of asthma. Although asthma is now regarded as a disease characterized by airway inflammation (11), this concept does not presently translate into criteria which can be readily used for the definition or detection of asthma. Therefore, the most reliable method for determining the presence of asthma for epidemiological purposes remains a carefully taken history, accompanied by objective evidence of variable or reversible airflow obstruction.

The degree of "reversibility" required to diagnose asthma is somewhat arbitrarily defined, for example, a 20% increase in FEV_1 or peak expiratory flow rate occurring either spontaneously or with treatment (12). However, some adult patients with obstructive lung disease due to smoking have symptomatic and objectively documented variations in airflow, although they do not usually show reversibility to normal lung function. On the other hand, an asthmatic who smokes, or who works in a highly polluted atmosphere, may develop less reversible disease. Furthermore, some asthmatics develop irreversible or very poorly reversible disease despite being lifelong nonsmokers (13).

Even in childhood, where adult chronic obstructive lung disease does not confuse the clinical presentation, asthma is not clearly defined (14). Pediatricians usually separate bronchiolitis from asthma (15), as symptoms of bronchiolitis rarely respond to bronchodilator or steroid therapy, yet the clinical features of bronchiolitis in some children are very like those of asthma, and the subsequent course may be similar (16), leading some to recommend that infants with recurrent bronchiolitis should be considered asthmatic (17). Children with cystic fibrosis may develop labile airways with variable airflow rates consistent with asthma (18). Nocturnal or postexercise cough is a common presentation of asthma in childhood (19), but may be misdiagnosed as due to bronchitis or infection.

Several recent studies of the epidemiology of asthma have combined a symptom questionnaire with some means to assess airway responsiveness objectively. Rather than define asthma as the coexistence of relevant symptoms and increased airway responsiveness, it seems wise, in light of present knowledge, to describe these characteristics as separate yet closely related aspects of "asthma."

MORBIDITY FROM ASTHMA

Secular Trends in Childhood

Despite difficulties in precisely defining the condition, studies of the prevalence of "asthma" in childhood in different countries have yielded some remarkably consistent findings. In the United Kingdom (8,20), Canada (21,22), the United States (23), Australia (9,24), and New Zealand (25), ***between 10 and 20%*** of children aged seven to ten years have had significant recurrent respiratory symptoms suggesting asthma. Selected prevalence studies from these and other countries are listed in Table 1.

While recent studies report prevalence rates for asthma considerably higher than rates determined two or three decades ago (26-30), differences in methodology, definitions, and acceptance of the term "asthma" make the true increase in prevalence difficult to quantitate. For example, in New Zealand, a prevalence rate for "asthma" of 0.2% was determined in 1958 from school medical examinations (31); in 1961 a questionnaire mailed to parents yielded a prevalence rate of 1.9% in 5-16-year-old students (31); in 1968, a school survey revealed that 7.1% of 11-13-year-old children had at some time required treatment for asthma (26); in 1973, 5% of 9-year-old children had rhonchi on chest auscultation on the day of examination (27); and in 1979, 7.4% of 7-year-old children were reported to have asthma, while a further 4.8% had a history of wheezing with atopic features strongly suggestive of a diagnosis of asthma, making a total cumulative prevalence of probable asthma of 12.2% (32); a further 22.6%, who reported wheezing and who had weaker or no evidence for an associated atopic disease, were classified as possibly having asthma.

Comparison of some studies suggests that the prevalence of wheezing in childhood has in fact been fairly stable but that recurrent wheezing is now increasingly recognized as asthma. Two early studies in general practices in England found at least 20% of children had had one or more attacks of wheezing during their first 10 years of life (33,34). In Melbourne in 1969, 19.1% of 7-year-old children had had recurrent episodes of wheezing (24). In New Zealand in 1973, 23% of 9-year-old children had a history of one or more attacks of wheezing (27). Among another group of 9-year-old New Zealand children studied in 1981-1982, 18.1% had had more than three wheezing episodes in a year (25). Data from the 1982 Tyneside study of 7-year-old children (81), recalculated to allow for the underestimate of the prevalence of preschool symptoms, suggests that at least 15% had experienced symptoms of asthma, as had 20.5% of 9-year-old Canadian children studied in 1986-1987 (22). Each of these studies found that some two-thirds of wheezing children had not been given the diagnosis of

TABLE 1 Selected Studies of the Prevalence of Asthma and Wheezing in Children in 7 Countries

Country	Year published	Age	Prevalence	Reference
NEW ZEALAND				
Lower Hutt	1969	11–13	7.1% asthma	26
Lower Hutt	1974	9	5% rhonchi, 23% wheeze	27
Lower Hutt	1983	11–13	13.5% asthma	28
Dunedin	1987	9	18.1% wheeze (3/year or more)	25
AUSTRALIA				
Melbourne	1969	7	19.1% wheeze, 11.4% >5 episodes	24
Various cities	1972	6–15	12% male, 8% female	116
Busselton, WA	1974	6–17	6.3% asthma, 14% wheeze	155
South Australia	1986	8	27.4% cumulative (asthma+wheeze)	156
New South Wales	1987	8–10	12.4% asthma, 24.3% wheeze	9
UNITED KINGDOM				
Aberdeen	1969	10–15	4.8%	47
National	1969	11	3.5% asthma, 8.8% wheeze (total 12.3%)	29
Various cities	1972	6–15	9% males, 5% female	116
Tyneside	1983	7	9.3% current, 11.1% cumulative	8
London	1983	9	11.1% current, 18.2% cumulative	20
National	1987	7, 11, 16	current 8.3%, 4.7%, 3.5%, respectively cumulative 18.3%, 21.9%, 24.7%	83
UNITED STATES				
Boston	1980	5–9	9.2% persistent wheeze	23
Baltimore	1982	Gds 1, 6	7.2% current, 10.5% cumulative	46
National	1987	6–11	7.6% asthma and wheeze with colds	37
CANADA				
Hamilton	1986	7–10	4.4% asthma, 21.2% wheezing most days	21
East Halton	1988	9	20.5% wheezing (3/year or more)	22
SWEDEN				
Stockholm	1954	7–14	1.37%	157
NORWAY				
Oslo	1985	7–15	1.6% current, 3.7% cumulative, 9% wheeze	118

"asthma," and so a change in diagnostic fashion could greatly alter the prevalence of reported asthma. In the Tyneside study (8), 96% of children finally considered by the investigators to have asthma were identified by the question "Does your child have attacks of wheezing?"; this question could profitably be used in all future prevalence studies to achieve standardization of methodology.

Other studies, however, suggest that the prevalence of childhood asthma in developed countries has increased. In Birmingham, England, the prevalences of reported "asthma" in studies conducted ten years apart were 1.8% and 2.3%, respectively (30,35). In New Zealand, studies in the same two intermediate schools using identical methodology conducted nine years apart, yielded prevalence rates of "asthma" in 11-13 year olds of 7.1% in 1970 (26) and 13.5% in 1979 (28). A change in attitude toward the diagnostic label "asthma" in addition to change in the ethnic mix of the population in both of these studies combined to cast some doubt on the validity of the extent of the apparent increase in prevalence. In each case, the earlier study underestimated the true prevalence of asthma by not making enquiry regarding "wheezing" or "wheezy bronchitis." A study of general practice consultations in England and Wales at an interval of 10 years (36) suggested that there had been a genuine increase in prevalence of asthma between 1971 and 1981 across all ages; only in the 5-14-year-old age range was there any likelihood that some of the increased prevalence of "asthma" could be explained by diagnostic transfer as reflected in a reduction in prevalence of "acute bronchitis." In the United States, the reported prevalence among children 6 to 11 years old of ever having asthma increased significantly from 4.8% to 7.6% between the first (1971-1974) and second (1976-1980) National Health and Nutrition Examination Surveys (37). In each survey, "asthma" included recurrent wheezing not associated with colds along with physician-diagnosed asthma, making it most unlikely that the 58% increase in prevalence was due simply to a greater acceptance of the label "asthma." On balance, there does appear to have been a real increase in the prevalence of childhood asthma, but the degree is not easily verified, nor the cause known (38).

Substantial increases of recorded hospital admissions for asthma in children in many countries suggest that either prevalence or severity has increased (39). In the United States, admissions for asthma in some regions have increased as much as 300% (40), while nationally, the rate of hospitalization for children under 15 years with asthma increased by at least 145% between 1970 and 1984 (41). Similar increases have been seen in New Zealand (42) and England (43) where admissions increased 167% in 5-14-year-old children over an 8-year period. This rise is partially explained by a doubling of the readmission rate (40,44), suggesting an increase in frequency of severe episodes, but the increase in first admissions also strongly suggests an increase in prevalence.

The increase in hospital admissions for asthma has occurred in the face of a general decline in admission rates for respiratory conditions, and in spite of a considerable increase in the use of antiasthmatic medications (40) suggesting asthma has indeed increased in severity. Dawson (45) reviewed admissions for asthma to one New Zealand pediatric unit over a 20-year period. Not only did the annual number of admissions rise dramatically from 21 (in 17 patients) in 1965 to 186 (122 patients) in 1975 and 609 (374 patients) in 1985, but the severity on admission, as judged by a retrospective scoring system based on wheezing, pulse rate and accessory muscle use also increased considerably between 1975 and 1985.

Risk Factors for Childhood Asthma

Evidence from epidemiological studies indicates that in addition to genetic influences, several environmental factors which cause airway inflammation (irritants, infection, allergic hypersensitivity) may be associated with the development of asthma in children, while psychosocial factors probably are not important.

Genetic Factors

Current evidence indicates the probability that an inherited predisposition to airway hyperresponsiveness and superimposed environmental factors interact to produce the clinical syndrome of asthma. When an atopic predisposition is also inherited, conditions are highly favorable to the emergence of asthma as a clinical condition. The genetics of asthma are more fully discussed in Chapter 4.

Gender

Almost all studies of the prevalence of "asthma" in children have found a male preponderance, ranging from 1.6:1 (46) in the United States to over 2:1 (26) in New Zealand. This ratio is age related, as shown in an Aberdeen study (47) where in 10 year olds, the ratio was 3.3:1, and decreased steadily with each year of age to 1.3:1 in 14-15-year-old adolescents. The male predominance appears related to a greater degree of bronchial lability and not to a greater prevalence of atopy in males (48). The strikingly higher M:F ratio for diagnosed asthma highlights a probable diagnostic bias, namely that wheezing in boys may be more likely to be termed "asthma" than is wheezing in girls.

Ethnicity

Differences in prevalence between races may be due to both genetic and environmental factors. Among children of different races living in the same environment, the prevalence of respiratory symptoms may be very similar. For example, in a large ethnically mixed population in London, England, there were no significant differences in the proportions with a history of wheezing illness between children of European (15%), African (18%), or Indian (17%) extraction, although the European children reported a higher prevalence of croup, whooping cough, and bronchitis (49). The increased prevalence of atopic disease and asthma in Tokelauan Island children relocated in New Zealand, whose prevalence rates now equal those of European New Zealand children, further suggests that environmental factors dominate any genetic differences in the risk of developing asthma (50). In the United States, however, the prevalence of asthma is consistently 50% higher among black children than white children. In a Baltimore study (46), the prevalence in black first-graders was 12.0% while in their white classmates it was 7.9%; in sixth-grade children it was 11.2% and 8.8%, respectively; further, data from the National Health and Nutrition Examination Surveys (37) reports a prevalence of 9.4% in black children compared with 6.2% in white children. This persistent difference suggests significant genetic or ethnic factors influencing expression of asthma, but it is not possible to fully exclude differences in life-style affecting environmental factors despite residence in the same community.

Migration

Migration of children from a rural to an urban environment appears to substantially increase the likelihood of developing asthma. In South Africa, 3.17% of Xhosa children residents of Capetown, but only 0.14% of Xhosa children remaining in rural Transkei, demonstrated exercise-induced asthma (51). More than 25% of children relocated from the Tokelauan Islands in the Pacific to New Zealand had asthma, compared with only 11% of their peers who remained on the islands (50). Such differences are unlikely to be genetic or ethnic in origin, but suggest an added environmental factor resulting in increased expression of asthma symptoms in the new location. Both changes in microbiological flora (and its treatment) and in allergen exposure have been suggested as explanations of these observations.

In some studies, skin tests were more often positive in urban than rural populations (52). The prevalence rates of rhinitis and eczema in Tokelauan Islanders living in New Zealand were 28.3% and 8.5%, respectively, compared with 13.7% and 0.1% in their peers living on the islands (50), suggesting that allergens in the new environment were more potent sensitizing agents, and so may be significant factors in the initiation of asthma as well as provoking rhinitis and eczema.

Atopy

Not only is the expression of asthma in children related to the presence of atopy whether documented by skin tests (53) or elevated serum IgE levels (54), but the persistence of symptoms of wheezing into later childhood is very strongly associated with atopy. A follow-up study of the Tasmanian birth cohort study (55) showed that the presence of atopy manifested by hayfever and eczema in a seven-year-old child with wheeze was associated with a fourfold increase in risk of persistence of asthma to age 20 (56). The likelihood of persistence of asthma may depend on the nature of the allergen sensitivity. In a 5-year follow-up study of 9-14-year-old children in Melbourne, Australia (57), remission of asthma was more likely to occur in those who were sensitive to a perennial allergen, to which they became hyposensitized, for example, house dust mite, whereas sensitivity to intermittent seasonal allergen such as grass pollens was associated with more persistent clinical asthma and immunological hypersensitivity.

Atopic Australian children have an increased risk of having airway hyperresponsiveness, especially those with sensitivity to more than one allergen group (58,59). The severity of the airway hyperresponsiveness increased with the severity of atopy. While this study did not provide any clear evidence for a direct causal link between atopy and airway hyperresponsiveness, there may be a common link in their development. Allergy and asthma is reviewed fully in Chapter 6.

Parental Smoking

There is relatively little information directly relating parental smoking with wheezing illness or asthma in children, but a considerable body of data exist linking parental, especially maternal, smoking with reduction of pulmonary function in older children (60,61) and lower respiratory tract illness in young children (62-64). The latter is of particular interest in view of the reported association between early lower respiratory tract illness and the development of asthma.

The effect of parental respiratory symptoms must be taken into account when interpreting childhood symptoms. Although symptoms were consistently higher in children of current smoking families than nonsmoking families in the Tucson study (65), the correlation between respiratory symptoms in children and the smoking habits of parents was no longer significant when parental symptoms were controlled for.

Cogswell et al. (66) followed a cohort of high-risk children born to parents at least one of whom was atopic. At age 1 year there was no difference in the prevalence of wheezing in children of parents who did or did not smoke at that time, but by age 5 years, 62% of parents who smoked had children who had experienced episodes of wheeze compared with 37% in families where the parents did not smoke. On the other hand, in a longitudinal New Zealand study of 1265 children (62), occurrence of lower respiratory tract illness in the first year of life was significantly related to maternal smoking, with a dose-response relationship and no effect of family socioeconomic status, but the relationship was equivocal at two years and absent at three years. However, in that study children with diagnosed asthma were excluded from this analysis, and as the diagnosis of asthma is made more frequently with increasing age in childhood, this omission could significantly diminish an association. In another study (67), the prevalence of parent-reported asthma in children aged 0-17 years was increased from 5.0% to 7.7% if the mother smoked, and the prevalence of "functionally impairing" (i.e., severe) asthma was doubled (from 1.1% to 2.2%).

A British study showed a positive correlation between parental (especially maternal) smoking and frequent cough in nonsmoking 8-19 year olds, again irrespective of socioeconomic status, and more obvious in younger children (68). The prevalence of frequent cough in children of nonsmoking parents was 35% (boys) and 32% (girls), compared with 42% and 40% if one parent smoked, and 48% and 52% if two parents smoked. As childhood cough is often a manifestation of covert asthma (19), associated with increased airway responsiveness to nonspecific stimuli, this could be further indirect evidence linking parental smoking with asthma.

There is strong evidence for impairment of pulmonary function in children exposed to maternal smoking (60,61). That this might relate to development of asthma was suggested by the study of Ekwo and colleagues (69), who showed small differences in the degree of change in lung function (FEV_1, flow at 75% vital capacity, and maximal midexpiratory flow rate) after inhaled isoproterenol in children of smokers and nonsmokers. The greater increase suggested impaired pulmonary function and/or greater airway lability in children of smoking parents. However Weiss et al. (70) recalculated the differences in responsiveness as a percentage of the baseline prebronchodilator values and found the small changes did not achieve statistical significance.

The role of passive smoking in the development of symptoms of childhood asthma has been more clearly defined in studies from Boston. In a study of 650 children aged 5 to 9 years, 9.2% of whom had persistent wheezing, Weiss et al. found parental cigarette smoking was linearly related to the occurrence of persistent wheeze (23). Current persistent wheeze occurred in 1.85% of children from households where neither parent smoked, 6.85% of children from households with one parent currently smoking, and 11.8% of children from households with two parents currently smoking. This trend was independent of the parental history of wheezing, and was associated with a reduction in lung function in these children. Similar results, including reduced pulmonary function, were found in children, especially female children, of smoking mothers in Pennsylvania (71). The Boston group also found a relationship between increased airway responsiveness and maternal smoking in 21 subjects with asthma but not in 265 nonasthmatic subjects, even though maternal smoking in the latter group was associated with reduced lung function (60).

Lower Respiratory Tract Infections

Studies associating early childhood respiratory infection with later development of wheezing illness and adult chronic airflow obstruction have been reviewed by Samet et al. (72), who concluded that the considerable potential for recall bias invalidated the results of many of these investigations. However, those studies which were considered reliable do suggest that lower respiratory tract infections in early childhood have a lasting effect on respiratory symptoms and pulmonary function in childhood (64,72-75).

Children with bronchiolitis due to the respiratory syncytial virus (RSV) showed a greater exercise lability than did control children with the same degree of atopy (76). In a follow-up study of Canadian children ten years after their hospital admission for bronchiolitis, a positive methacholine test was found in 57% (77). Similarly, symptoms of wheezing were more common in Tyneside children who had RSV bronchiolitis, although the prevalence of recognized and treated asthma did not differ from that of a control group (16). The Tyneside RSV bronchiolitis group also showed greater lability to exercise and to histamine challenge, with a threefold increased prevalence of airway hyperresponsiveness, but no significant difference in the prevalence of atopy. These studies again raise the question as to whether "bronchiolitis," at least in some of these children, might be asthma; the findings emerging from follow-up would then be expected features of asthma rather than evidence that bronchiolitis has incited asthma. Similar findings have been reported after "croup" (78) and again the same explanation is plausible.

A 7-year follow-up of 200 children with lower respiratory tract infections in infancy (79,80), showed that those children subsequently had an increased prevalence of cough, wheeze, use of medication, absences from school, and consultations with general practitioners compared with controls. They also showed increased airway responsiveness to exercise and reduced pulmonary function, but no difference in the prevalence of atopy. One might argue that these children had pre-existing or potential airway hyperresponsiveness which predisposed them to more severe and symptomatic lower respiratory tract infections. For example, children said to have "bronchitis" before age 5 who were then subsequently found at age 11 and 14 to have symptoms consistent with asthma, may well have had asthma before age 5, but their symptoms were attributed to "bronchitis" at that time (81). This hypothesis could also fit the Boston data (23) where children with persistent wheezing were more likely to report an early lower respiratory tract infection. The overall evidence that early lower respiratory tract infection is a significant risk factor for development of asthma is still somewhat uncertain. Rigorously controlled longitudinal studies, which include measurements of airway responsiveness from infancy through to adulthood, are required to clarify this question.

Psychosocial Factors

There is no consistent psychological profile of the asthmatic child nor is an association between socioeconomic class and asthma established. Asthmatic children in Aberdeen, Scotland were reported to have a higher mean IQ than the general population, although children with severe asthma were mostly from the lower socioeconomic classes (47). In other studies, asthma was more common in children of socioeconomic classes I and II (82). In the United Kingdom national sample, asthma was reported to be more frequent among children from nonmanual than manual laboring social classes (29), but the prevalence of wheezy bronchitis showed no such class difference. In part, these findings may have been biased by greater medical access of the higher social classes, increasing the likelihood of recognition and diagnosis of asthma. Anderson et al's. (83) recent review of risk factors for asthma in British children found a striking similarity in the prevalence of asthma in different social strata. While the prevalence of asthma may not be clearly associated with socioeconomic status, clinical manifestations and subsequent effects (e.g., school absenteeism) may differ among socioeconomic groups (20,46).

Asthma Symptoms and Airway Responsiveness in Childhood

Children with obvious or frequent symptoms of asthma almost invariably have airway hyperresponsiveness to histamine or methacholine (6-9,84). These children also have frequent variation in peak flow measurements. However, a substantial number of children with airway hyperresponsiveness to methacholine or histamine have no current or past symptoms suggestive of asthma. This finding is consistent among studies in New Zealand (7), Australia (9), Canada (22), the United States (85), and the United Kingdom (8), and was similar in degree whether the challenge was performed using histamine (8,9), methacholine (7,22), or hyperventilation with cold air (85). On the other hand, occasional children with a history of current symptoms strongly suggesting asthma (wheezing, cough, chest tightness on exercise) do not have demonstrable nonspecific airway hyperresponsiveness (7-9,22). Although overall there is a good correlation between asthmalike symptoms and the presence of airway hyperresponsiveness, the measurement has not proven highly specific or sensitive in epidemiologic studies, and is less useful in this context than it is in assessing severity and understanding mechanisms of asthma (86).

In a New Zealand longitudinal study of a birth cohort of 1037 children (25), the cumulative prevalence of symptoms of wheezing, whether or not recognized as asthma, was determined by responses to a questionnaire administered by a physician to parents of 9-year-old children, while airway responsiveness was assessed using an abbreviated validated methacholine inhalation challenge test (7). The correlation between symptoms and airway hyperresponsiveness defined as a 20% fall in FEV_1 at a provoking concentration of methacholine of 8 mg/ml or less ($PC_{20}FEV_1 < 8$ mg/ml) was high in those with chronic or frequent symptoms requiring treatment (79%), but an increased $PC_{20}FEV_1$ was found in only 39% of those with a history of less than 12 wheezing episodes per annum, even though asthma was current (episodes within the last 12 months) in the majority of these children. On the other hand, 32 of 480 children (6.7%) who had never had recurrent respiratory symptoms, showed increased airway responsiveness to methacholine (Table 2).

Among 2,363 New South Wales school children aged 8-11 years (9,58,59), 17.9% had hyperresponsive airways, defined as a $PD_{20}FEV_1$ of less than 7.8 μmol by the Yan method (87). However, 6.7% of the cohort had hyperresponsiveness without current or past respiratory symptoms, while 5.6% had had a diagnosis of asthma but did not show airway hyperresponsiveness. All children with $PD_{20}FEV_1$ less than 0.1 μmol had wheeze and all but one had diagnosed asthma, whereas of 77% of children with $PD_{20}FEV_1$ between 0.1 and 0.8 μmols had a history of wheeze and 64% had diagnosed asthma, while 81% had at least one respiratory symptom (wheeze, exercise wheeze, or night cough). The total prevalence of airway hyperresponsiveness at 17.9% was higher than the prevalence of diagnosed asthma (12.8%) but less than the prevalence of wheezing (24.3%) or of any respiratory symptom (33.9%). The association between symptoms and airway hyperresponsiveness was highly significant ($p < 0.001$) and the $PD_{20}FEV_1$ of those children with diagnosed asthma and respiratory symptoms was significantly lower (1.17 μmols) than the $PD_{20}FEV_1$ in hyperresponsive children without symptoms, or in children with wheezing not diagnosed as asthma.

TABLE 2 Correlation Between Cumulative Prevalence of Symptoms of Asthma and Airway Responsiveness in 9-Year-Old Children Enrolled in the Dunedin Multidisciplinary Health and Development Research Study, New Zealand

	Cumulative symptoms		Current airway hyperresponsiveness	
	n	%	n	%
Chronic severe asthma	3	0.4	3	100.0
Frequent asthma (regular therapy)	31	3.8	24	77.4
Infrequent asthma (3-12 episodes/year)	113	13.9	44	38.9
Trivial asthma (1-2 episodes/year)	92	11.3	20	21.7
Cough/bronchitis	94	11.6	11	11.7
No symptoms to age 9	480	59.0	32	6.7
Total	813	100.0	132	16.2

[a]Defined as $PC_{20}FEV_1$ to methacholine less than 8 mg/ml by abbreviated method (Ref. 7).

Factors associated with development of airway hyperresponsiveness in the New South Wales study (58,59) included a history of early respiratory illness, a history of asthma in either parent, and atopy, the latter being the most important. If all three factors were present, there was a sixfold increased risk of moderate or severe airway hyperresponsiveness ($PD_{20}FEV_1 < 0.8$ μmols), suggesting that infections in early childhood and exposure to environmental aeroallergens superimpose a risk on the inherited ability for airways to become hyperresponsive. In that study, the prevalence of airway hyperresponsiveness was higher in an inland region where grass pollen was the dominant allergen and lower in a coastal region where house dust mite sensitivity was more common. In contrast, in New Zealand children, skin sensitivity to the house dust mite was associated with a fivefold risk of developing airway hyperresponsiveness by age 13, whereas grass pollen sensitivity alone was not a significant risk factor either for hyperresponsiveness or for asthma symptoms (88).

Progression of Childhood Asthma into Adult Life

A number of studies suggest that respiratory illness, including asthma in childhood, can result in chronic airways disease in the adult (89). Colley et al. (73) followed up a group of British children born in 1946, and found increased prevalence of cough and sputum at age 20 and 25 years in those whose parents had reported early childhood infections. However, the followup was comprised of fewer than 50% of the original sample, and the results were confounded by the effect of smoking. Burrows et al. (90) showed that adults with chronic bronchitis or impaired airway function had a greater likelihood of a history of childhood respiratory problems, mainly "asthma-bronchitis," but because the data were retrospective and subject to preferential recall bias, the association was not regarded as certain. In those in the age range of 20-44 years, more than twice as many with a history of childhood respiratory trouble (CRT) reported frequent wheeze compared with those without CRT (8.6% vs. 3.8%), and there was a strikingly high prevalence of a history of any wheeze (62.9%) among those with CRT compared with 33.7% in those without CRT.

The finding that childhood bronchitis, which now would be more readily termed asthma, increased respiratory symptoms and impaired lung function in later life has been reported in follow-up of the longitudinal Australian study initiated by Williams and McNicol (24). They found no significant features which would distinguish children with an illness termed "bronchitis" from those with "wheezy bronchitis" or "asthma," and stated that these conditions were all one entity–asthma. Martin et al. (91) found that more than half of the children with infrequent wheezing in childhood were wheeze free in early adult life, while most of the remainder continued to have infrequent wheezing. Only 20% of those with frequent wheezing in childhood stopped wheezing in adolescence, but almost half noted considerable improvement in symptoms by age 21 years. Almost all children with persistent wheezing in childhood continued to wheeze into adult life, but most were improved. At followup at age 21, both asthma and smoking contributed to chronic sputum production, but the association with asthma was stronger (92). Those with more frequent wheezing persisting to age 21 had a higher frequency of abnormalities of pulmonary function (93). Further follow-up at age 28 (94) confirmed the predictive value of persistent wheeze at age 14 which indicated the likely persistence of symptoms to age 28 years, with no substantial change in the pattern of symptoms between ages 21 and 28 years.

Blair, following up a London childhood asthmatic population seen in general practice, noted similar findings (95,96). After 20 years, 21% of children with asthma (defined as at least three episodes of paroxysmal dyspnea with wheezing) seen originally before age 12 had had continuous asthma into adult life, and a further 27% had recurrent asthma after a symptom-free period of three or more years in adolescence. The remaining 52% without persistent wheeze comprised 24% with occasional wheezing but no disability, and 28% who were totally wheeze free, of whom a third showed reduced pulmonary function and increased airway lability. Hence the great majority of children with diagnosed significant asthma before age 12 continue to show asthmatic features in adult life.

These recent studies are similar to earlier studies by Rackemann and Edwards (97) of follow-up of childhood asthma in the United States. Of 449 patients seen and treated by the authors before age 13 (82.1% of whom were atopic), only 30% were completely symptom free and leading normal lives 20 years later.

It is possible that childhood asthma not only predisposes to continuing asthma in adults, but also acts as a direct risk factor for smoking-related chronic obstructive pulmonary disease (COPD). Airway hyperresponsiveness which usually accompanies childhood asthma may be associated with a greater tendency to airflow obstruction in smoking adults, and a more rapid progression of chronic lung disease in adults. However, further longitudinal studies are required to prove this hypothesis.

Asthma in Adulthood

There are relatively few community studies of the prevalence and characteristics of asthma in adults. The difficulties of obtaining a random sample in a noncaptive population of adults are much greater than in childhood where schools make ideal sampling frames. Furthermore, the identification of asthma is more difficult in older subjects in whom asthma symptoms may be confused with symptoms due to airway obstruction caused by smoking-related diseases (3). Dodge and Burrows (98) have clearly shown the very different prevalence figures found for "physician-diagnosed asthma" compared with "wheezing" in all age groups. For example, in the 20-24-year-old Tucson population, 5% had asthma, 12% had attacks of shortness of breath with wheeze, 25% had wheeze even without colds, and 42% had experienced wheezing with colds. It would seem unlikely that in this age group there was a major component of chronic bronchitis and emphysema, and that the majority of the symptomatic subjects had asthma. In older subjects, however, most diagnosed as having asthma also carried the diagnosis of chronic bronchitis or emphysema, and differentiation may be difficult without detailed investigation and a prolonged test of reversibility. Selected studies of the prevalence of "asthma" in adulthood are summarized in Table 3.

The incidence of asthma in adult life has been little studied, but some data allow calculation of incidence (new cases of the disease). In the follow-up of asthmatic children in Melbourne into adulthood, 15 of 82 "control" 14-year-old adolescents had developed symptoms of asthma by age 21, an incidence of 18.3% in 7 years or 2.6% per annum (91). A study in Connecticut found an incidence rate of 1.4% in 6 years, or 0.2% per annum (99), similar to that found in the Tecumseh study which reported an incidence of 1% in 4 years, or 0.25% per annum (100).

Measurements of airway responsiveness in adults appear to be no more specific or sensitive than they are in children for confirming the diagnosis of asthma. In a study of 654 Italian adults aged 15-64 years, the difference in methacholine responsiveness between those with obvious histories of asthma and those with no history was not well defined, although the difference in mean airway responsiveness between the two groups was highly significant (101). In another study of 18-64 year olds in England, 14% had increased airway hyperresponsiveness to histamine; airway hyperresponsiveness was associated with age, smoking (the effect of which increased with age), and atopy (the effect of which decreased with age) (102). Airway hyperresponsiveness was least obvious in the 35-44-year-old subjects and increased in older and younger subjects. Clear correlations have been found between the presence of airway hyperresponsiveness and chronic respiratory symptoms in adults (103,104), but the presence of airway hyperresponsiveness is not specific for asthma. Cockroft (105) showed in a population of 20-29-year-old college students that the distribution of airway hyperresponsiveness was unimodal with asthmatic subjects forming a subgroup within the hyperresponsiveness distribution tail rather than a separate distribution peak.

Asthma may be significantly underdiagnosed in adults. One third of adult asthmatic patients attending a hospital outpatient clinic were not diagnosed on referral as having asthma (106). Over 40% of a geriatric population in Wales demonstrated a 15% or greater increase in peak expiratory flow rate 5 min after inhaled salbutamol, but only 6% of the patients were being treated for asthma (107). Dyspnea and poor lung function may be incorrectly ascribed to chronic bronchitis or cardiac failure in the elderly.

TABLE 3 Selected Studies of the Prevalence of Asthma and Wheezing in Adults

Country	Year published	Age	Prevalence	Reference
NEW ZEALAND				
Dunedine	1979	all	current 4.2%, cumulative 6.2%	158
AUSTRALIA				
Busselton, WA	1987	18–88	5.9% current (symptoms + AHR)	159
UNITED STATES				
Tecumseh, MI	1962	all	4.1% certain, 10.2% total	160
Glenwood, CO	1971	20–69	3.6% male, 1.2% female	161
Tecumseh, MI	1974	all	12.3% male, 11.4% female	162
Tucson, AZ	1980	>20	3.0–7.9% asthma, depend. age, sex >30% wheezing most ages	98
Lebanon, CT	1984	>7	5.6% asthma, 21.3% wheeze	99
CANADA				
Saskatoon	1983	20–29	2.7% current, 9.3% cumulative	105

The rate of decline of lung function in adults with asthma has been found to be related both to the presence of airway hyperresponsiveness and the degree of airflow limitation, but the effect of smoking on these data could not be assessed in this study (108).

Factors Affecting the Expression of Adult Asthma

"Westernization"

In contrast to findings in developed countries, the prevalence of asthma in children in some developing countries is considerably lower than the prevalence in adults, and the age of onset of asthma in such countries is often over 20 years. Among the South Fore people of Papua, New Guinea, the point prevalence of asthma in children in the 1970s was nil, and the adult prevalence only 0.28% (109). A decade later, the prevalence in children was 0.6%, but a striking 7.3% in adults over 20 years (110). Changes in the prevalence of house dust mite in the environment may be important (111) although these people do not suffer other allergic diseases such as rhinitis or dermatitis.

Severe asthma, provoked by factors which previously were benign—exercise, stress, infection—now occurs in these people who have been shown to have a high level of allergy to the house dust mite. This group had a four- to fivefold greater mite density in blanket dust than that found in a similar village which has not experienced a dramatic increase in asthma prevalence (112,113). That the house dust mite is relevant to the development of asthma and airway hyperresponsiveness is suggested by several studies. We have shown that mite sensitivity is associated with a fivefold relative risk for the development of asthma in New Zealand children (88), while Platts-Mills et al. (114) showed that airway hyperresponsiveness diminished on avoidance of the mite. The adult asthma in the Papuan people has become increasingly severe and is associated with a very high mortality rate; 28% have died in 10 years (113).

A vast array of environmental substances exist in developed societies whose effects on airway responsiveness are as yet virtually unknown, and which could potentially be equally as important as the house dust mite in inducing asthma, for example, food preservatives, coloring agents, building materials, industrial wastes, vehicle emissions, pesticides and other agricultural products, and many more.

Occupation

The increasing number of recognized occupational causes of asthma are reviewed in Chapter 7. The prevalence of occupational asthma depends not only on the nature of the inciting agent, but also on the circumstances of exposure. In some industries, 30% of workers or more develop asthma (e.g., animal handlers and workers with proteolytic enzymes), whereas lower rates occur with other agents (e.g., 5% with isocyanates and 4% with western red cedar). Occupational asthma may account for a significant part of the total burden of asthma in a population—some 15% of all cases of asthma in Japan are attributed to occupational causes (115).

Climate

Differences in prevalence of asthma in regions of differing climates have not been widely explored. Cullen compared chest disorders in children in various regions of Australasia and the United Kingdom, and contrary to prior expectations found a higher prevalence of bronchitis and asthma in warmer compared with cooler regions (116). A recent study comparing asthma in children living in a temperate region of New Zealand with children in Southern Ontario, Canada, with its much greater climatic extremes, found no significant differences in the prevalence of symptoms (22). The prevalence of asthma in dry desert climates (98,117) is similar to that found in moist temperate zones. The much lower reported prevalence rates for asthma in some countries with considerably cooler temperatures, for instance in Scandinavia (118) could relate in part to methodological differences or to other factors such as diet, rather than be due primarily to differences in climate.

That climate does affect the expression of asthma is evident from reports of epidemics of severe asthma and increased hospital admissions during or following weather changes. Outbreaks of asthma were associated with thunderstorms in Melbourne, Australia (119) and in Birmingham, England (120). A correlation was shown between asthma admissions in Birmingham and daily spore counts measured 60 km away in Derby (121). The dependence of some fungi on the weather for spore release (e.g., Didymella) gives credence to the association of fungal aeroallergens with epidemics of clinical asthma, similar to that seen in countries experiencing ragweed seasons (122). It is likely that the effects of weather changes on asthma are largely related to the indirect effects on local allergens (e.g., fungal spores, pollens, or house dust mite populations) rather than to direct cold or irritant effects on the airways. However, the correlation between increased emergency presentations with asthma and climatic change in Bermuda (123) should be noted, as Bermuda has little air pollution and pollen counts are low all year. Asthma attendances increased with lower relative humidity, lower ambient air temperature, and winds from the northeast ocean with no appreciable aeroallergens, suggesting a more direct effect of climatic factors on the expression of asthma.

Evidence for Increasing Severity of Asthma

Data relating to hospital admissions for asthma (39-44), and to the use of antiasthma drugs in several countries (124,125), suggests that either the prevalence or severity of asthma, or both, have increased over the last decade. The increase in admissions does not seem to be due to earlier presentation of patients with milder asthma; a retrospective study of emergency room data on pulse rate and respiratory rate of patients attending with acute asthma over 10 years showed no significant difference in the degree of distress indicated by these variables (126). The increased use of bronchodilator medications (beta sympathomimetic and theophylline) and inhaled corticosteroids in New Zealand, Australia, and the United Kingdom between 1975 and 1981, seen most markedly in New Zealand (124), could reflect increased severity of asthma, improved treatment of asthma, or greater use of these drugs in other airway diseases. However, a community survey of antiasthma drug use in New Zealand in 1984 found that 80% of prescriptions for salbutamol, the most commonly prescribed bronchodilator drug in New Zealand, were for patients verified by the investigators as having asthma rather than chronic bronchitis and/or emphysema (125). The same study found that, despite the considerable increase in sales of inhaled corticosteroid aerosols over recent years, that therapy was still underutilized in that only 42% of subjects with daily symptoms of asthma were prescribed inhaled corticosteroids. The increase in sales of antiasthma drugs then has not necessarily been the result of improved treatment of asthma. It seems likely that a considerable part of the increase may relate to an increase in the prevalence and/or severity of the disease.

MORTALITY FROM ASTHMA

Secular Trends

Asthma is rarely fatal, and changes in mortality rates are generally too small to be useful in studying the epidemiology of the disease. On two occasions in the last three decades, however, significant changes in reported asthma mortality have occurred; these have been widely discussed and their meaning debated (127-130). Between 1964 and 1966, reported asthma mortality in England and Wales, Australia, and New Zealand increased substantially, especially in young people in whom it increased three or fourfold. This increase has been variously attributed to a direct toxic effect of high-dose sympathomimetic bronchodilator drugs (131), to delay in obtaining more effective treatment due to overreliance on symptomatic relief from bronchodilator therapy (132), to increased or unusual exposure to aeroallergens (133), or to diagnostic transfer as the availability of potent bronchodilator aerosols enhanced recognition of asthma (128). This latter explanation is scarcely plausible in young people for whom the mortality rates changed most abruptly, as nonasthmatic causes of wheezing in 15-34 year olds are few. Over the next decade, despite continued use of aerosol bronchodilators, mortality rates declined to pre-epidemic levels in the United Kingdom and in Australia, although the rate in New Zealand remained somewhat elevated. The second "epidemic" of asthma mortality, first noted anecdotally in New Zealand in 1977 and later confirmed by national statistics, took mortality in young people in the late 1970s and early 1980s to even higher rates than experienced in the earlier epidemic (over 4.0 per 100,000 in the 5-34-year-old population (134). Changes in asthma mortality in other countries over the last decade have been much more gradual and at a lower level than in New Zealand (135,136), but it appears that the second "wave" of asthma mortality has not been confined to New Zealand (Table 4).

In the United Kingdom, Burney showed a significant increase in mortality in young people occurring between 1974 and 1985 (137), and in Canada, mortality in 5-34 year olds more than doubled, from 0.2 per 100,000 in 1974 to 0.5 per 100,000 in 1984 (138). In the United States asthma mortality rates also doubled from 0.15 to 0.36 per 100,000 in this age group (136). The increase there, as in New Zealand, has been more obvious in non-whites than whites and in younger rather than older persons (139).

Trends in mortality in older subjects are harder to verify for reasons which are discussed below, but there has been a substantial increase in reported mortality in all age groups in many countries in the last 10 years, only a part of which can be explained by changes in classification and coding of deaths.

Validation of Statistics

The questions to be answered regarding trends in asthma mortality are whether they are real or artefactual; if real, what is their basis (140)? The accuracy of national asthma mortality statistics depends on the accuracy of physician certification of the cause of death, and the extent to which false positive and false negative reporting of asthma mortality may occur (141). National statistics will also be influenced by periodic changes in the rules governing the statistical coding of death certificates. The accuracy of certification of death due to asthma has been studied in two major investigations into asthma deaths, the first in two regions of England (142), and the second in New Zealand (134) with similar results.

Between 1981 and 1983, the Asthma Task Force of the Medical Research Council of New Zealand reviewed the deaths of all 492 people for whom the word "asthma" or a derivative was recorded somewhere in Part I of the death certificate or on the coroner's report (134). After detailed information was obtained by questionnaire from relatives and doctors, and hospital records and autopsy results (where available) were studied, 66.9% of these deaths were accepted by the medical reviewing panel as being due to asthma (141). A comparison of the final coding of these deaths by the reviewing panel and by the New Zealand National Health Statistics Centre, which generally use only death certificate information their basis for coding, showed that agreement was high, indeed 100% in persons aged less than 35 years, but the accuracy of certification and the subsequent statistical coding declined with increasing age (Table 5). Inac-

TABLE 4 Annual Mortality Rates from Asthma in 5-34 Year Olds in Eight Countries, 1970-1984 (Rate per 100,000 population)

	1970	1971	1972	1973	1974	1975	1976	1977	1978	1979	1980	1981	1982	1983	1984	1985
United States	0.34	0.27	0.26	0.24	0.20	0.22	0.19	0.17	0.21	0.22	0.26	0.29	0.35	0.36	0.31	0.37
Canada	0.21	0.18	0.21	0.22	0.32	0.31	0.36	0.33	0.28	0.31	0.44	0.46	0.45	0.50	0.50	0.42
England/Wales	0.82	0.84	0.80	0.66	0.53	0.59	0.52	0.61	0.68	0.68	0.68	0.91	0.82	0.90	0.81	0.88
Australia	1.29	1.21	1.04	1.18	1.42	0.78	0.81	0.98	0.93	0.87	0.94	1.10	1.03	0.95	1.28	1.37
New Zealand	1.81	1.91	2.40	1.49	1.32	1.42	2.02	3.64	2.96	4.12	3.46	3.27	3.14	2.28	2.57	1.85
Japan	0.99	0.85	0.67	0.54	0.48	0.44	0.46	0.42	0.33	0.33	0.36	0.40	0.39	0.47	0.39	0.53
West Germany	0.41	0.41	0.50	0.54	0.49	0.49	0.66	0.63	0.70	0.78	0.85	0.83	0.86	0.84	0.80	0.86
France	0.15	0.21	0.23	0.18	0.17	0.26	0.26	0.20	0.28	0.19	0.27	0.29	0.31	0.26	0.37	–

TABLE 5 Relationship of Accuracy of Certification and Coding of Asthma Deaths to Age at Death, New Zealand, August 1981–July 1983

Age (years)	Deaths certified as due to asthma[a]	Deaths coded by National Health Statistics Centre as due to asthma	Verified asthma deaths[b]	Verified asthma deaths (% of certified)	Verified asthma deaths (% of coded)
0–14	18	17	17	94.4	100.0
15–34	72	71	71	98.6	100.0
35–44	39	37	33	84.6	89.2
45–54	68	62	56	82.4	90.3
55–64	93	83	64	69.6	77.1
65–69	52	45	30	56.6	66.7
70+	150	116	58	38.7	50.0
Total	492	431	329	66.9	74.6
15–64	272	253	224	82.7	88.5

[a]"Asthma" in Part I of death certificate or coroner's report.
[b]As judged by reviewing panel of National Asthma Mortality Study.
Source: Reprinted with permission from Ref. 141.

curacies in certification and subsequent statistical coding of apparent "asthma" deaths were due largely to false positive reporting associated with three factors. Some patients said to have died from asthma had never suffered from asthma but rather had chronic airflow obstruction due to chronic bronchitis and/or emphysema. A second group of patients had had asthma in earlier life, but their dominant lung disease at death was chronic bronchitis and/or emphysema related to smoking, with no recent evidence of reversibility of airflow obstruction sufficient to be termed asthma. A third group of patients with true asthma died of other causes, for example, myocardial ischemia, but were coded as asthma deaths because the word "asthma" was included in the lowest entry in Part I of the death certificate rather than being entered more appropriately in Part II as another condition suffered by the deceased but not contributing directly to death. In all, 26% of all "asthma" deaths coded as such by the National Health Statistics Centre according to information available to that office, were not accepted as due to asthma by the reviewing panel of the Task Force.

In England, the review of accuracy of certification in 15-64 year olds investigated in the British Thoracic Association study (143) found a net overestimate of asthma mortality of 13%. Relatively more false negatives and fewer false positives were identified in England compared with New Zealand, although overall both countries had an identical net overestimate of asthma mortality when groups were matched for age (144), indicating that the higher New Zealand mortality rate was not due to reduced accuracy of certification.

The classification of the cause of death in the manner described by the World Health Organization (WHO) requires coding of the disease or injury which initiated the train of morbid events leading directly to death (145). The condition entered on the lowest used line of Part I of the death certificate is selected for statistical coding unless it is highly improbable that this condition gave rise to all the conditions entered above it. If more than one condition is entered on the lowest used line in Part I, and all could be considered an underlying cause of conditions in the lines above, the first mentioned condition is used for coding. The rules governing the 9th Revision allow that acute circulatory diseases, myocardial ischemia, ischemic heart disease, cardiac failure, and dysrhythmia are acceptable as possible Part I sequences arising from asthma. These coding rules, if not understood by the certifying doctor, lead to inaccuracies in statistical coding. While in some instances an acute cardiac event is the terminal episode of a severe attack of asthma, evidence that asthma predisposes to these diseases is slight, therefore death from myocardial ischemia in an asthmatic, unless occurring at the height of a severe attack of asthma with profound hypoxemia, should not be attributable to asthma and the term asthma would rightly be entered in Part II of the death certificate.

In the main, errors in certification result in false positive reporting of asthma deaths rather than false negative reporting. The false negative rate cannot be accurately determined unless all cases dying of some form of cardiorespiratory disorder are carefully evaluated. This would be an onerous and difficult undertaking. However, in a regional study within New Zealand, a very low rate of false negative reporting of asthma deaths was found in young people, again verifying that 5-34 year olds represent a suitable group for longitudinal study of trends (130).

The introduction in 1979 of the 9th revision of the WHO International Classification of Diseases (ICD) and associated rulings caused temporary confusion in analysis of trends in mortality. Under the new ICD9 rules, deaths certified as due to asthma, but with mention of bronchitis, previously coded under ICD8 to bronchitis, were now coded to asthma (145). In older age groups, this caused an apparent increase in asthma mortality of 35% or more (146). However, in the 5-34 year age range, the effect of the introduction of ICD9 was negligible, and trends through 1979 in this group can be accepted as valid (147). Furthermore, although the 1979 change in ICD produced a significant step increase in reported asthma mortality across the whole age group, this does not explain the subsequent upward trends in mortality rates in many countries. An increase in either severity or prevalence, a reduction in efficacy of treatment, or an adverse effect of treatment, may be suggested as the cause(s) of the increase in asthma mortality seen in many countries, as it seems unlikely that changes in diagnostic fashion, accuracy of certification, or coding rules can explain the significant changes in mortality in young people.

Risk Factors for Mortality

Studies of death from asthma (134,142,148) have allowed us to draw a characterization of patients who are at higher risk of dying of their disease (149). Identifiable risk factors for death included age, race, psychosocial factors, previous history of severe or life-threatening attacks, previous hospital admissions and emergency room visits, and discontinuity of physician care (142). An increased risk of death was not associated with age of onset of asthma, family history of asthma, and smoking habits.

The age group most highly represented in the New Zealand National Asthma Mortality Study, the only study to include a whole population, was the decade 15-24 years (134). The epidemic of asthma mortality that swept through the United Kingdom, Australia, and New Zealand in the 1960s had also been most evident in young people (127). Case histories in this age group frequently suggested that removal of parental care coupled with rebelliousness against medical and parental authority resulted in less reliable self-care and reduced compliance with therapy.

There was a higher mortality rate among nonwhites in New Zealand; the mortality rates for Maori (18.9/100,000) and Pacific Island polynesians (9.4/

100,000) were, respectively, 5.6 and 2.8 times higher than the rate for Europeans (3.4/100,000) (134). Similar higher mortality rates are evident among black compared with white children in the United States (139). Differing attitudes to medical care, and cultural and economic barriers to good quality medical care, may explain part of this difference.

In the Auckland, New Zealand case-control study (150), psychosocial factors (problems clearly documented by hospital or general practice records, and in the main comprising depression, recent family bereavement, and recent unemployment) were associated in adults with a relative risk of dying of 3.5 compared with hospital controls with asthma of similar severity. Half of the deaths in children under 15 years old identified in the New Zealand national study were associated with disturbed home and family relationships resulting in less attention being given to the child's asthma (151). Similar findings have been reported by Strunk et al. in a case-controlled series of childhood asthma deaths in the United States (152).

A history of previous life-threatening attacks of asthma (attacks resulting in altered consciousness or hypercapnia) was associated with a relative risk of dying of 3.8 compared with hospital controls (150). A recent hospital admission (within one year) carried a 16-fold increased risk of a fatal outcome, and one or more emergency room visits in the last year with an 8-fold relative risk, compared with control asthmatics in the community whose disease was otherwise of similar severity (150).

Aspects of medical management identifiable as risk factors included the prescription of three or more different classes of drugs for asthma, and low scores for adequacy of prescribed drug therapy, as evaluated by a panel of experienced respiratory physicians (150).

Overall, the dominant lesson from the English (153), American (148), and New Zealand (134,150,154) studies of asthma mortality is that a fatal outcome is associated with inadequate assessment and inappropriate treatment of severe asthma, with overreliance on palliative bronchodilator therapy and insufficient use of corticosteroid therapy because of inadequate appreciation of the persistent inflammatory nature of severe asthma.

REFERENCES

1. *Webster's Third New International Dictionary*. Merriam Co., Chicago, 1976.
2. Gross NJ. What is this thing called love?—or, defining asthma. Am Rev Respir Dis 1980; 121:203-204.
3. Fletcher CM, Pride NB. Definitions of emphysema, chronic bronchitis, asthma, and airflow obstruction: 25 years on from the Ciba symposium. Thorax 1984; 39:81-85.

4. Scadding JG. Definition and clinical categories of asthma. In: *Asthma*. Clark TJH, Godfrey S, eds. London: Chapman and Hall, 1983, p 5.
5. Venables KM, Burge PS, Davison AG, Newman Taylor AJ. Peak flow rate records in surveys: reproducibility of observers' reports. Thorax 1984; 39:828–832.
6. Hargreave FE, Ryan G, Thomson NC, O'Byrne PM, Latimer K, Juniper EF, Dolovich J. Bronchial responsiveness to histamine or methacholine in asthma: measurement and clinical significance. J Allergy Clin Immunol 1981;68:347–355.
7. Sears MR, Jones DT, Holdaway MD, Hewitt CJ, Flannery ME, Herbison GP, Silva PA. The prevalence of bronchial reactivity to inhaled methacholine in New Zealand children. Thorax 1986;41:283–289.
8. Lee DA, Winslow NR, Speight ANP, Hey EN. Prevalence and spectrum of asthma in childhood. Br Med J 1983;286:1256–1258.
9. Salome CM, Peat JK, Britton WJ, Woolcock AJ. Bronchial hyperresponsiveness in two populations of Australian schoolchildren. I. Relation to respiratory symptoms and diagnosed asthma. Clin Allergy 1987; 17:271–281.
10. Enarson DA, Vedal S, Schulzer M, Dybuncio A, Chan-Yeung M. Asthma, asthmalike symptoms, chronic bronchitis, and the degree of bronchial hyperresponsiveness in epidemiological surveys. Am Rev Respir Dis 1987; 136:613–617.
11. Holgate ST, Beasley R, Twentyman OP. The pathogenesis and significance of bronchial hyperresponsiveness in airways disease. Clin Sci 1987; 73: 561–572.
12. Editorial. Airflow limitation–reversible or irreversible? Lancet 1988; 1: 26–27.
13. Brown PJ, Greville HW, Finucane KE. Asthma and irreversible airflow obstruction. Thorax 1984;39:131–136.
14. Anderson HR. Respiratory disease in childhood. Br Med Bull 1986; 42: 167–171.
15. Henderson FW, Clyde WA, Collier AM, Denny FW. The etiologic and epidemiologic spectrum of bronchiolitis in pediatric practice. J Pediatr 1979;95:183–190.
16. Pullan CR, Hey EN. Wheezing, asthma, and pulmonary dysfunction 10 years after infection with respiratory syncytial virus in infancy. Br Med J 1982;284:1665–1669.
17. Tabachnik E, Levison H. Infantile bronchial asthma. J Allergy Clin Immunol 1981;76:339–347.
18. Hordvik NL, Konig P, Morris D, Krentz C, Barbero J. A longitudinal study of bronchodilator responsiveness in cystic fibrosis. Am Rev Respir Dis 1985; 131:889–893.
19. Konig P. Hidden asthma in childhood. Am J Dis Child 1981; 135:1053–1055.
20. Anderson HR, Bailey PA, Cooper JS, Palmer JC, West S. Morbidity and school absence caused by asthma and wheezing illness. Arch Dis Child 1983;58:777–784.

21. Kerigan AT, Goldsmith CH, Pengelly LD. A three year cohort study of the role of environmental factors in respiratory health of children in Hamilton, Ontario. Am Rev Respir Dis 1986; 133:987-993.
22. Fitzgerald JM, Sears MR, Roberts RS, Morris MM, Fester DA, Hargreave FE. Symptoms of asthma and airway hyperresponsiveness to methacholine in a population of Canadian schoolchildren. Am. Rev Respir Dis 1988; 137: 285.
23. Weiss ST, Tager IB, Speizer FE, Rosner B. Persistent wheeze. Its relation to respiratory illness, cigarette smoking, and level of pulmonary function in a population sample of children. Am Rev Respir Dis 1980; 122:697-707.
24. Williams H, McNicol KN. Prevalence, natural history and relationship of wheezy bronchitis and asthma in children: an epidemiological study. Br Med J 1969; 4:321-325.
25. Jones DT, Sears MR, Holdaway MD, Hewitt CJ, Flannery EM, Herbison GP, Silva PA. Asthma in New Zealand children. Br J Dis Chest 1987; 81: 332-340.
26. Milne GA. The incidence of asthma in Lower Hutt. NZ Med J 1969: 70: 27-9.
27. Anyon CP, Kiddle GB. The prevalence of wheezy children in Lower Hutt. NZ Med J 1974; 79:822-823.
28. Mitchell EA. Increasing prevalence of asthma in children. NZ Med J 1983; 96:463-464.
29. Peckham C, Butler N. A national study of asthma in childhood. J Epidemiol Comm Health 1978; 32:79-85.
30. Smith JM. Prevalence and natural history of asthma in school children. Br Med J 1961; 1:711-3.
31. Blanc ADG. The prevalence of asthma. In: *So You Have Asthma*! Charles C Thomas, Springfield, IL, pp. 181-194.
32. Sears MR, Jones DT, Silva PA, Simpson H, Williams SM. Asthma in seven year old children: a report from the Dunedin Multidisciplinary Child Development Study. NZ Med J 1982; 95:533-536.
33. Fry J. Acute wheezy chests. Clinical patterns and natural history. Br Med J 1961; 1:227-232.
34. Goodall JF. The natural history of common respiratory infection in children and some principles in its management. III. J Roy Coll Gen Pract 1958; 1:51-59.
35. Smith JM, Harding IK, Cumming G. The changing prevalence of asthma in school children. Clin Allergy 1971; 1:57-61.
36. Fleming DM. Prevalence of asthma and hayfever in England and Wales. Br Med J 1987; 294:279-283.
37. Gergen PJ, Mullally DI, Evans R III. National survey of prevalence of asthma among children in the United States, 1976 to 1980. Pediatrics 1988; 81:1-7.
38. Burr ML. Is asthma increasing? J Epidemiol Comm Health 1987; 41:185-189.

39. Mitchell EA. International trends in hospital admissions rates for asthma. Arch Dis Child 1985; 60:376-378.
40. Mullally DI, Howard WA, Hubbard TJ, Grauman JS, Cohen SG. Increased hospitalizations for asthma among children in the Washington, D.C. area during 1961-1981. Ann Allergy 1984; 53:15-19.
41. Halfon N, Newacheck PW. Trends in the hospitalization for acute childhood asthma, 1970-84. Am J Public Health 1986; 76:1308-1311.
42. Jackson RT, Mitchell EA. Trends in hospital admission rates and drug treatment of asthma in New Zealand. NZ Med J 1983; 96:727-729.
43. Anderson HR, Bailey P, and West S. Trends in the hospital care of acute childhood asthma 1970-8: a regional study. Br Med J 1980; 281:1191-1194.
44. Mitchell EA, Cutler DR. Paediatric admissions to Auckland Hospital for asthma from 1970-1980. NZ Med J 1984; 97:67-70.
45. Dawson KP. The severity of asthma in children admitted to hospital: a 20 year review. NZ Med J 1987; 100:520-521.
46. Mak H, Johnston P, Abbey H, Talamo RC. Prevalence of asthma and health service utilization of asthmatic children in an inner city. J Allergy Clin Immunol 1982; 70:367-372.
47. Dawson B, Horobin G, Illsley R, Mitchell R. A survey of childhood asthma in Aberdeen. Lancet 1969; 1:827-830.
48. Verity CM, VanHeule B, Carswell F, Hughes AO. Bronchial lability and skin reactivity in siblings of asthmatic children. Arch Dis Child 1984; 59:871-876.
49. Johnston IDA, Bland JM, Anderson HR. Ethnic variation in respiratory morbidity and lung function in childhood. Thorax 1987; 42:542-548.
50. Waite DA, Eyles EF, Tonkin SL, O'Donnell TV. Asthma prevalence in Tokelauan children in two environments. Clin Allergy 1980; 10:71-5.
51. Van Niekerk CH, Weinberg EG, Shore SC, Heese H de V, Van Schalkwyk DJ. Prevalence of asthma: a comparative study of urban and rural Xhosa children. Clin Allergy 1979; 9:319-24.
52. Turner KJ, Dowse GK, Stewart GA, Alpers MP. Studies on bronchial hyperreactivity, allergic responsiveness and asthma in rural and urban children of the highlands of Papua New Guinea. J Allergy Clin Immunol 1986; 77: 558-66.
53. Zimmerman B, Feanny S, Reisman J, Hak H, Rashed N, McLaughlin FJ, Levison H. Allergy in asthma. 1. The dose relationship of allergy to severity of childhood asthma. J Allergy Clin Immunol 1988; 81:63-70.
54. Stempel DA, Clyde WA, Henderson FW, Collier AM. Serum IgE levels and the clinical expression of respiratory illness. J Pediatr 1980; 97:185-190.
55. Gibson HB, Silverstone H, Gandevia B, Hall GJL. Respiratory disorders in seven-year-old children in Tasmania. Aims, methods and administration of the survey. Med J Aust 1969; 2:201-205.
56. Giles GG, Gibson HB, Lickiss N, Shaw K. Respiratory symptoms in Tasmanian adolescents: a follow up of the 1961 birth cohort. Aust NZ Med 1984; 14:631-637.

57. Hill DJ, Hosking CS, Shelton MJ, Turner MW. Growing out of asthma: clinical and immunological changes over 5 years. Lancet 1981; 2:1359-1362.
58. Peat JK, Britton WJ, Salome CM, Woolcock AJ. Bronchial hyperresponsiveness in two populations of Australian schoolchildren. II. Relative importance of associated factors. Clin Allergy 1987; 17:283-290.
59. Peat JK, Britton WJ, Salome CM, Woolcock AJ. Bronchial hyperresponsiveness in two populations of Australian schoolchildren. III. Effect of exposure to environmental allergens. Clin Allergy 1987; 17:291-300.
60. O'Connor GT, Weiss ST, Tager IB, Speizer FE. The effect of passive smoking on pulmonary function and nonspecific bronchial responsiveness in a population-based sample of children and young adults. Am Rev Respir Dis 1987; 135:800-804.
61. Tager IB, Weiss ST, Munoz A, Rosner B, Speizer FE. Longitudinal study of the effects of maternal smoking on pulmonary function in children. N Engl J Med 1983; 309:699-703.
62. Fergusson DM, Horwood LJ, Shannon FT, Taylor B. Parental smoking and lower respiratory illness in the first three years of life. J Epidemiol Comm Health 1981; 35:180-184.
63. Harlap S, Davies AM. Infant admissions to hospital and maternal smoking. Lancet 1974; 1:529-532.
64. Leeder SR, Corkhill R, Irwig LM, Holland WW, Colley JRT. Influence of family factors on the incidence of lower respiratory illness during the first year of life. Br J Prev Soc Med 1976; 30:203-212.
65. Lebowitz MD, Burrows B. Respiratory symptoms related to smoking habits of family adults. Chest 1976; 69:48-50.
66. Cogswell JJ, Mitchell EB, Alexander J. Parental smoking, breast feeding, and respiratory infection in development of allergic diseases. Arch Dis Child 1987; 62:338-344.
67. Gortmaker SL, Walker DK, Jacobs FH, Ruch-Ross H. Parental smoking and the risk of childhood asthma. Am J Public Health 1982; 72:574-579.
68. Charlton A. Children's coughs related to parental smoking. Br Med J 1984; 288:1647-1651.
69. Ekwo EE, Weinberger MM, Lachenbruch PA, Huntley WH. Relationship of parental smoking and gas cooking to respiratory disease in children. Chest 1983; 84:662-668.
70. Weiss ST, Tager IB, Speizer FE. Passive smoking. Its relationship to respiratory symptoms, pulmonary function and nonspecific bronchial responsiveness. Chest 1983; 84:651.
71. Vedal S, Schenker MB, Samet JM, Speizer FE. Risk factors for childhood respiratory disease. Analysis of pulmonary function. Am Rev Respir Dis 1984; 130:187-192.
72. Samet JM, Tager IB, Speizer FE. The relationship between respiratory illness in childhood and chronic air-flow obstruction in adulthood. Am Rev Respir Dis 1983; 127:508-523.

73. Colley JRT, Douglas JWB, Reid DD. Respiratory disease in young adults: influence of early childhood lower respiratory tract illness, social class, air pollution, and smoking. Br Med J 1973;3:195-198.
74. Kiernan KE, Colley JRT, Douglas JWB, Reid DD. Chronic cough in young adults in relation to smoking habits, childhood environment and chest illness. Respiration 1976;33:236-244.
75. Colley JR, Holland WW, Leeder SR, Corkhill RT. Respiratory function of infants in relation to subsequent respiratory disease: an epidemiological study. Bull Eur Physiopathol Respir 1976;12:651-657.
76. Sims DG, Downham MAPS, Gardner PS, Webb JKG, Weightman D. Study of 8-year-old children with a history of respiratory syncytial virus bronchiolitis in infancy. Br Med J 1978;1:11-14.
77. Gurwitz D, Mindorff C, Levison H. Increased incidence of bronchial reactivity in children with a history of bronchiolitis. J Pediatr 1981;98:551-555.
78. Gurwitz D, Corey M, Levison H. Pulmonary function and bronchial reactivity in children after croup. Am Rev Respir Dis 1980;122:95-99.
79. Mok JYQ, Simpson H. Symptoms, atopy, and bronchial reactivity after lower respiratory infection in infancy. Arch Dis Child 1984;59:299-305.
80. Mok JYQ, Simpson H. Outcome for acute bronchitis, bronchiolitis, and pneumonia in infancy. Arch Dis Child 1984;59:306-309.
81. Holland WW, Bailey P, Bland JM. Long-term consequences of respiratory disease in infancy. J Epidemiol Comm Health 1978;32:256-259.
82. Peat JK, Woolcock AJ, Leeder SR, Blackburn CRB. Asthma and bronchitis in Sydney schoolchildren. II. The effect of social factors and smoking on prevalence. Am J Epidemiol 1980;111:728-735.
83. Anderson HR, Bland JM, Peckham CS. Risk factors for asthma up to 16 years of age: evidence from a national study. Chest 1987;91:127S-130S.
84. Hopp RJ, Bewtra AK, Nair NM, Watt GD, Townley RG. Methacholine inhalation challenge studies in a selected pediatric population. Am Rev Respir Dis 1986;134:994-998.
85. Weiss ST, Tager IB, Weiss JW, Munoz A, Speizer FE, Ingram RH. Airways responsiveness in a population sample of adults and children. Am Rev Respir Dis 1984;129:898-902.
86. Hargreave FE, Ryan G, Thompson NC, O'Byrne PM, Latimer K, Juniper EF. Bronchial responsiveness to histamine or methacholine in asthma: measurement and clinical significance. Eur J Respir Dis 1982; (Suppl) 121:79-88.
87. Yan K, Salome C, Woolcock AJ. Rapid method for measurement of bronchial responsiveness. Thorax 1983;38:760-765.
88. Sears MR, Herbison GP, Holdaway MD, Hewitt CJ, Flannery EM, Silva PA. The relative risks of allergy to grass pollen, house dust mite and cat dander in the development of childhood asthma. Am Rev Respir Dis 1988; 137:239.
89. Burrows B, Lebowitz MD, Knudson RJ. Epidemiologic evidence that childhood problems predispose to airways disease in the adult (an association

between adult and pediatric respiratory disorders). Pediat Res 1977; 11: 218-220.

90. Burrows B, Knudson RJ, Lebowitz MD. The relationship of childhood respiratory illness to adult obstructive airway disease. Am Rev Respir Dis 1977; 115:751-760.
91. Martin AJ, McLennan LA, Landau LI, Phelan PD. The natural history of childhood asthma to adult life. Br Med J 1980; 1:1397-1400.
92. Martin AJ, Landau LI, Phelan PD. Asthma from childhood to age 21: the patient and his disease. Br Med J 1982; 284:380-382.
93. Martin AJ, Landau LI, Phelan PD. Lung function in young adults who had asthma in childhood. Am Rev Respir Dis 1980; 122:609-616.
94. Kelly WJW, Hudson I, Phelan PD, Pain MCP, Olinsky A. Childhood asthma in adult life: a further study at 28 years of age. Br Med J 1987; 294:1059-1062.
95. Blair H. Natural history of childhood asthma. Arch Dis Child 1977; 52: 613-619.
96. Blair H. The wheezy child. J Roy Soc Med 1979; 72:42-48.
97. Rackemann FM, Edwards MC. Asthma in children. A follow-up study of 688 patients after an interval of twenty years. N Engl J Med 1952; 246: 815-823.
98. Dodge RR, Burrows B. The prevalence of asthma and asthma-like symptoms in a general population sample. Am Rev Respir Dis 1980; 122:567-575.
99. Schachter EN, Doyle CA, Beck GJ. A prospective study of asthma in a rural community. Chest 1984; 85:623-630.
100. Broder I, Higgins MW, Mathews KP, Keller JB. Epidemiology of asthma and allergic rhinitis in a total community, Tecumseh, Michigan. IV. Natural history. J Allergy Clin Immunol 1974; 54:100-110.
101. Cerveri I, Bruschi C, Zoia MC, Zanon P, Maccarini L, Grassi M, Rampulla C. Distribution of bronchial nonspecific reactivity in the general population. Chest 1988; 93:26-30.
102. Burney PGJ, Britton JR, Chinn S, Tattersfield AEM, Papacosta AO, Kelson MC, Anderson F, Corfield DR. Descriptive epidemiology of bronchial reactivity in an adult population: results from a community study. Thorax 1987; 38:38-44.
103. Ricjken B, Schouten JP, Weiss ST, Speizer FE, van der Lende R. The relationship of nonspecific bronchial responsiveness to respiratory symptoms in a random population sample. Am Rev Respir Dis 1987; 136:62-68.
104. Sparrow D, O'Connor G, Colton T, Barry CL, Weiss ST. The relationship of nonspecific bronchial responsiveness to the occurrence of respiratory symptoms and decreased levels of pulmonary function. The normative aging study. Am Rev Respir Dis 1987; 135:1255-1260.
105. Cockroft DW, Berscheid BA, Murdock KY. Unimodal distribution of bronchial responsiveness to inhaled histamine in a random human population. Chest 1983; 83:751-754.

106. Stellman JL, Spicer JE, Cayton RM. Morbidity from chronic asthma. Thorax 1982;37:218-221.
107. Banerjee DK, Lee GS, Malik SK, Daly S. Underdiagnosis of asthma in the elderly. Br J Dis Chest 1987;81:23-29.
108. Peat JK, Woolcock AJ, Cullen K. Rate of decline of lung function in subjects with asthma. Eur J Respir Dis 1987;70:171-179.
109. Anderson HR. The epidemiological and allergic features of asthma in the New Guinea Highlands. Clin Allergy 1974;4:171-183.
110. Woolcock AJ, Dowse GK, Temple K, Stanley H, Alpers MP, Turner KJ. The prevalence of asthma in the South Fore people of Papua New Guinea. A method for field studies of bronchial reactivity. Eur J Respir Dis 1983; 64:571-581.
111. Dowse GK, Turner KJ, Stewart GA, Alpers MP, Woolcock AJ. The association between *Dermataphagoides* mites and the increasing prevalence of asthma in village communities within the Papua New Guinea highlands. J Allergy Clin Immunol 1985;75:75-83.
112. Turner KJ. Changing prevalence of asthma in developing countries. In: *Highlights in Asthmology*. Michel FB, Bousqet J, Godard P, eds. Springer-Verlag, New York, 1987; pp 37-43.
113. Woolcock AJ, Alpers MP, Hurry VM. An epidemic of asthma in Papua New Guinea? Aust NZ J Med 1988; 18:544.
114. Platts-Mills TAE, Mitchell EB, Nock P, Tovey ER, Moszoro H, Williams SR. Reduction of bronchial hyperreactivity during prolonged allergen avoidance. Lancet 1982; 2:675-677.
115. Kobayashi S. Different aspects of occupational asthma in Japan. In: *Occupational Asthma*. Fraser CA, ed. Van Nostrand Reinhold, New York, 1980; pp 229-244.
116. Cullen KJ. Climate and chest disorders in schoolchildren. Br Med J 1972; 4:65-67.
117. Ellul-Micallef R, Al-Ali S. The spectrum of bronchial asthma in Kuwait. Clin Allergy 1984; 14:509-517.
118. Skarpaas IJK, Gulsvik A. Prevalence of bronchial asthma and respiratory symptoms in schoolchildren in Oslo. Allergy 1985;40:295-299.
119. Egan P. Weather or not. Med J Aust 1985; 142:330.
120. Packe GE, Archer P St J, Ayres JG. Asthma and the weather. Lancet 1983; 1:281.
121. Brown HM, Jackson F. Asthma and the weather. Lancet 2:630.
122. Salvaggio JE, Kundar VG. New Orleans epidemic asthma: relationship between outbreaks and influx of ragweed pollen. J Allergy 1968;41:90.
123. Carey MJ, Cordon I. Asthma and climatic conditions: experience from Bermuda, an isolated island community. Br Med J 1986; 293:843-844.
124. Keating G, Mitchell EA, Jackson R, Beaglehole R, Rea H. Trends in sales of drugs for asthma in New Zealand, Australia and the United Kingdom, 1975-81. Br Med J 1984;289:348-51.
125. Sinclair BL, Clark DWJ, Sears MR. Use of anti-asthma drugs in New Zealand. Thorax 1987;42:670-5.

126. Rea H, Sears M, Mitchell E, Garrett J, Mulder J, Anderson R. Is asthma becoming more severe? Thorax 1987; 42:736.
127. Speizer FE, Doll R, Heaf P. Observations on recent increase in mortality from asthma. Br Med J 1968; 1:335-339.
128. Esdaile JM, Feinstein AR, Horwitz RI. A reappraisal of the United Kingdom epidemic of fatal asthma. Arch Intern Med 1987; 147:543-549.
129. Gandevia B. Pressurised sympathomimetic aerosols and their lack of relationship to asthma mortality in Australia. Med J Aust 1973; 1:273-277.
130. Jackson RT, Beaglehole R, Rea HH, Sutherland DC. Mortality from asthma: a new epidemic in New Zealand. Br Med J 1982; 285:771-4.
131. Stolley PD, Schinnar R. Association between asthma mortality and isoproterenol aerosols: a review. Prev Med 1978; 7:519-38.
132. Beaupre A. Death in asthma. Eur J Respir Dis 1987; 70:259-260.
133. Jenkins PF, Mullins J, Davies BH, Williams DA. The possible role of aeroallergens in the epidemic of asthma deaths. Clin Allergy 1980; 11:611-620.
134. Sears MR, Rea HH, Beaglehole R, Gillies AJD, Holst PE, O'Donnell TV, Rothwell RPG, Sutherland DC. Asthma mortality in New Zealand: a two year national study. NZ Med J 1985; 98:271-5.
135. Buist AS. Is asthma mortality increasing? Chest 1988; 93:449-450.
136. Robin ED. Death from bronchial asthma. Chest 1988; 93:614-618.
137. Burney PGJ. Asthma mortality in England and Wales: evidence for a further increase, 1974-1984. Lancet 1986; 2:323-326.
138. Mao Y, Semenciw R, Morrison H, MacWilliam L, Davies J, Wigle D. Increased rates of illness and death from asthma in Canada. Can Med Assoc J 1987; 137:620-624.
139. Sly RM. Mortality from asthma in children 1979-1984. Ann Allergy 1988; 60:433-442.
140. Sears MR. Increasing asthma mortality—fact or artefact? J Allergy Clin Immunol (in press)
141. Sears MR, Rea HH, de Boer G, Beaglehole R, Gillies AJD, Holst PE, O'Donnell TV, Rothwell RPG. Accuracy of certification of deaths due to asthma. A national study. Am J Epidemiol 1986; 124:1004-1011.
142. British Thoracic Association. Death from asthma in two regions of England. Br Med J 1982; 285:1251-1255.
143. A subcommittee of the BTA Research Committee. Accuracy of death certificates in bronchial asthma. Thorax 1984; 39:505-9.
144. Sears MR, Rea HH, Rothwell RPG, O'Donnell TV, Holst PE, Gillies AJD, Beaglehole R. Asthma mortality: comparison between New Zealand and England. Br Med J 1986; 293:1342-1345.
145. World Health Organisation. Manual of the international statistical classificiation of diseases, injuries and cases of death: based on the recommendations of the ninth revision conference, 1975. Vol 1. Geneva, World Health Organisation.
146. Stewart CJ, Nunn AJ. Are asthma mortality rates changing? Br J Dis Chest 1985; 79:229-234.

147. Jackson R, Sears MR, Beaglehole R, Rea HH. International trends in asthma mortality 1970–1985. Chest (in press)
148. Barger LW, Vollmer WM, Felt RW, Buist AS. Further investigation into the recent increase in asthma death rates: a review of 41 asthma deaths in Oregon in 1982. Ann Allergy 1988; 60:31–39.
149. Buist AS, Sears MR, Reid LM, Boushet HA, Spector SL, Sheffer AL. Asthma mortality: trends and determinants. Am Rev Respir Dis 1987; 136:1037–1039.
150. Rea HH, Scragg R, Jackson R, Beaglehole R, Fenwick J, Sutherland DC. A case-control study of deaths from asthma. Thorax 1986; 41:833–839.
151. Sears MR, Rea HH, Fenwick J, Beaglehole R, Gillies AJD, Holst PE, O'Donnell TV, Rothwell RPG, Sutherland DC. Deaths from asthma in New Zealand. Arch Dis Child 1986; 61:6–10.
152. Strunk RC, Mrazek DA, Fuhrmann GSW, LaBrecque JF. Physiological and psychological characteristics associated with deaths due to asthma in childhood: a case-controlled study. J Am Med Assoc 1985; 254:1193–1198.
153. Johnson AJ, Nunn AJ, Somner AR, Stableforth DE, Stewart CJ. Circumstances of death from asthma. Br Med J 1984; 288:1870–1872.
154. Rea HH, Sears MR, Beaglehole R, Jackson RT, Gillies AJD, O'Donnell TV, Holst PE, Rothwell RPG. Lessons from the national asthma mortality study: circumstances surrounding death. NZ Med J 1987; 100:10–13.
155. Turner KJ, Rosman DL, OMahony J. Prevalence and familial association of atopic diseases and its relationship to serum IgE levels in 1061 school children and their families. Int Arch Allergy 1979; 47:650–664.
156. Crockett AJ, Ruffin RE, Schembri DA, Alpers JH. The prevalence rate of respiratory symptoms in schoolchildren from two South Australian rural communities. Aust NZJ Med 1986; 16:653–657.
157. Kraepelien S. The frequency of bronchial asthma in Swedish school children. Acta Paediatr Scand 1954; 43(Suppl 100):149–153.

3

Genetics of Asthma

RUSSELL J. HOPP and ROBERT G. TOWNLEY

Creighton University School of Medicine
Omaha, Nebraska

INTRODUCTION

Historical Perspective and Observational Studies

Asthma has been associated with familial or genetic factors for centuries. In 1868 Salter (1) noted that siblings in the same family could be asthmatic. An extensive study of family histories of 504 allergic subjects was reported in 1916 by Cooke and Vander Veer (2). Since a number of the subjects had asthma their observations are pertinent. Nearly 50% had positive family histories compared with fewer than 15% for the 76 normal subjects. It was later noted by Clarke et al. (3) that "the atopic shock tissues (bronchial and upper respiratory) are subject to separate hereditary influences." The concept that allergic and non-allergic triggers could be involved with asthma was discussed by Rackemann (4). Bray (5) reviewed the literature to 1930 and suggested that the tendency to develop asthma was inherited. This is akin to our present concept of airway hyperresponsiveness having a genetic basis (6) while the clinical condition of asthma is a complex interaction of genetic and environmental components.

Genetics of IgE Production

At the current time it seems reasonable to suggest that the presence of an atopic disease, such as allergic rhinitis, has a strong genetic determination. This is based, in large part, on studies showing that IgE is regulated by precise genetic mecha-

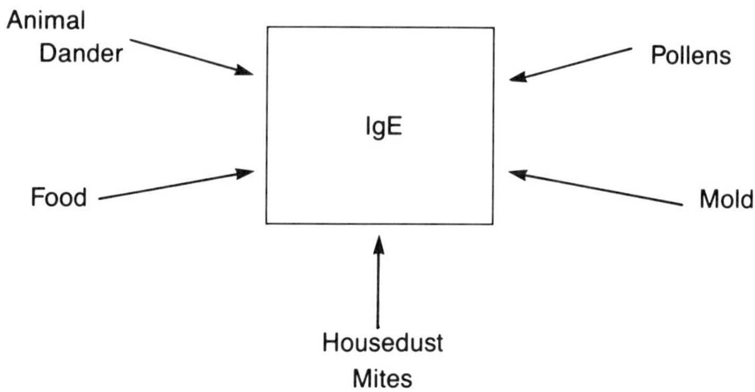

FIGURE 1 Theoretical schema for the IgE-mediated rhinitis.

nisms. Marsh et al. (7) have shown high IgE levels to be determined by two recessive alleles and Gerrard et al. (8), using a segregation analysis, suggested a regulatory locus with a recessive homozygote results in high levels of IgE. Since it is well known that individuals can be atopic, yet have a low serum IgE level, a recent study investigating the genetic component of IgE hyperresponsiveness was based on three definitive criteria. In this report by Cookson and Hopkin (9), subjects in nuclear and extended families were labeled as atopic if the subject had an IgE level greater than two standard deviations above the mean, if they had one or more positive skin tests, or if they had one or more positive radioallergosorbent IgE tests (RAST). Their analysis suggested that the inclination to develop atopy is inherited as an autosomal dominant trait. Using this reasoning it is possible to represent allergic rhinitis as in Figure 1.

Asthma as a Genetic Disease

A similar approach to asthma has not proved to be as straightforward. A hypothetical model (Fig. 2) suggests that while IgE has a potential role in the aggravation of asthma, it is likely not the primary defect. The high prevalence of atopy in young asthmatics, compared with adult-onset asthmatics, might suggest that allergic asthma and allergic nonasthmatic diseases is one disease complex and intrinsic (nonallergic) asthma is a separate disease, but with each having enough clinical overlap to provide similar presentations. Alternatively, the potential for IgE sensitization and asthma are closely linked, but separate diseases. At the present time, tools are not available to adequately distinguish between these possibilities.

A major problem in asthma studies, genetic or otherwise, is the lack of a precise definition for the condition. As depicted in Figure 2, asthma appears

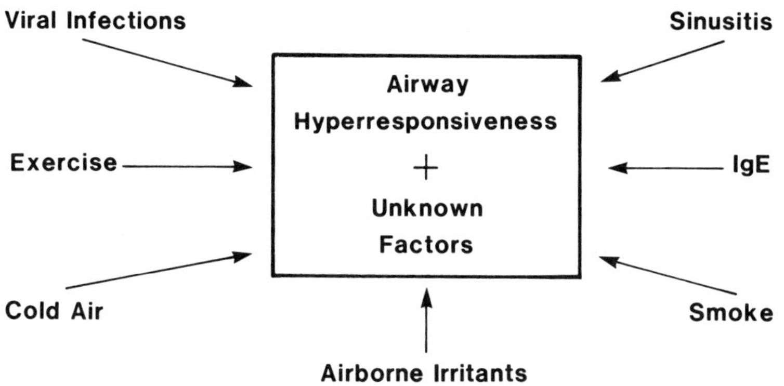

FIGURE 2 Proposed schema for bronchial asthma.

to result from a close association of increased airway responsiveness and as yet unspecified factors. It was previously thought that measuring the degree of airway responsiveness could be used as a diagnostic test for asthma. The absence of nonspecific bronchial reactivity, using histamine or methacholine, can generally qualify an individual as being a current nonasthmatic. However, the opposite may not be true.

Despite the fact that asthma is well-recognized clinically, epidemiological studies have shown that symptoms compatible with asthma do not always correlate with physician diagnosis or the presence of airway hyperresponsiveness (10). The lack of a definitive diagnostic criteria or a biochemical marker for asthma has made advances in genetic analysis shorthanded when it comes to trying to unravel the etiology of the disease.

GENETIC STUDIES USING THE DIAGNOSIS OF ASTHMA

Family Studies

There have been many attempts to investigate allergic diseases and asthma using family and twin studies. One approach uses a reasonable definition of asthma to ascertain a proband, and then studies the nuclear families of the asthmatic. The most extensive use of this technique has been performed by Sibbald and Turner-Warwick. In their earliest report (11) they selected allergic and nonallergic asthmatic probands from a clinic population. Asthma was defined by episodic wheezing, responsive to bronchodilators, or by improvement in airways obstruction on follow-up visits. A positive response to one or more prick skin tests defined the subject as atopic. Information about first-degree relatives was obtained from the proband.

In the families of allergic asthmatics, the risk for siblings of the proband to also be asthmatic increased when one or both parents were asthmatic. Allergic histories in siblings increased as the parents histories of these diseases increased. In the families of the nonallergic asthmatic, there were fewer atopic or asthma familial associations. Comparison of the two family types showed that the allergic asthmatics' families had more asthma and allergic histories compared with the nuclear families with a nonallergic asthmatic as the proband. In a subsequent review, Sibbald (12) reported that the presence of asthma was higher in the parents and offspring of asthmatics, compared with the siblings of the proband. The conclusion drawn from a study by Sibbald et al. (13) was that atopic asthma appears to have a genetic basis and that atopic risk factors enhance the development of asthma.

A further study using asthmatic children and a control group was undertaken by Sibbald et al. (13) using similar criteria and methods (11). There was a significant difference in family histories of asthma, hay fever, and eczema between the two groups. In the asthma families, more parents (of asthmatics) had asthma than did siblings of the asthmatics; in control families the parents and siblings were equally affected. Furthermore, the type of asthma (allergic vs. nonallergic) in the relatives of the probands was not associated with the atopic status of the proband. The authors concluded that atopy and asthma are inherited separately. Atopy may also influence or potentiate the development of asthma.

Similar findings were presented by Gerrard et al. (14). In a study of 176 families, using methods and definitions of asthma comparable to the reports of Sibbald et al. (11-13), the investigators found significant associations between asthma, hay fever, recurrent rhinitis, or bronchitis in parents and children. They suggested a heritable component to end-organ allergic hyperresponsiveness.

In a later report, Sibbald et al. (15) looked at the familial incidence of asthma in children with wheezy bronchitis. Their results suggested that both conditions shared similar backgrounds, with enhanced familial incidences of asthma. A current theory would be that wheezy bronchitis is asthma triggered by a viral illness, but the child, as yet, does not have a definite allergic history.

In a study by Leeder et al., 2000 children were evaluated for family factors associated with asthma and wheezy bronchitis (16). Their hypothesis was that if wheezy bronchitis was only mild asthma the familial factors would be the same. By the age of five years, asthma had been reported in about 3% of the children (boys > girls), while wheezy bronchitis was reported in approximately 21% of the children (boys > girls). The incidence of asthma and wheezy bronchitis was higher in a child if the parent(s) had a history of asthma or wheezing.

Twin Studies

Twins provide a suitable model for studying the hereditary and environmental influences on clinical states. An often cited study (17) was derived from nearly 7000 pairs collected in a Swedish Twin Registry. Questionnaire information was used for zygosity determination and asthma history. A diagnosis of current or former asthma was found in 3.8% of the population. The concordance rate for monozygous twins was 19%, but only 4% in dizygous twins. Other studies, which have been reviewed by Falliers et al. (18), reported concordance rates for asthma to be 30-80% for monozygous twins and 4 to 45% for nonidentical twins. The results of numerous twin studies suggest a hereditary component to the development of asthma. Based on a risk analysis of the Swedish twin data (19), it was estimated that a first-degree relative of an asthmatic has an increased risk of developing asthma.

HLA MARKERS IN ASTHMA

If asthma or atopy has a genetic cause or susceptibility it would be reasonable to investigate the association of different HLA types. Specific HLA loci have been associated with the atopic immune response to purified ragweed fractions (20). A similar approach has been investigated with asthma. This is limited, however, by the fact that the diagnosis of asthma in most studies was established by history, and not by using a biochemical or quantitative marker. The analysis may also be complicated by the fact that most young asthmatics are also atopic and HLA loci identified in studies may reflect the existence of two diseases. In an attempt to overcome this problem, investigation of a HLA association has been done using asthmatics without coexisting evidence for atopic disease. Table 1 summarizes the studies to date, that have attempted to identify HLA associations in asthmatics.

Several studies have used specific criteria to identify asthmatics. Rachelefsky et al. (33) used a positive response to a bronchodilator to identify their asthmatic population. The subjects were also atopic. There was a trend toward a greater frequency of HLA-A2 in the asthmatics. Using methacholine airway hyperresponsiveness as a marker, Easton et al. (34) confirmed an association between an HLA haplotype and atopy in nonasthmatics (who were siblings of asthmatics) hyperresponsive to methacholine as well as a HLA haplotype association in 10 families with a parent and child with atopic asthma.

Investigators have looked at B-lymphocyte antigen frequencies in asthmatics. The expression of the different B-cell antigens is dependent on HLA specificity. In one report (33), there was a strong association with a B-cell antigen Group 2 in individuals with asthma. In a study of 30 families with an asthmatic child as

TABLE 1

Author	Year	Asthma	HLA association	Reference
Thorsby	1971	Mixed	HL-A1, 8 HL-2, BB	21
Geerts	1975	Mixed	HL-A	22
Bruce	1976	Extrinsic	HLA-BW40	23
Brostoff	1976	Intrinsic	HLA-B W6	24
Wagatsuma	1976	Extrinsic	HLA association	25
Flaherty	1977	Intrinsic	No W4 or W6 association	26
Morris	1977	Mixed	HLA-B8, A1	27
Rachelefsky	1977	?	B8 (low), HLA-A2	28
Turton	1979	Mixed	No HLA association	29
Flaherty	1980	Mixed	No HLA association	30
Morris	1980	Mixed	No definite associations	31
Nakai	1982	Extrinsic	No HLA-A or B association	32

Extrinsic = + skin tests, Intrinsic = – skin tests, Mixed = Both +/–.

proband (35), the specificity of B-cell antigens was consistent with an association of their presence in asthmatics and HLA-A and HLA-B loci.

The presence of a HLA-D(DR) association with asthma is limited by the extensive laboratory evaluation necessary to delineate a possible relationship. Nakai et al. (32), using 23 allergic asthmatics, found no HLA-A,B,C association, but did find that 100% of the asthmatics demonstrated a MB3 antigen (includes DR4, DR5, and DRw9) compared with 72% of controls. A positive HLA-D(R) association was reported by Morris et al. (31). Further work in the association of HLA-D(R) antigens and asthma is needed.

The HLA studies make a reasonable argument for a genetic basis for asthma. The lack of a clear determination of HLA types as it relates to asthma, however, could be explained many ways: (1) a difference in allergic and nonallergic asthma; (2) several different HLA loci determine the susceptibility to asthma; (3) a susceptibility gene(s) must interact with yet unspecified environmental stimuli; (4) there is a delayed penetrance to the expression of a susceptibility gene.

GENETIC STUDIES USING QUANTITATIVE MEASURES OF AIRWAY RESPONSIVENESS

Family Studies

It is accepted that airway hyperresponsiveness is a necessary component to the definition of current asthma (Fig. 2). All current asthmatics have airway hyperresponsiveness to inhaled methacholine or histamine. The presence of a response to methacholine or histamine, however, does not in itself establish the diagnosis of asthma. Since there is no established or undisputed method of establishing a clinical diagnosis of asthma, it seems reasonable to employ a quantitative measurement of airway responsiveness as a marker. A number of studies, in both families and twins, have utilized measures of airway responsiveness to help establish a genetic link to asthma.

Rachelefsky et al. (33) previously reported HLA associations in individuals who respond to a bronchodilator. A positive response to a bronchodilator is generally considered an indicator of airway hyperresponsiveness. In their report of 30 families in which the child with asthma was also allergic, there was no HLA association, but there was an association with B-cell antigen Group 2. Easton et al. (34) did find an association between an HLA antigen and airway hyperresponsiveness.

There are two centers with extensive experience of measures of airway responsiveness in families. Townley et al. (6) published a report that showed airway hyperresponsiveness in asthma nuclear families, ascertained by the recruitment of an asthmatic proband (ages 6–25 years), and compared with families without an asthma/allergy family history. Probands from both families were excluded from the analysis. Further analysis of these families has confirmed the original observation (36,37).

In a similar investigation, Longo et al. (38) measured airway responsiveness to inhaled carbacholine in nonasthmatic parents of asthmatics, nonasthmatic controls, and current symptomatic asthmatics. They found that 10% of controls and 50% of parents of asthmatics had airway hyperresponsiveness in the same range as the current asthmatics (Fig. 3). There was no association between airway hyperresponsiveness and atopy, as determined by skin test response to six common antigens. They concluded that the airway hyperresponsiveness that exists in asthma families indicates an autosomal-dominant pattern of inheritance. Townley et al. (6) had previously reported the bimodal distribution of airway responsiveness in their studies of asthma families (Fig. 4) suggested a single biochemical or physical defect.

This pattern of airway hyperresponsiveness in nonasthmatic parents has also been reported by Hopp et al. (39) (Fig. 5), who demonstrated no significant association between nonspecific airway hyperresponsiveness and atopic status. This would further suggest that while IgE influences airway hyperresponsiveness (40), it does not singularly cause it. A recent report further confirms the familial aggregation of airway hyperresponsiveness. Clifford et al. (41) studied 50 children who had one parent with asthma. These children had a 50% increase in respiratory symptoms of cough, wheeze, and shortness of breath when compared with controls. Over 90% of the asthmatic parents had methacholine airway hyperresponsiveness, while 45% of the children had similar responses.

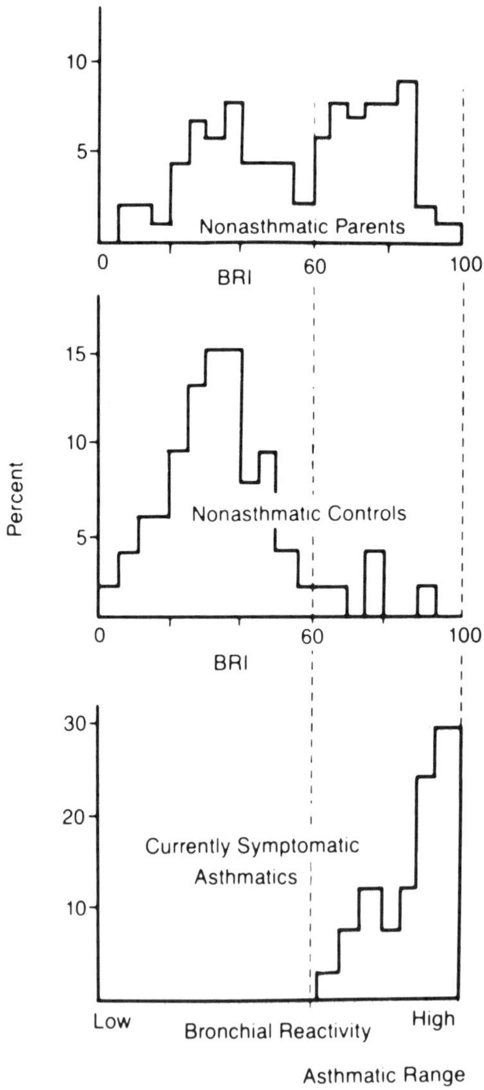

FIGURE 3 Frequency distribution of age-corrected methacholine airway responsiveness in normal individuals from control families and families with asthma. From Ref. 6.

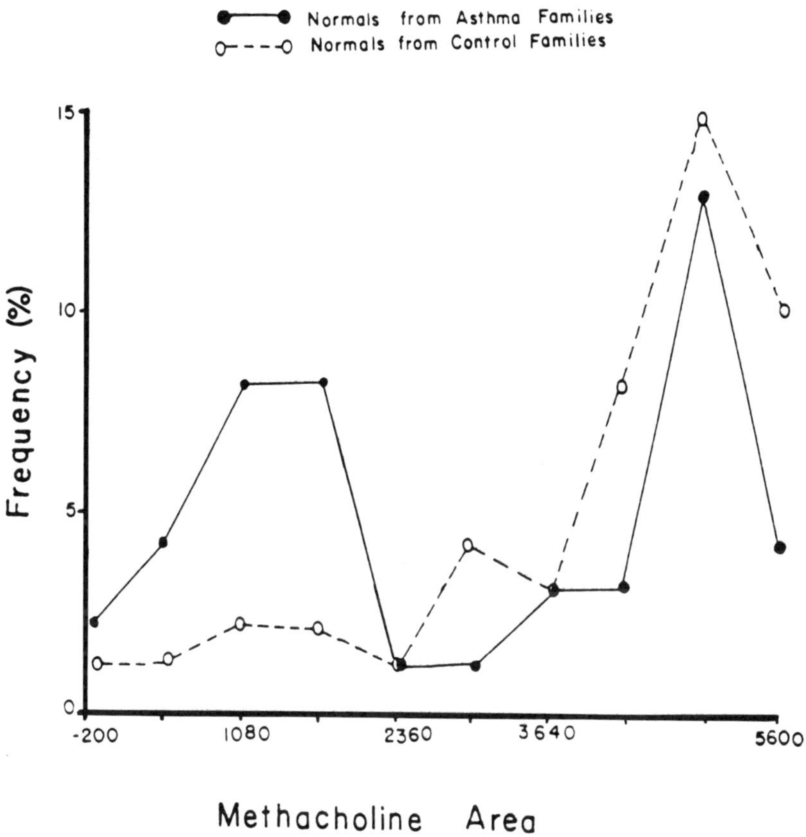

FIGURE 4 Distribution of methacholine airway responsiveness in non-asthmatic parents pairs who have a asthmatic child. From Ref. 39.

Bruderman et al. (42) recently investigated the degree of mechacholine airway hyperresponsiveness in parents of asthmatic children, parents of healthy children, and asthmatics. Airway responsiveness was assessed both by sensitivity, defined as the dose of methacholine inducing a 25% change in specific airway conductance (SGaw), and reactivity, defined as the slope of the dose-response line. There were 28 parents of asthmatics, 7 parents of healthy children, and 4 current asthmatics. The parents of the asthmatics were divided into two groups (Fig. 6). Group A (17 subjects) had allergic rhinitis or a decreased forced expiratory flow at 50% of vital capacity. The remaining 11 subjects (Group B) were not atopic and had normal baseline pulmonary function. The four asthmatics had the highest degree of both reactivity and sensitivity to metha-

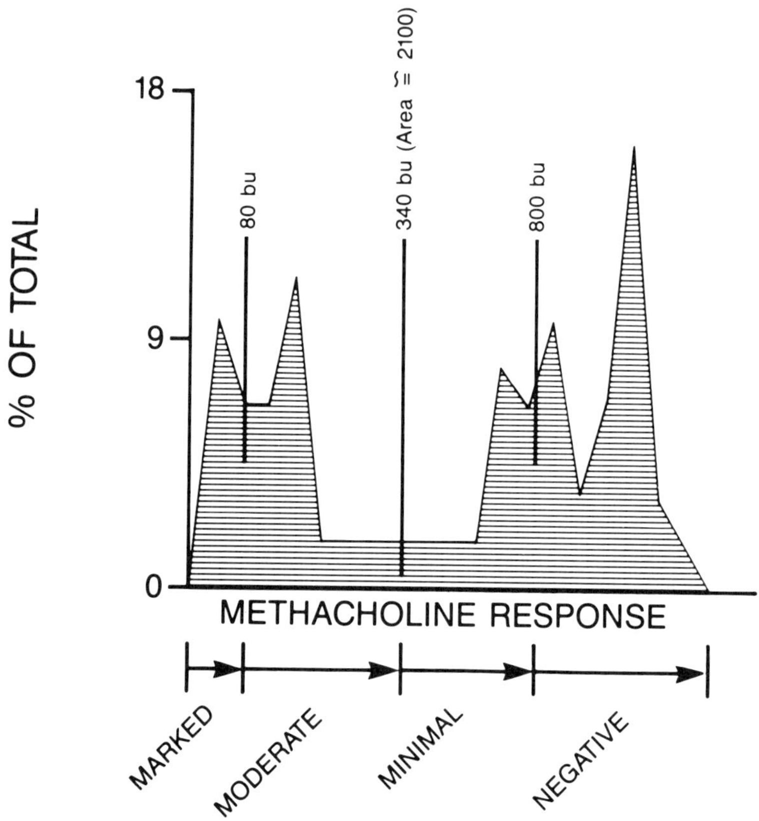

FIGURE 5 Distribution of carbacholine airway responsiveness in three studies groups. From Ref. 38.

choline (Fig. 6). The parents of healthy children did not have a response to the methacholine challenge. The Group A parents had a significant degree of sensitivity and reactivity, and three of these subjects subsequently developed asthma. Group B subjects had minimal reactivity and sensitivity, but more than the parents of healthy children. The mean percent decrease in SGaw for the Group A parents was 50 ± 32 and for the Group B parents 4.5 ± 1.5. This would again suggest (Fig. 6) the bimodal distribution of methacholine responses in parents of asthmatics as previously reported (37,38).

A segregation analysis of airway responsiveness to methacholine in nuclear families with and without asthma was reported by Townley et al. (43). They

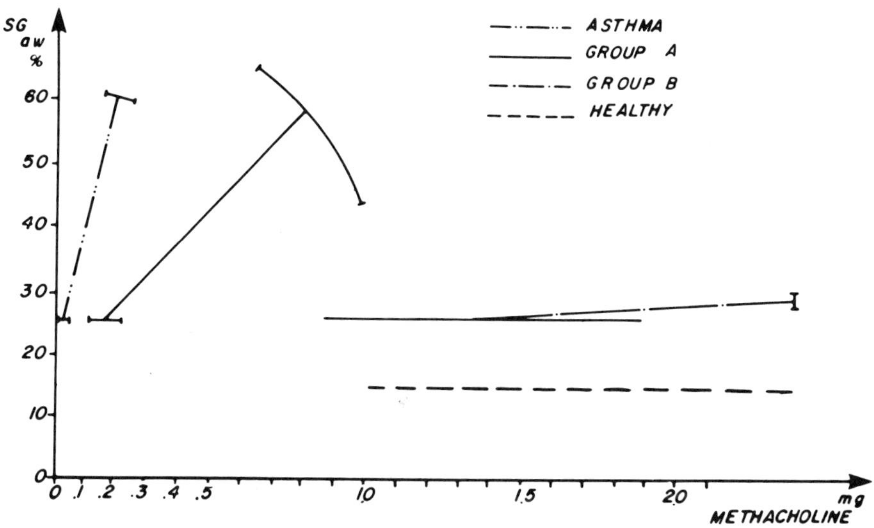

FIGURE 6 Mean dose responses lines for methacholine airway hyperresponsiveness in Group A parents, Group B parents, asthmatics and normal controls. From Ref. 42.

found a familial (possibly genetic) transmission of methacholine airway hyperresponsiveness.

The studies of airway hyperresponsiveness in parents and nuclear families of asthmatics have unanimously agreed that familial, possibly genetic, factors are involved in the genesis. Studies in random populations (44) have shown that the distribution of airway responsiveness is probably unimodal. Selected populations, however, have shown bimodal (6,37,38) distributions. It is clear that the results of studies of airway hyperresponsiveness are largely dependent on subject selection.

Other studies provide further insight into end-organ hyperresponsiveness. Bertrand et al. (45) speculated that there is an association between familial airway hyperresponsiveness, premature labor, and the development of long-term pulmonary problems in premature infants. Their study of children with a history of premature birth and respiratory distress indicate these children will have airway hyperresponsiveness. Airway hyperresponsiveness was also present in the mothers of the premature children. This suggests several possibilities. There may be a common hyperresponsiveness in uterine and airway smooth muscle. Females who have airway hyperresponsiveness also have uterine musculature that has enhanced responsiveness, resulting in susceptibility to premature labor. This is supported by the fact that medications used to stop premature labor are often the same ones used in asthma management.

The incidence of family histories of asthma in children with bronchpulmonary dysplasia is high (46). When born prematurely, these children have airway hyperresponsiveness and therefore, may be more susceptible to the influences of treatment, including oxygen and pressure ventilation.

Although methacholine and histamine challenge are the most sensitive indicators of airway hyperresponsiveness, other tests are available. Exercise challenges have been used to determine the degree of airway responsiveness in relatives of asthmatics. Konig and Godfrey (47) reported exercise challenge and skin test results in 65 first-degree relatives of 12 children with asthma. A positive index for airway hyperresponsiveness occurred in 10 of the 12 asthmatic children, 50% of family members with a current history of asthma, 33% of the family members with a past history of asthma, 40% with hay fever, and 32% of the healthy relatives. Overall, 28 of the 65 family members responded, while 48% of subjects with at least one positive skin test responded. Although a control group was not included, it is impressive that many nonasthmatic subjects responded to a challenge that generally is considered not to be as sensitive as methacholine.

In a similar study Konig and Godfrey (48) suggested the existence of a genetic background to airway hyperresponsiveness, based on the investigation of children with a past history of wheezy bronchitis. A current philosophy is that "wheezy bronchitis" is asthma predominantly triggered by viral infections. A similar genetic background would be expected.

The longitudinal study of pulmonary function and disease undertaken by Higgins and Keller (49) of residents in Tecumseh, Michigan, provides additional, although indirect, evidence for genetic factors in the development of various pulmonary conditions. Although airway responsiveness was not directly measured, there was significant correlation between FEV_1 values in first-degree relatives and between parents and children. They also found that prevalences of chronic bronchitis, asthma, and allergic rhinitis were higher in offspring when a parent(s) had the same condition.

In a review of autonomic abnormalities of cystic fibrosis, Davis (50) mentions that cholinergic dysfunction seen in asthmatics is also seen in healthy first-degree relatives of cystic fibrosis patients. These abnormal findings include pupillary dysfunction to carbacholine and airway hyperresponsiveness. Although not yet investigated in detail, this would suggest a genetic basis for the autonomic abnormalities seen in these two diseases.

The entire concept of airway hyperresponsiveness in asthmatics and their family members raises the equally intriguing question of why some nonasthmatic subjects fail to react when challenged with methacholine or histamine. All normal human bronchi or trachea, when suspended in a muscle bath, respond in a dose-dependent manner to histamine or methacholine (51). The reason non-asthmatic adult subjects fail to respond similarly to asthmatic subjects and many of their family members in vivo needs to be addressed.

A recent report may provide a partial answer. In this study of 10 normal infants, all responded to methacholine (52). This is consistent with the finding that the airways in young children are more responsive than in adults (53). Serial measurement of airway responsiveness from infancy to adulthood may help identify potential asthmatics. These individuals may fail to lose the airway hyperresponsiveness that appears to be present in infancy.

Twin Studies

Although there are limitations in using the twin model to examine the influence of heredity, genetic analysis of twins remains an accessible and practical method of estimating the weight of genetic influence on clinically measurable parameters. This is because members of a monozygous twin pair share a genotype and a relatively similar environment. By comparing clinical or laboratory parameters of a disease condition in monozygous twins (MZ) and dizygous twins (DZ), it is possible to provide evidence for the genetic determination of those parameters, under reasonable assumptions (54).

Comparison of intrapair correlation coefficients (r) provides an indicator of the role of heredity as a clinical marker of atopic disease or airway hyperresponsiveness. An estimate of heritability (H), 2(rMZ-rDZ), has been used (55). It provides an estimation of the contribution of heredity to the variance of the measured trait or marker. When H equals one, the variation in the measurement is due completely to heredity. As H approaches zero the measurement is presumed to be determined by environmental factors. In addition, pair and casewise (proband) concordance rates are commonly used to express the results of twin data (56).

It is well recognized that elevated levels of IgE are associated with allergic disease, and that total IgE is under genetic control. In a study (57) of IgE levels in young twins, including 61 MZ pairs and 47 DZ pairs, the intrapair correlation coefficient for the MZ pairs was 0.82 and 0.52 for the DZ pairs. The heritability estimate was 0.61. This value suggests an important genetic contribution to the total IgE level.

Measurements of airway responsiveness can be compared in twins. A twin study by Falliers et al. (18) reported that in the decade from 1960–1970, 11 asthmatics had a unaffected fraternal twin at home. During the same time period, three identical twin pairs were seen, all with asthma. An additional two pair of identical twins were found to be discordant for asthma diagnosis. All four were atopic and had similar IgE levels. Only the asthmatic twins responded to an exercise challenge. Both asthmatics responded to methacholine, as expected. Neither of the nonasthmatic twins had a methacholine response. They further suggested that longitudinal studies of identical twins discordant for asthma diagnosis would be valuable.

Konig and Godfrey (58) used a standardized exercise challenge to compare 8 identical (5 male pairs) and 7 nonidentical twin pairs (5 male-female, 1 male-male, 1 female-female). They found that 6 pairs of the MZ twins were concordant for exercise lability, while only one of the DZ pairs was concordant.

A methacholine inhalation challenge is a well-standardized and accepted method of measuring airway responsiveness. Parametric (numerical) measurements of airway responsiveness in each twin pair can be used to determine an intrapair correlation coefficient and a heritability index. In a studied group of 107 twin pairs (57), the 61 MZ pairs had a correlation coefficient for methacholine airway hyperresponsiveness of 0.67, while the 47 DZ pairs had a correlation coefficient of 0.34. The methacholine challenge in this study is presented using an area under the best-fit parabolic curve (58). The endpoint is a 35% fall in the FEV_1. The cumulative dose of methacholine is 800 bu. All subjects have a quantitative value for their challenge, even if there was a zero percent change by the last step (59). A determination of the heritability estimate for the methacholine airway hyperresponsiveness was 0.66. This provides support for a genetic influence on airway hyperresponsiveness.

A study by Zamel et al. (60), with 10 pairs of MZ and 10 pairs of DZ twins, did not find a major genetic influence to airway hyperresponsiveness. Response to methacholine was measured using an 11-step methacholine dose regimen. The 40% change in V_{40p} and the 20% fall in FEV_1 were both used as measured parameters. The step at which there was a 40% fall in V_{40p} or a 20% fall in FEV_1 was compared (between the twin pairs), and a mean intrapair difference determined. There was no significant difference between the MZ and DZ groups. The author had no explanation as to why there was not a better correlation in MZ twins compared with DZ twins. He suggested that a larger group of twins needed to be studied using their methodology prior to making definitive conclusions. This study was performed on healthy adults compared with the larger group of twins reported by Hopp et al. (57), who had asthmatic, allergic, and normal histories. This difference in populations may account for the disparity of the reported results. At the present time the report by Zamel et al. (60) provides pertinent information, but must be interpreted in view of the patient numbers and conditions. It should not be used as conclusive proof for the lack of a genetic component to airway hyperresponsiveness.

A recent report provides a unique insight into the genetic contribution to pulmonary function as reflected in twin studies. Ackerman et al. (61) investigated 39 twin pairs at a mean age of 11.4 months. Included were 25 MZ and 14 DZ pairs. A positive family history for asthma was found in 30% of the infants.

Pulmonary function in the infants was determined in a sleep state, and the measurements of maximal expiratory FRC (functional residual capacity) were performed with rapid chest compression. There was greater intrapair variation in pulmonary measurements between DZ twins compared with MZ twins. A similar finding had been previously shown in a large population of adult twins using standard pulmonary function testing (62).

GENETIC STUDIES USING BIOCHEMICAL MARKERS POSSIBLY ASSOCIATED WITH ASTHMA

Other biochemical markers have been studied to determine their connection with asthma. This may provide further support for a genetic background to asthma. A study from 1975 (63) investigated the association of 13 protein and blood enzyme markers in 127 asthmatic subjects and controls. There was a statistical difference in the distribution of $alpha_1$-antitrypsin types (more MS in the asthmatics) and the 6-GPD levels (approaching significance). They also found a possible difference in adenosine deaminase (ADA) levels between the two groups. A more definitive study in this regard was reported by Ronchetti et al. (64) in 1984, when they investigated the ADA phenotype in 291 children (1 month to 15 years) who had episodes of wheezing requiring medical intervention and compared them with 56 controls. They demonstrated that the frequency of ADA phenotype 2-1 (random population frequency: 1-1 = 83%, 2-2 = .5%, 2-1 = 16%) is significantly reduced in "wheezers" compared with controls. However, wheezy atopic children over 5 years old are more likely to be ADA phenotype 1. The genetic association of ADA phenotypes and asthma is, however, still not known.

Much attention has been directed toward the possible association of $alpha_1$-antitrypsin levels and types and asthma. There has been an association of Z heterozygote variants and deficient Pi types in steroid-dependent asthmatics (65). The association found to date would suggest an additive role of selected Pi types to the exacerbation of pre-existing asthma.

Additional studies have investigated the genetic link of other biochemical markers and asthma. Anton-Guirgis et al. (66) compared the immunoglobulin allotypes, Gm-Am and Km, in 33 asthma families and 11 control families. Methacholine airway responsiveness was determined in the members of the families. They found an association between methacholine airway responsiveness and different immunoglobulin allotypes, which suggested to them evidence for an incomplete genetic predisposition to allergic asthma.

In other reports Piessens et al. (67) found a high frequency of decreased haptoglobin levels in patients with asthma and/or rhinitis, and suggested this was a genetically determined reduction in haptoglobulin levels with a yet undetermined association with atopic or asthmatic conditions. Srivastava et al. (68)

found an association between the $C3^F$ (complement) gene and bronchial asthma. Brostoff et al. (24) reported that 13 of 26 intrinsic asthmatics had a low level of C2.

OCCUPATIONAL ASTHMA

At the present time it has not been conclusively established that airway hyperresponsiveness is a pre-existing phenomenon in the development of either nonoccupational or occupational asthma. Until studies of this type are performed, a strong argument for a genetic basis for asthma and airway hyperresponsiveness is incomplete. An additional body of information to be confirmed is whether there is evidence of familial histories of asthma in subjects who develop occupational asthma in comparison with workers who do not. Studies of this type in asthma have shown a family association. It seems feasible to suggest that subjects who develop occupational asthma to high-molecular-weight substances which is due to IgE sensitization, will have increased family histories, while an investigation of the family allergy and asthmatic histories in subjects with occupational asthma to low-molecular-weight substances, which is not obviously due to IgE sensitization would be enlightening.

A further argument against a genetic influence in occupational asthma, is that airway hyperresponsiveness, present during the acute problem, diminishes (or returns to "normal") after removal from the environment. Airway hyperresponsiveness in some instances does not completely return to normal after removal (69,70) and has been shown to increase again if the subject returns to the work place. Similarly, individuals with nonoccupational asthma have a diminished degree of airway hyperresponsiveness as time from last symptoms increases (71).

Asthma symptoms have been reported in subjects exposed to high levels of smoke, ammonia, or other airborne contaminants at work (72). Biopsy specimens from two subjects showed respiratory epithelial injury with chronic inflammatory response. This condition is probably similar to that seen in subjects with chronic bronchitis (73), in whom chronic bronchial inflammation exists. It would not be expected that allergic or asthmatic family histories would be markedly elevated in these subjects as they likely are a heterogeneous subject population, with variable allergic and families histories of asthma or allergies.

CONCLUSIONS

Most studies investigating the hereditary aspect of atopic (the genetic predisposition to develop IgE-mediated disease) asthma show that genetic factors influence the development of the clinical allergic state. Occurrence of asthma in population, family, and twin studies has been subjected to genetic analysis, and investigators have suggested that the inheritance of asthma does not fit a single gene Mendelian pattern, but more closely fits a polygenic pattern. The concept of the influence of a hereditary factor on the end organ separate from the atopic tendency itself is reported in studies suggesting the existence of a separate genetic localization factor for asthma. Studies of twins have revealed that the concordance of asthma is higher in monozygotic than dizygotic twins, but environmental factors are at least as important as genetic factors. Before further progress can be made it will be necessary to define and classify asthma more precisely. This precondition has not yet been met, but certain aspects of the inheritance of asthma have been examined. Although many studies have been done in humans, no association of asthma with a specific histocompatibility locus has been shown.

Airway hyperresponsiveness in siblings of asthmatic subjects suggests that genetic factors contribute to methacholine hyperresponsiveness.

To evaluate the familial nature of asthma and methacholine hyperresponsiveness, Townley et al. (6) studied 47 atopic and 26 nonatopic families. Atopic families had at least one child with current asthma. There was a total of 648 members in these families. In nonatopic families, 237 members had no reported history of asthma, hayfever, or atopic eczema for at least three generations. All probands were excluded for genetic analysis.

When the frequency of positive responses for the methacholine challenge in the normal subjects from atopic and nonatopic families was determined, two peaks or subpopulations were obtained in the atopic (asthma) families. In contrast, the normal subjects from nonatopic families have a single uniform distribution with no corresponding subpopulation of methacholine responders. The individuals with a positive test may be potential asthmatics.

We reported on 107 pairs of twins (61 monozygous and 46 dizygous). Included were histories of allergic disease and asthma, IgE antibody levels, methacholine airway responsiveness, and skin responses. The analysis (57) demonstrated that these characteristics were heritable traits and suggested a genetic contribution to their expression.

ACKNOWLEDGMENT

Supported in part by Grant No. HL-01508 from the National Heart, Lung and Blood Institute.

REFERENCES

1. Salter HH. *On Asthma: Its Pathology and Treatment*. London, Churchill, 1968, 2nd ed.
2. Cooke RA, Vander Veer A. J Immunol 1916; 1:201–305.

3. Clarke JA Jr, Donnally HH, Coca AF. Studies in specific hypersensitiveness XXXII. On the influence of heredity in atopy. J Immunol 1928; 15: 9–11.
4. Rackemann FM. Studies in asthma. Arch Int Med 1928;41:346–369.
5. Bray GW. The hereditary factor in asthma and other allergies. Br Med J 1930;1:384–387.
6. Townley RG, Bewtra AK, Nair NM, Brodkey FD, Watt GD, Burke KM. Methacholine inhalation challenge studies. J Allergy Clin Immunol 1979; 64(2):569–574.
7. Marsh D, Bias W, Ishizaka K. Genetic control of basal serum immunoglobin E level and its effect on specific sensitivity. Proc Natl Acad Sci 1974;71:3588–3592.
8. Gerrard JW, Rao DC, Morton NE. A genetic study of immunoglobulin E. Am J Hum Genet 1978;30:46–58.
9. Cookson WOCM, Hopkin JM. Dominant inheritance of atopic immunoglobulin-E responsiveness. Lancet 1988;i:86–88.
10. Enarson DA, Vedal S, Schulzer M, Dybuncio A, Chan-Yeung M. Asthma, asthmalike symptoms, chronic bronchitis, and the degree of bronchial hyperresponsiveness in epidemiologic surveys. Am Rev Resp Dis 1987; 136:613–617.
11. Sibbald B, Turner-Warwick M. Factors influencing the prevalence of asthma among first degree relatives of extrinsic and intrinsic asthmatics. Thorax 1979;34:332–337.
12. Sibbald B. Extrinsic and intrinsic asthma: Influence of classification on family history of asthma and allergic disease. Clin Allergy 1980; 10:313–318.
13. Sibbald B, Horn MEC, Brain EA, Gregg I. Genetic factors in childhood asthma. Thorax 1980;35:671–674.
14. Gerrard JW, Ko CG, Vickers P, Gerrard CD. The familial incidence of allergic disease. Ann Allergy 1976;36:10–15.
15. Sibbald B, Horn MEC, Gregg I. A family study of the genetic basis of asthma and wheezy bronchitis. Arch Dis Child 1980; 55:354–357.
16. Leeder SR, Corkhill RT, Irwig LM, Holland WW. Influence of family factors on asthma and wheezing during the first five years of life. Br J Prev Soc Med 1976;30:213–218.
17. Edfors-Lubs ML. Allergy in 7000 twin pairs. Acta Allergol (Kbh) 1971; 26:249–285.
18. Falliers CJ, de A Cardoso RR, Bane HN, Coffey R, Middleton E Jr. Discordant allergic manifestations in monozygotic twins: Genetic identity versus clinical, physiologic and biochemical differences. J Allergy 1971; 47:207–219.
19. E Lubs ML. Emperic risks for genetic counseling in families with allergy. Pediatrics 1972;80:26–31.
20. Marsh DG, Hsu SH, Hussain R, Meyers DA, Freidhoff LR, Bias WB. Genetics of human immune response to allergens. J Allergy Clin Immunol 1980;65:322–332.

21. Thorsby E, Lie SO. Relationship between the HL-A system and susceptibility to diseases. Transplant Proc 1971;3:1305–1307.
22. Geerts SJ, Pottgens H, Limburg M, Van Rood JJ. Predisposition for atopy or allergy linked to HL-A. Lancet 1975;i:461.
23. Bruce CA, Bias WB, Norman PS, Lichtenstein LM, Marsh DG. Studies of HLA antigen frequencies, IgE levels, and specific allergic sensitivities in patients having ragweed hayfever, with and without asthma. Clin Exp Immunol 1976;25:67–72.
24. Brostoff J, Mowbray JF, Kapoor A, Hollowell SJ, Rudolf M, Saunders KB. 80% of patients with intrinsic asthma are homozygous for HLA W6. Is intrinsic asthma a recessive disease? Lancet 1976;ii:872–873.
25. Wagatsuma Y, Yakura H, Nakayama E, Wakisaka A, Aizawa M, Miyata M, Matsuyama R, Sato M, Itakura K. Inheritance of asthma in families and its linkage to HLA haplotypes. Acta Allergol (Kbh) 1976;31:455–462.
26. Flaherty DK, Geller M, Bach FH, Reed CE. Frequency of W4 and W6 antigens in perennial, nonallergic asthmatics. J Allergy Clin Immunol 1977; 60:236–237.
27. Morris MJ, Vaughan H, Lane DJ, Morris PJ. HLA in asthma. Monogr Allergy 1977; 11:30–34.
28. Rachelefsky GS, Terasaki PI, Katz RM, Siegel SC. B lymphocyte and histocompatibility antigens in extrinsic asthma. Monogr Allergy 1977; 11:35.
29. Turton CWG, Morris L, Buckingham JA, Lawler SD, Turner-Warwick M. Histocompatibility antigens in asthma: Population and family studies. Thorax 1979;34:670–676.
30. Flaherty DK, Geller M, Surfus JE, Leo GM, Reed CE, Rankin J. HLA antigen frequencies and natural history in Alternaria-sensitive and perennial nonallergic asthmatics. J Allergy Clin Immunol 1980; 66:408–416.
31. Morris MJ, Faux JA, Ting PJ, Morris PJ, Lane DJ. HLA-A, B and C and HLA-DR antigens in intrinsic and allergic asthma. Clin Allergy 1980; 10: 173–179.
32. Nakai Y, Kano T, Moriuchi J, Wakisake A, Aizawa M, Tsuneta H, Togashi K, Sakiyama Y, Wagatsuma Y, Matsumoto S. Association between the MB system and asthma in the Japanese. Hum Immunol 1982; 4:265–270.
33. Rachelefsky G, Park MS, Sieges S, Terasaki PI, Katz R, Saito S. Strong association between B-lymphocyte group-2 specificity and asthma. Lancet 1976;ii:1042–1044.
34. Easton J, Brady R, Kaplan M, Terasaki PI, Glovsky M. Studies on the relationship of bronchial hyperreactivity to methacholine and HLA haplotypes in asthmatic families. J Allergy Clin Immunol 1978; 61:158.
35. Saito S, Terasaki PI, Rachelefsky GS, Park MS, Mickey MR. B-lymphocyte haplotypes in asthma families. Transplant Proc 1977; 9 (Suppl 1):127–132.
36. Hopp RJ, Bewtra AK, Nair NM, Watt GD, Townley RG. Methacholine inhalation challenge studies in a selected pediatric population. Am Rev Respir Dis 1986; 134:994–998.

37. Hopp RJ, Townley RG. Evidence that bronchial reactivity may be inherited. Pediatr Res 1985; 19(2):248a.
38. Longo G, Strinati R, Poli F, Fumi F. Genetic factors in nonspecific bronchial hyperreactivity. Am J Dis Child 1989; 141:331-334.
39. Hopp RJ, Bewtra AK, Nair N, Townley R. Bronchial reactivity patterns in nonasthmatic parents of asthmatics. Ann Allergy 1988; 61:184-186.
40. Crockcroft DW, Murdock KY, Berscheid BA. Relationship between atopy and bronchial responsiveness to histamine in a random population. Ann Allergy 1984; 53:26-29.
41. Clifford RD, Pugsley A, Radford M, Holgate ST. Symptoms, atopy, and bronchial response to methacholine in parents with asthma and their children. Arch Dis Child 1987; 62:66-73.
42. Bruderman I, Cohen R, Schachor J, Horowitz I. Bronchial response to methacholine in parents of asthmatic children. Chest 1987; 91(2):210-213.
43. Townley RG, Bewtra A, Wilson AF, Hopp RJ, Elston RC, Nair N, Watt GD. Segregation analysis of bronchial response to methacholine inhalation challenge in families with and without asthma. J Allergy Clin Immunol 1986; 77:101-107.
44. Crockcroft DW, Berscheid BA, Murdock KY. Unimodal distribution of bronchial responsiveness to inhaled histamine in a random human population. Chest 1983; 83:751-754.
45. Bertrand JM, Riley SP, Popkin J, Coates AL. The long-term pulmonary sequelae of prematurity: The role of familial airway hyperreactivity and the respiratory distress syndrome. N Engl J Med 1985; 312:742-745.
46. Nickerson BG, Taussig LM. Family history of asthma in infants with bronchopulmonary dysplasia. Pediatrics 1980; 65:1140-1144.
47. Konig P, Godfrey S. Prevalence of exercise-induced bronchial lability in families of children with asthma. Arch Dis Child 1973; 48:513-518.
48. Konig P, Godfrey S. Genetics of wheezy children assessed by exercise-induced bronchial lability. Arch Dis Child 1974; 49:242.
49. Higgins M, Keller J. Familial occurrence of chronic respiratory disease and familial resemblance in ventilatory capacity. J Chron Dis 1975; 28:239-251.
50. Davis PB. Physiologic implications of the autonomic aberrations in cystic fibrosis. Horm Metabol Res 1986; 18:217-220.
51. Vincenc KS, Black J, Armour CL, Donnelly PD, Woolcock AJ. Comparison of in vivo and in vitro responses to histamine in human airways. Am Rev Resp Dis 1983; 128:875-879.
52. Tepper RS. Airway reactivity in infants: A positive response to methacholine and metaproterenol. J Appl Physiol 1987; 62:1155-1159.
53. Hopp R, Bewtra A, Nair NM, Townley R. Effect of age on methacholine response. J Allergy Clin Immunol 1985; 76:609-613.
54. Haseman JK, Elston RC. An estimation of genetic variance from twin data. Behav Genet 1970; 1:11-19.

55. Woolf CA. *Principles of Biometry*. Princeton D. Van Nostrand Co. Inc., 1968, pp. 230–231.
56. Allen G, Harvald B, Shields J. Measures of twin concordance. Acta Genet Basel 1967; 17:475–481.
57. Hopp RJ, Bewtra AK, Watt GD, Nair NM, Townley RG. Genetic analysis of allergic disease in twins. J Allergy Clin Immunol 1984; 73:265–270.
58. Konig P, Godfrey S. Exercise-induced bronchial lability in monozygotic (identical) and dizygotic (nonidentical) twins. J Allergy Clin Immunol 1974; 54:280–287.
59. Hopp RJ, Weiss SJ, Nair NM, Bewtra AK, Townley RG. Interpretation of the results of methacholine inhalation challenge tests. J Allergy Clin Immunol 1987; 80:821–830.
60. Zamel N, Leroux M, Vanderdoelen JL. Airway response to inhaled methacholine in healthy nonsmoking twins. J Appl Physiol 1984; 56:936–939.
61. Ackerman V, Long V, Hui C, Eigen H, Tepper R. Evaluation of pulmonary function in twin infants. Am Rev Resp Dis 1988; 137(Suppl):406.
62. Redline S, Tishler PV, Lewitter FI, Tager IB, Munoz A, Speizer FE. Assessment of genetic and nongenetic influences on pulmonary function. Am Rev Resp Dis 1987; 135:217–222.
63. Mano K, Harada S, Miyahara H, Miyamoto T, Horiuchi Y. The distribution of polymorphic traits in atopic asthmatic patients. Acta Allergol (Kbh) 1975; 30:80–88.
64. Ronchetti R, Lucarini N, Lucarelli P, Martinez F, Macri F, Carapella E, Bottini E. A genetic basis for heterogeneity of asthma syndrome in pediatric ages: Adenosine deaminase phenotypes. J Allergy Clin Immunol 1984; 74:81–84.
65. Arnaud P, Chapuis-Cellier C, Souillet G, Carron R, Wilson GB, Creyssel R, Fudenberg HH. High frequency of deficient Pi phenotypes of alpha-1-antitrypsin in nonatopic infantile asthma. Trans Assoc Am Physicians 1976; 89:205–214.
66. Anton-Guirgis H, Townley RG, Schanfield MS. Methacholine inhalation and Gm allotypes in familial asthma. J Asthma 1984; 21:1–8.
67. Piessens MF, Marien G, Stevens E. Decreased haptoglobin levels in respiratory allergy. Clin Allergy 1984; 14:287–293.
68. Srivastava N, Gupta SP, Srivastava LM. Association between C3 complement types and bronchial asthma. Hum Hered 1985; 35:263–264.
69. Lam S, Wong R, Yeung M. Nonspecific bronchial reactivity in occupational asthma. J Allergy Clin Immunol 1979; 63:28–34.
70. Hudson P, Cartier A, Pineau L, Lafrance M, St-Aubin JJ, Dubois JY, Malo JL. Follow-up of occupational asthma caused by crab and various agents. J Allergy Clin Immunol 1985; 76:688–694.
71. Townley RG, Ryo UY, Miller-Kolotkin B, Kang B. Bronchial sensitivity to methacholine in current and former asthmatic and allergic rhinitis patients and control subjects. J Allergy Clin Immunol 1975; 56:429–442.

72. Brooks SM, Weiss MA, Berstein IL. Reactive airways dysfunction syndrome (RADS). Persistent airways hyperreactivity after high level irritant exposure. Chest 1985; 88:376–384.
73. Bahous J, Cartier A, Ouimet G, Pineau L, Malo J-L. Nonallergic bronchial hyperexcitability in chronic bronchitis. Am Rev Resp Dis 1984; 129:216–220.

4

Airway Hyperresponsiveness and Asthma

JEAN-LUC MALO and PIERRE TESSIER

Hôpital du Sacré-Coeur
Montreal, Quebec, Canada

INTRODUCTION

The expression "airway hyperresponsiveness" refers to increased sensitivity of the airways to a variety of stimuli. This results in airway smooth muscle contraction, an increase in mucus secretion, and inflammation (edema, vasodilatation, influx of inflammatory cells, and release of mediators). This causes symptoms such as cough, shortness of breath, and wheezing.

Asthma (from the Greek word meaning "panting" or "difficulty in breathing") is a condition characterized by widespread narrowing of the airways, which is partly or completely reversible either spontaneously or as a result of therapy; and airway hyperresponsiveness (1,2). These two characteristics of the definition are interrelated. It is known that there is a relationship between the degree of airway hyperresponsiveness to a bronchoconstrictor agent and the daily fluctuations in airway caliber as documented by swings in peak expiratory flow rates (PEFR). Significant fluctuations in PEFR are generally seen in individuals with greater airway hyperresponsiveness (3), whereas asthmatic subjects with mild airway hyperresponsiveness demonstrate lesser fluctuations (3,4). There is, furthermore, a relationship between the bronchoconstrictor response to a pharmacological agent and the effect of an inhaled bronchodilator (5). Both features of the definition thus are mirror images of the same reality.

The expression "airway hyperresponsiveness" is generally reserved for increased bronchospastic reaction to nonspecific stimuli as opposed to bronchospastic reactions that may occur after exposure to specific sensitizing stimuli (common allergens, occupational agents). Whereas only a percentage (close to 50%) of the general asthmatic population will demonstrate atopy (6) and have a bronchospastic reaction after exposure to at least one inhaled allergen, virtually all current asthmatic subjects will demonstrate airway hyperresponsiveness after exposure to nonspecific stimuli.

HISTORICAL BACKGROUND

Several early authors have noted that asthmatic subjects are likely to report symptoms when exposed to stimuli such as exercise, cold air, dust, fumes, or heavy smell. In his ***Treatise of the Asthma***, Sir John Floyer (7) mentions that:

> During the fit of the Asthma, the smoak of tobacco is so offensive that it very much staitens the Breath, if it be smoaked the first day of the fit, and much endangers a suffocation.

Other nonspecific factors such as emotions have also been recognized as causing asthma. Laënnec (8) in his ***Traité de l'Auscultation médiate*** summarized it as follows:

> De ces faits et de ces rapprochements je crois pouvoir conclure que la plupart des attaques d'asthme, quoique dues à plusieurs causes réunies, le sont principalement à une altération primitive et momentanée de l'influence nerveuse" (Because of this, I believe I can conclude that most asthma attacks, although caused by several factors, are primarily instigated by a short-lived alteration of a nervous nature).

In 1921, Alexander and Paddock (9) reported changes in breathing in asthmatic subjects, absent in normal subjects after injecting pilocarpine. It is thought that Dautrebande and Philippot (10) were the first to use an inhaled bronchoconstrictor agent derived from acetylcholine to induce bronchoconstriction in humans. Curry (11), Tiffeneau and Beauvallet (12), and De Vries et al. (13) later proposed the use of histamine and acetylcholine derivatives in the assessment of airway responsiveness. Standardized procedures for challenges with pharmacological agents were introduced more recently (14,15) and thorough reviews of the subject have been published elsewhere (16-19).

Although assessment of airway hyperresponsiveness with pharmacological agents is still the gold standard, interest in other means has been growing over the last few years. As a result of several studies into the mechanisms of exercise-induced asthma (20-22), it has been proposed that hyperventilation of room temperature or unconditioned air be used as a means of assessing airway hyperresponsiveness (23-26). More recently, inhalation of hypo- and hyperosmolar

TABLE 1 Stimuli Used to Measure Airway Responsiveness

1. Pharmacological agents:
Acetylcholine and derivatives (carbachol, methacholine)
Histamine
Prostaglandins
Leukotrienes (LTO_4, LTD_4, LTE_4
Bradykinin
Platelet activating factor (PAF)
2. Physical agents
Exercise
Hyperventilation of unconditioned or conditioned air
3. Chemical agents
Hypotonic solutions
Hypertonic solutions

solutions (27,28) and of a variety of other agents listed in Table 1 has also been proposed for the evaluation of airway hyperresponsiveness.

MECHANISMS OF AIRWAY HYPERRESPONSIVENESS

The complexity of the anatomical structures and physiological reactions that control airway tone is such that, in spite of major effort, the precise mechanisms causing airway hyperresponsiveness remain unknown.

As discussed in another chapter and in a recent review (29), heredity and environment can both play a role in airway hyperresponsiveness and asthma. Airway responsiveness is increased in relatives of asthmatic subjects, and a closer association of asthma is found in monozygotic, as opposed to dizygotic, twins. However, even in the former instance, the concordance is low. The effect of environment is supported by the observation that airway responsiveness can be elevated in populations that are heavily exposed to an allergenic product. Furthermore, some occupational agents such as isocyanates, to which subjects had never been previously exposed, can induce airway hyperresponsiveness in 5-10% of exposed workers.

The possible mechanisms causing airway hyperresponsiveness include:

Reduction in Airway Caliber

Resistance to flow is inversely proportional to the fourth power of radius in small airways where the flow is laminar and to an even higher power in larger airways where turbulent flow is present. Therefore, reduction in caliber of an

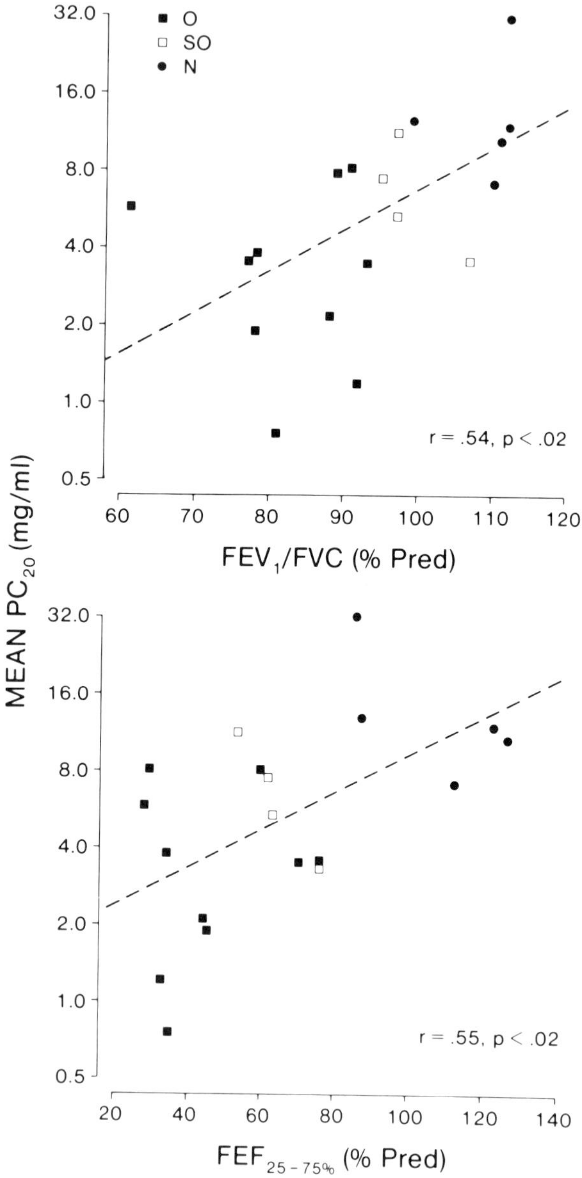

FIGURE 1 Relationship between FEV_1/FVC (% predicted) and FEF 25–75% (% predicted) on the left and right abscissas, respectively, and mean PC_{20} (mg/ml) to histamine and methacholine on the ordinate. The dotted lines are the regression lines. The correlation coefficients and the levels of significance are given. Obstructed (closed squares), slightly obstructed (open squares), and non-obstructed (closed circles) subjects. From Ref. 32.

already contracted airway leads to a larger increase in airway resistance compared with the reduction in caliber of an airway that was initially normal. Most studies have shown an inverse correlation between airway caliber and airway responsiveness in both normal subjects (31) and those with asthma (15) or chronic bronchitis (32) (Figs. 1, 2). However, the role of airway caliber on airway hyperresponsiveness as assessed by the r^2 obtained from linear regression analysis is only approximately 25%. Some asthmatic subjects can demonstrate severe airway hyperresponsiveness with almost normal airway caliber, whereas subjects with chronic obstructive bronchitis having marked airway obstruction may demonstrate mild airway hyperresponsiveness. Consequently, the relationship between airway caliber and airway hyperresponsiveness based on the geometry of the airways and the physical properties of inhaled air cannot be retained as one primary mechanism explaining airway hyperresponsiveness.

Abnormalities of the Airway Smooth Muscle

Chronic asthma can result in hypertrophy and hyperplasia of the airway smooth muscle (33). These abnormalities may lead to more significant airway obstruc-

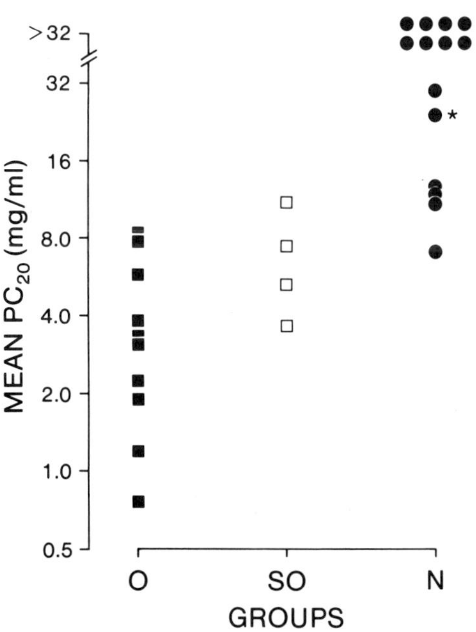

FIGURE 2 Mean PC_{20} results to histamine and methacholine for the obstructed (SO), and nonobstructed (NO) groups (* = value obtained for histamine, as the result for methacholine was > 32 mg/ml). From Ref. 32.

tion after exposure to a stimulus. However, several studies summarized by Hargreave and coworkers (34) have shown *no* relationship between the level of airway hyperresponsiveness as assessed in vivo as opposed to in vitro on isolated tracheal or bronchial smooth muscle. In all of these studies, the contractile response was assessed by isometric tension (i.e., the force measured during a contraction at a constant muscular length). As pointed out by Macklem (35), no study has evaluated the isotonic response (i.e., the force measured during a contraction when the muscle reduces its length at a constant force). Also, the role of muscle hypertrophy does not account for the transient increase in airway hyperresponsiveness after a viral infection or exposure to an irritant agent.

In sensitized animals, the speed of bronchial shortening and relaxation in vitro is altered even in the absence of muscular hypertrophy (36). It is also possible that the airway smooth muscle acts as a single unit, a myogenic tonus, and contractile activity is spontaneous. An alteration in the mechanical properties of the bronchial smooth muscle could therefore be responsible for airway hyperresponsiveness (37). This abnormality could be taking place in different locations: the cellular membrane and its electric excitability threshold; the excitation-contraction coupling mechanism of the cell; the contractile apparatus (actin, myosin, ATPase) or the cellular metabolism of calcium.

Finally, based on the finding that histamine dose-response curves reach a plateau in normal subjects but not in asthmatic subjects (38), Macklem (35) suggested that the abnormality of the airway smooth muscle might be the airway *hypo*responsiveness found in normal subjects and not the airway hyperresponsiveness of asthmatic subjects.

Abnormalities of the Airway Mucosa

Based on the observation that viral infections can induce airway hyperresponsiveness, possibly through epithelial damage, Hogg (39) proposed that an increase in permeability of the airway mucosa could facilitate access of bronchoconstricting agents to irritant receptors and to the airway smooth muscle, thus inducing airway hyperresponsiveness. However, this attractive hypothesis was not confirmed by the same group of investigators (40) who showed that the airway mucosal permeability of asthmatic subjects with airway hyperresponsiveness was not impaired, and that asymptomatic smokers can have increased mucosal permeability without demonstrating airway hyperresponsiveness.

Abnormalities of the Autonomic Nervous System

Airway autonomic innervation has three components: the parasympathetic, the sympathetic, and the nonadrenergic noncholinergic systems.

The Parasympathetic System

The parasympathetic system exerts its effect through the release of acetylcholine that activates muscarinic postjunctional receptors, thus inducing airway smooth muscle contraction and glandular secretion. Parasympathetic bronchoconstrictive reflexes are mediated by the vagus nerve. They originate from nerve endings of afferent neurones in the bronchi when these are activated by thermal, physical, or chemical stimuli. Administration of anticholinergic agents can reduce or, in certain subjects, even abolish airway responses to histamine, exercise, and hyperventilation. However, by analyzing all of these studies testing the role of this system in airway hyperresponsiveness, Nadel and coworkers (41) concluded that the parasympathetic contribution is still controversial, although it may have a significant effect in some asthmatic subjects. Therefore, an excess of parasympathetic activity cannot, in itself, explain airway hyperresponsiveness.

The Sympathetic System

Although there are very few sympathetic fibers in the airways, the adrenergic system has some influence on airway caliber. Its effect is probably mediated by systemic catecholamines influencing alpha (bronchoconstrictor) and beta (bronchodilator) receptors. Human lungs are rich in beta-$_2$ receptors demonstrated by the significant bronchodilator efficacy of beta-$_2$-adrenergic agents. Szentivanyi (42) originally proposed that the beta-adrenergic receptors might be less responsive in asthmatic subjects. It is now evident, as summarized by Nadel and coworkers (41) that a less than normal function of beta-adrenergic receptors is unlikely to explain the airway hyperresponsiveness observed in asthma.

Ingestion of clonidine, a selective alpha-$_2$-adrenergic agent, can reduce the activity of the sympathetic system and increase airway hyperresponsiveness to histamine. However, the role of the adrenergic system is probably minor (43). On the one hand, it has been shown that phenylephrine, an alpha agonist, does not alter airway caliber when its effect is isolated by blocking cholinergic and beta-adrenergic activities (44). On the other hand, prazosin, which is a selective alpha-adrenergic antagonist, has only a minor effect on airway hyperresponsiveness induced by histamine (45).

The Nonadrenergic Noncholinergic System

The presence of a nonadrenergic noncholinergic system was originally demonstrated by Richardson and Beland (46) and shown to be functionally active in humans (47). As the neurotransmitter (hypothetically a neuropeptide) has not been identified, it has not been possible to clarify the role of this system in airway hyperresponsiveness.

Barnes (48) recently proposed that nonmyelinated C-fibers may be stimulated by the release of inflammatory mediators, which, by an axon antidromic reflex, could activate the afferent branches and cause bronchoconstriction. This interesting hypothesis requires more study if it is to be considered as a possible mechanism of airway hyperresponsiveness.

Inflammation

Pathological evidence from postmortem and biopsy studies, as well as the results derived from bronchoalveolar lavage and bronchial brushings have demonstrated that airway inflammation is important in the pathogenesis of asthma. Influx of eosinophils and mast cells, as well as a thickening of the basal membrane and mucosal desquamation has been demonstrated. An animal model has shown that exposure to ozone leads to epithelial damage, an influx of neutrophils (49, 50). Exposure of humans to ozone can also cause airway hyperresponsiveness and an influx of neutrophils. Studies of individuals sensitized to toluene diisocyanate (TDI) have shown an influx of hemophils and eosinophils in those subjects who develop late asthmatic reactions (51) which are associated with airway hyperresponsiveness (52). Several mediators of the inflammatory cascade such as leukotrienes (LTB_4, LTO_4, LTD_4), prostaglandins ($PGF2\alpha$), and platelet activating factor (PAF) are potent bronchoconstrictors and add weight to the evidence for a major role of inflammation in the mechanism of airway hyperresponsiveness.

MEANS OF ASSESSING AIRWAY HYPERRESPONSIVENESS

The level of airway responsiveness to a stimulus is measured by exposing subjects to the stimulus and measuring his response. All challenge tests are performed this way and the different methods make use of that same principle. The various modalities that have been proposed for these tests can be explained by: differences in the selected stimulus, the mode of administration, the dose, and the method of assessing the response.

Pharmacological Methods

Agents

The most widely used method for assessing airway hyperresponsiveness is through the nebulization of a variety of pharmacological agents. The most commonly used are histamine or cholinergic agonists. Histamine can act in two different ways: it can have a direct effect on the histaminic receptors of the bronchial smooth muscle (53) or it can stimulate irritant receptors in the bronchi through the vagus (54). Acetylcholine, acetylbetamethylcholine (methacholine), and carbaminoylcholine (carbachol) exert their bronchoconstrictor effect directly on the muscarinic receptors of the bronchial muscle. Both histamine and methacholine result in similar responses on a mg/ml basis. However, histamine causes more side effects (such as cough and flushing) particularly in higher concentrations and, for this reason, cannot be used in concentrations > 32 mg/ml. Methacholine can be used safely in concentrations up to 256 mg/ml.

Modes of Administration

Deposition of the aerosol in the bronchial tree is dependent on its geometry, on the physical properties of the particles (diameter), and on the ventilatory pattern. Although it is possible to measure the quantity of the nebulized bronchoconstrictor agent, it is difficult to know which proportion actually enters the airways.

Aerosol can be administered by either of two methods: (1) the aerosol is generated (continuously or noncontinuously) or (2) the aerosol is stored in a reservoir. With continuously generated aerosol, the subject inhales the flow at tidal volume breathing for a determined period of time. The administration of progressively increasing doses can be carried out either by varying the duration of exposure or, more often, by increasing the concentration of the bronchoconstrictor agent. An estimation of inhaled doses can be obtained if the output of the nebulizer and the duration of exposure are known. The aerosol can also be generated noncontinuously. A device known as a dosimeter limits the duration of nebulization, and times the release in relation to the slow inspiratory capacity manoeuvres (14). Two methods of generating aerosols are commonly used in North America and Europe: one using the dosimeter (14) and the other one using the Wright's nebulizer at tidal volume breathing (15). Both methods give comparable results (55,56).

As mentioned above, the two most important technical factors conditioning the response are the output of the nebulizer and the duration of inhalation. Nebulizers should be calibrated by weighing them before and after a fixed period of nebulization, because the output may vary from one nebulizer to another. Furthermore, the recorded output should be checked periodically. Comparison of responses obtained with different inhalers can be made by adjusting for the varying output. After nebulizing phosphate buffer saline and assessing airway caliber (to be used as the baseline value), double concentrations of histamine or methacholine are inhaled and airway caliber is assessed between each nebulization.

The stored aerosol technique is used mainly in France and is based on the works of Tiffeneau (12). A reservoir is filled with a fixed concentration of the bronchoconstrictor agent. The volume of inhaled aerosol determines the approximate dose. No direct comparison of the response obtained with this method to the continuous aerosol methods described above has been made.

Assessment of the Response

Several functional indices of airway caliber can be used. The most widely used is the FEV_1 (forad expiratory volume in 1 second). This test is effort dependent, but its reproducibility is high and the apparatus, simple and portable. There was great interest several years ago in the partial (initiated from tidal volume) and complete (initiated from total lung capacity) flow-volume curves assessed at low lung volumes (near residual volume). However, these indices have a poor reproducibility, which precludes their clinical use. The assessment of lung or airway resistance/conductance is effort independent. However, the reproducibility is less satisfactory than FEV_1 (Fig. 3). Furthermore, if tested with body plethysmography, it requires more complex, less portable, and more expensive apparatus. The introduction of oscillometry (57,58) may allow easier assessment of resistance.

All these methods have advantages and inconveniences. Assessment of FEV_1 is most useful for clinical purposes. However, assessment of resistance might be preferable for research purposes because its greater sensitivity, and in less cooperative subjects such as children (58).

Drawing the Dose–Response Curve

The shape of dose-response curves to histamine is sigmoid in normal subjects. The plateau observed at higher doses is absent in asthmatic subjects (38,53) (Fig. 4). Dose-response curves can be characterized in several ways: the threshold dose, at which a significant response is initiated (originally called "sensitivity" by Tiffeneau); the slope of the dose-response curve beyond the threshold point (originally called "reactivity" by Tiffeneau); an arbitrary point beyond the threshold point, which is the provocative dose or concentration, ordinarily set at a 20% fall for FEV_1 (PC_{20}) and 35, 40, 50, or 100% for lung or airway resistance. Both "sensitivity" and "reactivity" as well as the indices derived from the dose-response curve are significantly different in normal and asthmatic subjects (59-61).

Dose-response curves can be drawn on a logarithmic scale, as for standard pharmacological dose-response curves. Although this is preferred on a theoretical basis because of the wide range of doses used for pharmacological challenges, Cockcroft and coauthors (62) showed that, in practice, the use of a linear scale would not change significantly the results of PC_{20}. A cumulative or noncumulative scale can be used. Due to the kinetics of recovery from bronchoconstriction to histamine and methacholine (63) and because the inhalation tests are performed without waiting for functional recovery between each dose, both agents have a cumulative bronchospastic effect. However, the assessment of PC_{20} is only slightly, if at all, affected regardless of the method for recording results (cumulative or noncumulative) (64).

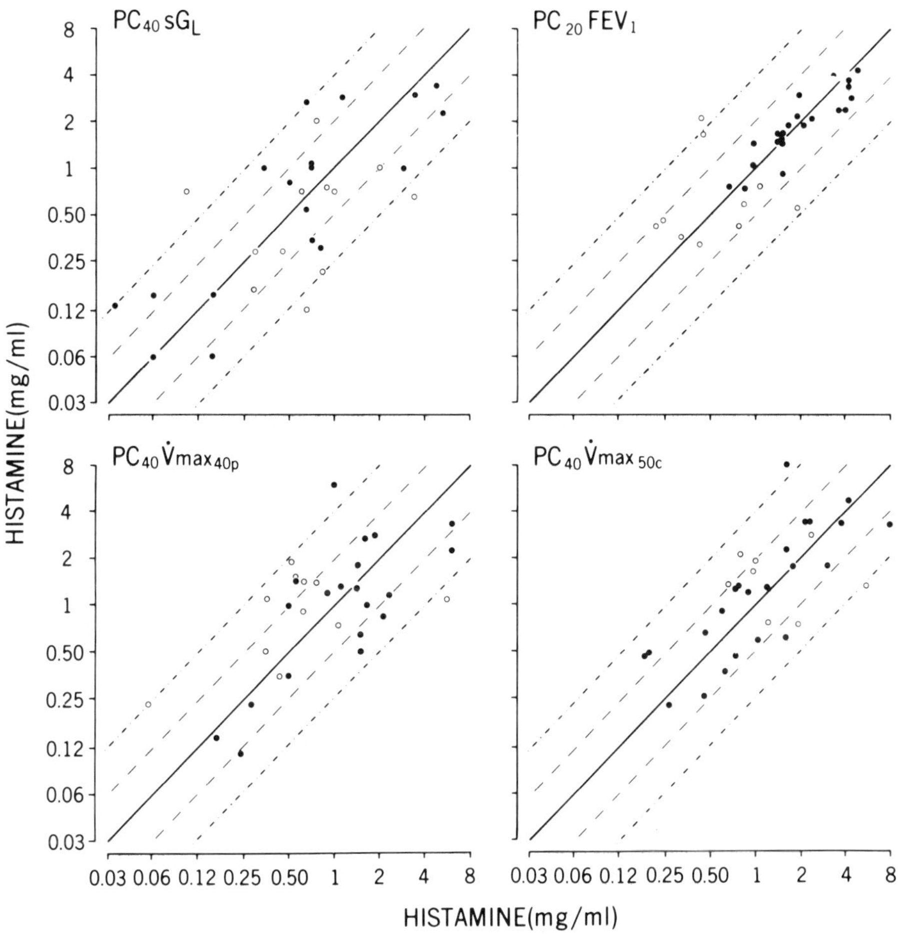

FIGURE 3 Reproducibility of the provocative concentration (PC) as assessed at a 20% fall in FEV_1 (PC_{20} FEV_1) and at a 40% change (PC_{40}) for the other functional indices. (SG_L = specific lung conductance; V_{max} 40p = maximal partial expiratory flow rate at 40% of forced vital capacity; V_{max} 50c = maximal complete expiratory flow rate assessed at 50% of forced vital capacity). Each point represents the results of two consecutive visits in a group of 18 asthmatic subjects in a clinical steady state. The continuous line is the line of identity whereas the interrupted lines represent single twofold and fourfold concentration differences from the line of identity. Closed circles represent the visits done in a functional steady state (i.e., 5% or less and 20% or less variations in baseline FEV_1 and other functional indices, respectively). Open circles represent visits done in a functional unsteady state (6–10% and 21–50% changes in baseline FEV_1 and other functional indices, respectively). Obtained from data of Ref. 65.

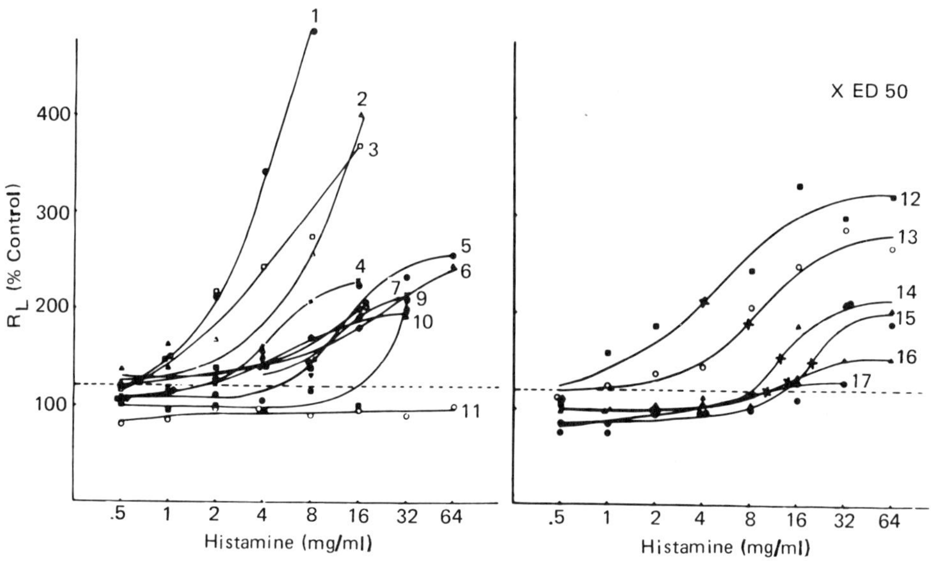

FIGURE 4 Dose-response curves to inhaled histamine in 17 normal individuals. Subjects 12 to 17 are those for whom a significant plateau of response was demonstrated. The X on the individual curves represent the ED_{50}, i.e., the dose of histamine producing 50% of the maximum response. Dotted lines indicates the level of RL at which the threshold dose was determined. From Ref. 53.

In selecting the index derived from the dose-response curve, several criteria should be taken into account: sensitivity, specificity, between-day reproducibility, and clinical usefulness. Indices such as PC_{40}, airway resistance, or conductance are more sensitive than PC_{20} FEV_1 (65,66). The latter is more specific in separating the normal from the asthmatic state and has a better reproducibility (59,65) (Fig. 3). However, the inspiration to total lung capacity (volume history) needed to perform the FEV_1 manoeuvre can induce bronchodilatation and modify the response to a bronchoconstrictor agent. The use of FEV_1 instead of lung resistance or conductance can slightly diminish the sensitivity of the test (66). However, the bronchoconstrictive effect of the forced expiratory manoeuvre in itself, which is observed mostly in more severe asthmatic subjects, can counteract this effect (67). The between-day reproducibility of PC_{20} is ±1 to 1.6 single twofold concentration interval (65,68) in stable asthmatic subjects with similar FEV_1 and assessed at the same time of the day.

Biologic Factors Affecting the Response

The distribution of PC_{20} in a random population seems to be unimodal (69). Abnormal airway responsiveness assessed by PC_{20} is present in approximately

10–15% of a random population, including normal individuals and subjects with asthma or other respiratory diseases (70,71). Even though it has been suggested that asthma can exist without airway hyperresponsiveness (72), virtually all current asthmatic subjects react to a concentration below 16 mg/ml of histamine or methacholine. Only 8% of normal subjects (nonsmokers with no personal or familial atopic history and without respiratory symptoms) have a $PC_{20} \leqslant 16$ mg/ml (31).

As discussed above, baseline airway caliber influences airway hyperresponsiveness. Therefore, the presence of airway hyperresponsiveness subjects with reduced airway caliber does not mean that they have asthma. However, such presence in a subject with an FEV_1 value > 80% predicted normal is indicative of asthma. Gender does not seem to influence airway hyperresponsiveness, but it has not yet been determined whether age has any effect (31,73). Circadian variations of airway hyperresponsiveness have been described, but this is highly variable from one subject to another (74,75). Tachyphylaxis to histamine occurs in subjects with mild airway hyperresponsiveness, if the test is repeated immediately after functional recovery (76) although this is not the case in subjects with more severe airway hyperresponsiveness (77–79).

Smoking, even though producing no symptoms of chronic bronchitis, can increase airway responsiveness. This effect can be demonstrated with sensitive indices though not with PC_{20} (80,81). Airway hyperresponsiveness assessed by PC_{20} has been documented in smokers with symptoms of chronic bronchitis, almost exclusively in those affected with bronchial obstruction (32) (Fig. 2). Rhinitis is also associated with mild airway hyperresponsiveness overlapping the asthmatic range, particularly if indices not requiring maximum forced expiratory manoeuvres, such as FEV_1 are used (82). Several respiratory conditions such as chronic bronchiectasis, sarcoidosis, pulmonary fibrosis (16–19,83) and left cardiac failure (84,85) are also associated with airway hyperresponsiveness.

Pretreatment with several medications can alter airway hyperresponsiveness. Inhaled beta-$_2$-adrenergic agents are the most powerful. Inhaled atropinic agents have an effect on methacholine challenges, but much less so on histamine-inhalation challenges. Oral antihistamines have a significant blocking effect on histamine-induced bronchoconstriction. Sodium cromoglycate does not inhibit histamine-induced bronchoconstriction (78), whereas theophylline has a minimal effect (79). Chronic use of inhaled steroids can reduce airway hyperresponsiveness (86,87).

Exposure to pollutants such as ozone can increase airway hyperresponsiveness. The effect is generally shortlived and is seen only by using sensitive indices of measurement (88). The same applies to respiratory viral infections (89). These effects are generally not shown by using PC_{20} (90). Bronchoconstriction induced by nonspecific stimuli such as exercise and hyperventilation of dry cold air (91) have no significant effect on airway hyperresponsiveness. The effect of hyperosmolar solutions is minimal and shortlived (92).

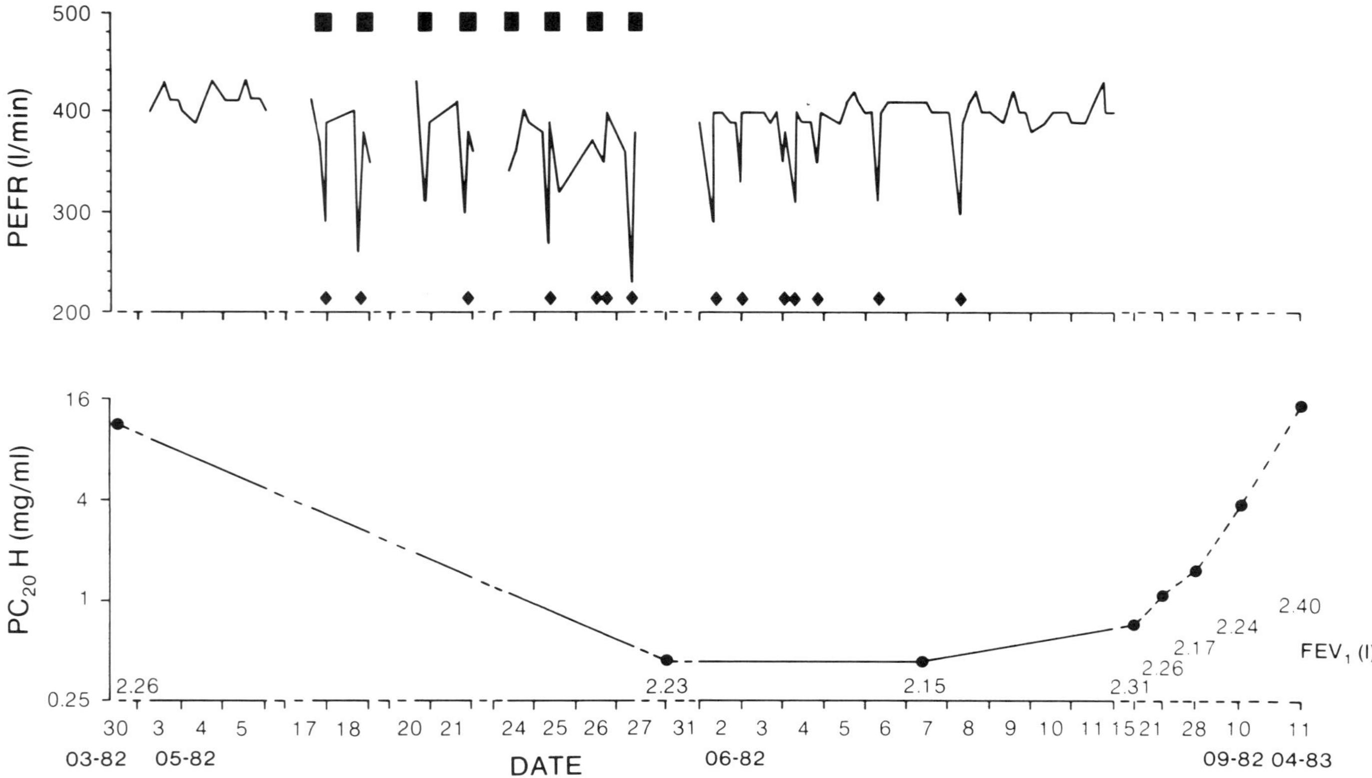

FIGURE 5 Combined monitoring of peak expiratory flow rate (PEFR) (upper panel) and PC_{20} H (PC_{20} histamine) (lower panel) in the same subject before and after return to work. Squares represent the time spent at work, whereas lozenges illustrate the use of inhaled salbutamol (albuterol). Baseline FEV_1 values before each histamine inhalation test are illustrated. They vary by no more than 6% from one test to another. Prolonged changes in PC_{20} H are shown after an exposure for only 8 days to the sensitizing agent (crab boiling water) at work. From Ref. 94.

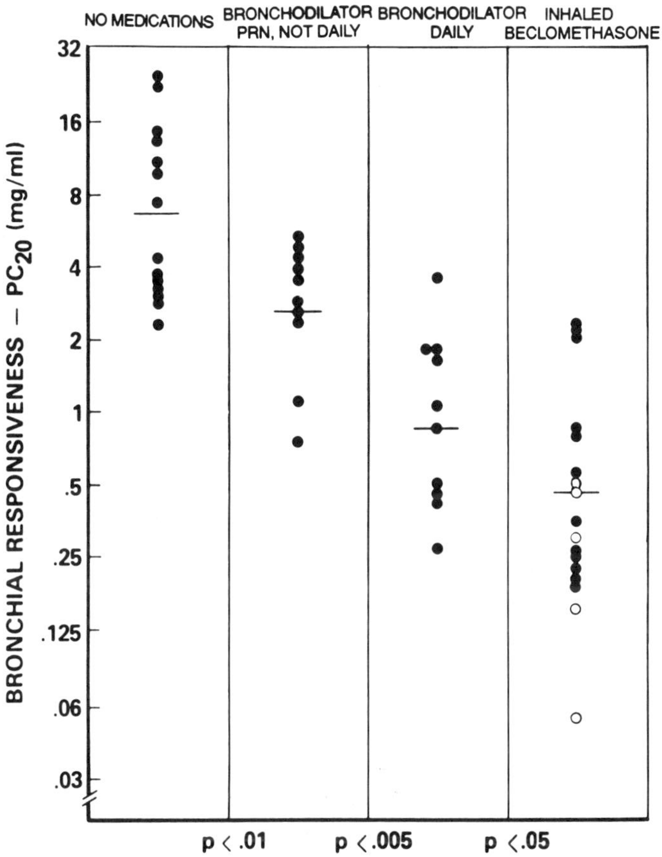

FIGURE 6 Relationship of PC_{20} (expressed as a mean of the results obtained with histamine and methacholine) to minimum medications required to control symptoms of asthma. Bars represent the mean PC_{20} in each treatment group. Open circles are those patients whose baseline FEV_1 was reduced to between 60 and 70% (and which rose to above 80% after salbutamol 200 μg given after the test). From Ref. 105.

Whereas pollutants and viral infections have a relatively small effect on airway hyperresponsiveness, allergens and occupational sensitizing agents have a more pronounced and long-term effect (Fig. 5). Through inhalation challenges in the laboratory, Cartier and coworkers (52) have demonstrated that late, as opposed to isolated immediate bronchoconstrictive reactions, due to inhaled allergens can markedly alter airway hyperresponsiveness. Such changes can also occur after exposure to common environmental allergens (93). Occupational sensitizing agents also have the same effect (94) in the laboratory and in the work place (Fig. 5).

Finally, airway responsiveness to common inhaled allergens depends both on the degree of airway hyperresponsiveness and the immunological reactivity evaluated by the quantification of specific IgE or the immediate skin reaction to one allergen. This relationship was first described by Tiffeneau (95). Consequently, the degree of airway hyperresponsiveness and the diameter of skin reaction to common inhaled allergens can be used as predictors of the immediate bronchospastic reaction (96,97).

Clinical Usefulness

A diagnosis of asthma can often be made with a history of typical symptoms and demonstrated by reversible airflow obstruction. However, asthmatic subjects are often seen at a time when they are asymptomatic. Also, the origin of respiratory symptoms can be difficult to determine. Physicians are not good predictors of airway hyperresponsiveness as assessed by pharmacological challenges. Disagreements between physicians' diagnosis and the results of the methacholine test can occur in as many as 40% of patients (98). Nearly 60% of subjects with respiratory symptoms of uncertain etiology will demonstrate airway hyperresponsiveness as assessed by histamine inhalation (99). There is little association between specific responses to a respiratory questionnaire and airway hyperresponsiveness to pharmacological agents in epidemiological studies (100–104). The categorization of respiratory symptoms under a specific name does not seem to be useful in identifying subjects with airway hyperresponsiveness. Dyspnea, chest tightness, cough, and wheezing may well be experienced differently from one subject to another. Subjects may therefore use a different term for each of these symptoms. The presence of airway hyperresponsiveness in a subject with respiratory symptoms does not confirm a diagnosis of asthma. As noted above, subjects with chronic bronchitis, especially those with bronchial obstruction (32), and rhinitis (15,82) can show airway hyperresponsiveness.

The assessment of airway hyperresponsiveness is useful in determining the need for medication in asthma (105) (Fig. 6). It can be particularly useful in those individuals who are poor perceivers of their symptoms. Finally, the assessment of airway hyperresponsiveness is instrumental in the investigation of occupational asthma (106) (as discussed in another chapter of this book) and in the assessment of impairment/disability (107).

Exercise

Historical Background

In his treatise on asthma, Sir John Floyer describes exercise-induced bronchoconstriction (7):

All violent exercise makes the asthmatic to breathe short . . . and if the exercise be continued it occasions a fit.

Herxheimer later identified the level of ventilation as the principal stimulus to exercise-induced asthma (108). In 1975, Godfrey published a thorough review of the technical factors affecting exercise-induced asthma such as the duration, the type of exercise, and the time course of the response (109). Edmunds (110) showed that exercise-induced bronchoconstriction gives rise to a refractory period during which a second challenge causes a smaller response. Studies in the pathogenesis of exercise-induced asthma have outlined the role of conditioning of the inspiratory air in determining the reaction (20-22), and have led to the development of tests using hyperventilation of unconditioned air as the stimulus (23,24).

Exercise as a Challenge Test

Depending on the selected group and the duration and the type of exercise, the prevalence of exercise-induced asthma can vary from 60 to 80% (109). Unlike pharmacological agents, exercise has the advantage of being a natural stimulus. Methods for exercise challenge tests were recently reviewed (111-113). Table 2, slightly modified from Hargreave and coworkers (114), lists the advantages and disadvantages of exercise as a challenge test in comparison to standard pharmacological procedures and hyperventilation. Subjects have to be carefully selected, because exercise results in cardiovascular stress. Exercise is an "all or nothing" type of test. Indeed, progressive doses cannot be administered. Exercise refractoriness has been described in a significant number of asthmatic subjects

TABLE 2 Tests Used for the Measurement of Airway Responsiveness: Advantages and Disadvantages

	Histamine/ methacholine	Exercise	Hyperventilation of unconditioned air
Stimulus	Artificial	Natural	Natural
Dose–response curve	Yes	No	Yes
Sensitivity	High	Moderate	Moderate
Reproducibility	High	Low	High
Clinical usefulness	High	Moderate	Moderate
Cooperation of patient	Little	Moderate	Much
Technical aspects	Simple	Variable	Variable
Equipment cost	Low	Variable	Variable
Research tool	Variable	Moderate	High

Source: Modified from Ref. 114.

(15), which may occur through inhibitory prostagland release (115). The optimal duration of exercise is between 6 and 8 minutes. The intensity of bronchoconstriction is proportional to the severity of exercise as reflected by cardiac frequency and oxygen consumption. Although free running is the most bronchoconstrictive type of exercise (109), because the level of ventilation reached is greater, two types of exercise are frequently used in the laboratory, the cycle ergometer and the treadmill. Airway caliber is assessed before, and at regular intervals after, exercise. The temperature and humidity of inspired air have an effect on the magnitude of exercise-induced bronchoconstriction. Cold dry air produces larger bronchospastic reactions and, consequently, increases the sensitivity of the test.

Although exercise has the advantage of being a natural stimulus, it has several pitfalls. It is not as useful a test as are pharmacological agents. It cannot be administered in a dose-response fashion, and only the maximum response can be quantified. Its sensitivity is less than pharmacological agents (117,118). Its reproducibility may vary by 10–20% from one visit to another (119-121). The presence of exercise refractoriness limits its use to 4 hours after an initial test.

Hyperventilation of Unconditioned Air

The recent interest in the physiopathology of exercise-induced bronchoconstriction has led investigators to propose hyperventilation of unconditioned air as a means of investigating airway hyperresponsiveness (23,24).

Mechanisms

When a subject inhales air that is not fully saturated with water nor at body temperature, a process of conditioning of the inspired air in the airways takes place. This results in a loss of water and heat from the airways, which is proportional to the volume of air that is inhaled.

Different authors (122,123) have shown that significant bronchoconstriction can be obtained in asthmatic subjects by inhaling dry air at body temperature. After demonstrating the similarities between bronchoconstriction due to the inhalation of hypertonic saline and hyperventilation (123), Anderson proposed that hyperosmolarity of the airway mucosa was responsible for hyperventilation- and exercise-induced bronchoconstriction. However, further studies by Eschenbacher and Sheppard (122) suggest that both heat and water loss contributes to the bronchoconstriction induced by hyperventilation with dry air. The mechanism by which changes in temperature and/or osmolarity cause bronchoconstriction is still not clear.

Although bronchoconstriction following exercise and hyperventilation is assumed to be caused by equivalent stimuli, studies reviewed by Lockhart and colleagues (115) have shown that they may differ in several ways. For example, neutrophil chemotactic factor is released after exercise- but not after hyperventilation-induced bronchoconstriction. Furthermore, Noviski and coworkers (124) recently showed that for equivalent respiratory heat exchange, exercise caused more bronchoconstriction than hyperventilation, thus suggesting that exercise per se may contribute to bronchoconstriction.

Methodology

STIMULUS Room air or an already prepared mixture of dry and cold air is inhaled. Cold air can be obtained by passing room air over a heat exchanger containing a cooling agent, such as isopropyl alcohol, methanol, ethylene glycol, freon, or a mixture of ice and acetone. Whatever the condition of the inspired air, the most important factor determining the response is the level of ventilation. Several methods have been suggested for obtaining sufficient levels of ventilation. Deal and colleagues (25) as well as Phillips and coworkers (125) have proposed the use of a balloon that empties at the same rate as the level of expected ventilation. By attempting to keep the balloon filled, the subject maintains the desired level of ventilation. In other methods, a metronome or respiratory breath sounds are played for the subject, who follows the imposed rhythm. The amplitude of tidal volume is set by the technician performing the challenge.

Hyperventilation leads to hypocapnia, which can have two deleterious effects. First, it causes dizziness, headaches, and eventually, loss of consciousness and, second, it can induce bronchoconstriction in humans. Therefore, CO_2 is added to air to maintain isocapnia. This is done either by analyzing end tidal CO_2 and adding CO_2 or by giving an appropriate preset quantity.

Hyperventilation tests can be administered in one of two ways: either as a single level of ventilation, usually maximum ventilatory ventilation (MVV) (25,26), or on a dose-response curve when subjects are asked to inhale unconditioned air at progressively increasing levels of ventilation from tidal volume breathing to MVV (126).

ASSESSMENT OF RESPONSE The time-course of maximum response to hyperventilation generally occurs within 5 minutes after inhalation (127). The same indices used for other types of bronchial challenges can be used to measure the response.

DRAWING THE DOSE-RESPONSE CURVE The shape of the dose-response curve to hyperventilation is sigmoid without a plateau for asthmatic subjects (128) (Fig. 7). A plateau possibly cannot be reached because of the inability of achieving a sufficiently high level of ventilation. A small cumulative bronchospastic reaction has been documented when the test was performed with progressively increasing levels of ventilation (129). Expressing the results in terms of $\dot{V}E$ or respiratory heat exchange gives similar results (24,130). Indices such as the dose causing a 20% or 15% fall in FEV_1 (PD_{20} and PD_{15}) can be interpolated from the individual dose-response curve. The dose that causes a 10% fall in FEV_1 (PD_{10}) might yield imprecise results, as the threshold for the response

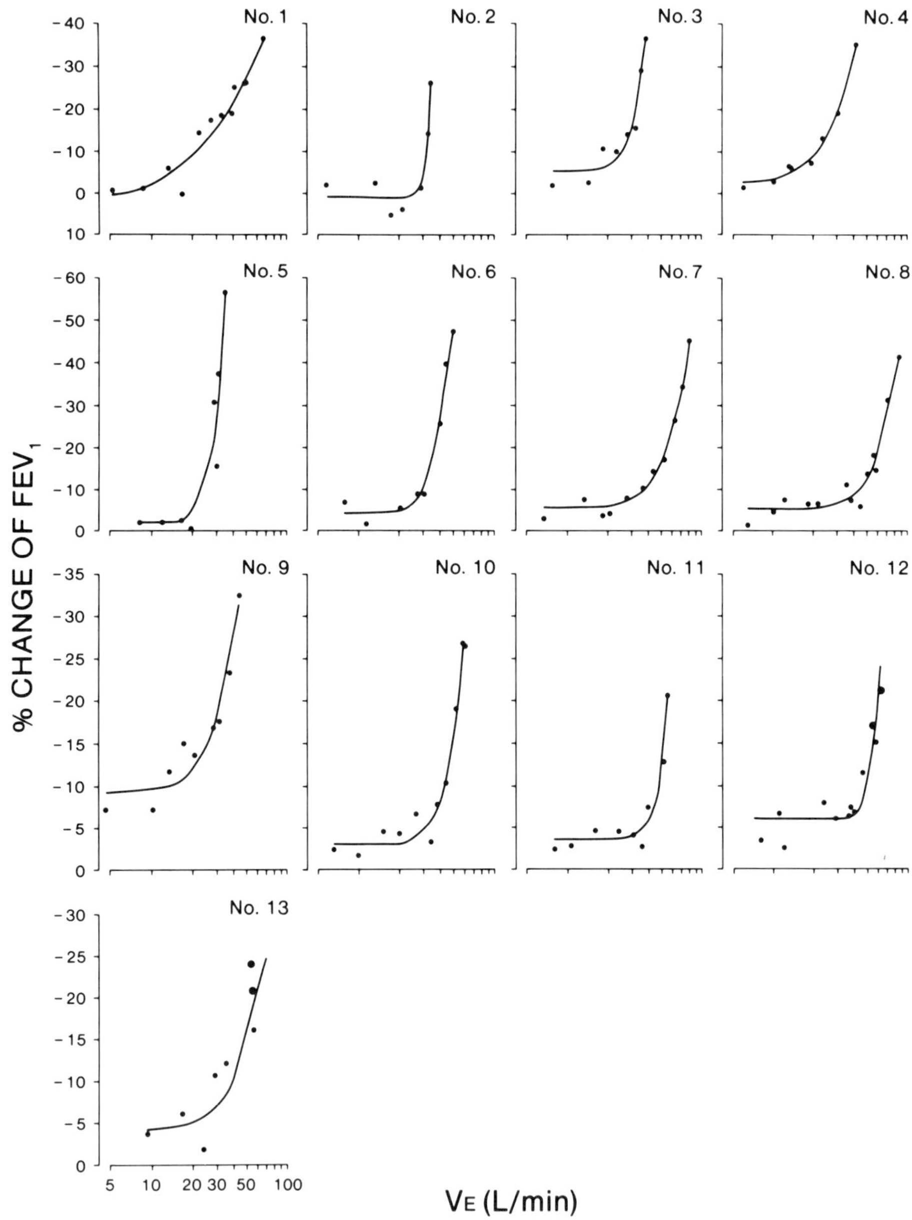

FIGURE 7 Dose-response curves for the 13 current asthmatic subjects. The best fit of the curves using the common pharmacologic logistic model is shown. For subjects 12 and 13, three maximal voluntary ventilatory periods were requested. The two extra periods are shown by open circles. From Ref. 128.

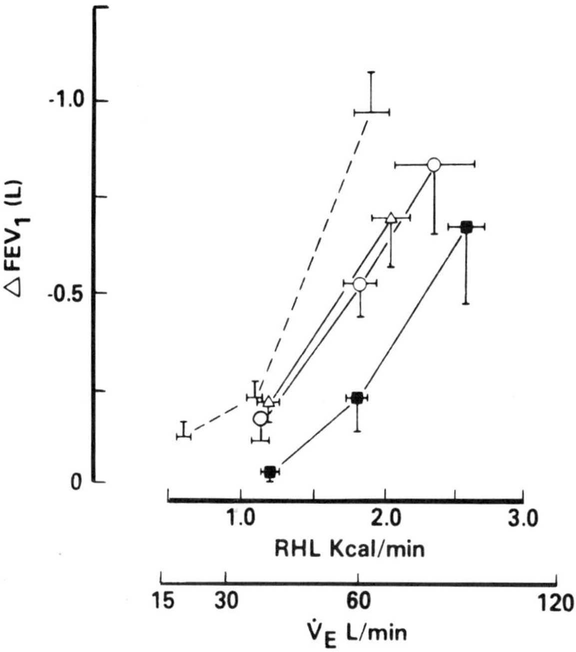

FIGURE 8 Dose-response relationships between respiratory heat loss (RHL) or minute ventilation (V_E) and changes in forced expiratory volume in one second (ΔFEV_1) after pretreatment with placebo (- - -), cromolyn sodium (Δ), terbutaline sulfate (○), and combined cromolyn and terbutaline (■). Data points are mean values and brackets represent ± 1 SEM. From Ref. 132.

is beyond 10% in some subjects (128). As the level of ventilation can theoretically vary from 5 to a little more than 100 L/min, expressing the results on a logarithmic or nonlogarithmic scale yields similar results.

BIOLOGICAL FACTORS AFFECTING THE RESPONSE The within-subject between-day reproducibility of the test among subjects with similar initial airway caliber is comparable to what has been found for pharmacological agents in terms of PD_{20} and PD_{15}. It corresponds to approximately one third of the hyperventilation scale (24). Using hyperventilation, subjects with chronic bronchitis will demonstrate airway hyperresponsiveness more rarely than with pharmacological agents (131). This can therefore be an advantage of hyperventilation over pharmacological agents in distinguishing asthma from chronic bronchitis. Inhaled beta-2 adrenergic agents, sodium cromoglycate, or even more so, a combination of both agents can block the bronchospastic reaction induced by hyperventilation (132) (Fig. 8), as can inhaled atropinic agents (133). Theophylline has a minor effect (134).

CLINICAL USEFULNESS Hyperventilation is a natural stimulus, which makes it useful in the assessment of the efficacy of a drug on airway hyperresponsiveness. This point is interesting as antiasthmatic medication needs assessment not only of its bronchodilator effect, but also of its effect on airway hyperresponsiveness (135). From a technical point of view, the factors that limit the effect of inhaled particles, for example, the output of the nebulizer and the deposition of inhaled particles, do not play a role when using hyperventilation. However, the apparatus needed for such tests is more complex than for pharmacological agents. A PD_{10} obtained with hyperventilation can be as sensitive as a PC_{20} using pharmacological agents to identify airway hyperresponsiveness. However, albeit more specific, a PD_{10} is less sensitive than a PC_{20}. These factors limit the clinical use of hyperventilation tests (23,99). Finally, this test requires cooperation from the subject, who is asked to breathe at progressively increasing levels of ventilation. The level which is reached is most often inferior to the theoretical obtainable value (24,99).

Hyper- and Hypo-osmolar Stimuli

Hyper- and hypo-osmolar solutions can cause bronchoconstriction (27,28). This test can be used in the assessment of airway hyperresponsiveness (136), although it has recently been shown that the results bear no relationship with the clinical status of asthma (137). The test has a satisfactory reproducibility (137), but no attempt has yet been made to standardize the test, which limits its use.

CONCLUSION

Although the mechanism of airway hyperresponsiveness is still debated and might well be multifactorial, its assessment has become routine procedure in clinical laboratories and epidemiological surveys. Even though the use of pharmacological agents is generally preferred for clinical assessment, other means such as hyperventilation, can be valuable research tools. Although the presence of airway hyperresponsiveness does not confirm a diagnosis of asthma, its presence in the absence of other respiratory conditions is highly suggestive of asthma.

It has recently been suggested (138) that better control of asthma, particularly by the use of inhaled steroids which reduce inflammation, can lead to a reduction in airway hyperresponsiveness; an interesting hypothesis, but one that requires confirmation in further studies. Just as it has been shown that preventive therapy for diabetes and hypertension can minimize long-term complications, it is possible that preventive therapy of asthma could diminish both airway hyperresponsiveness and the tendency toward fixed airway obstruction seen in a subset of subjects with asthma.

ACKNOWLEDGMENTS

Pierre Tessier is a research fellow of the Université de Montréal, supported by the Medical Research Council of Canada. We are grateful to Katherine Tallman for reviewing the manuscript.

REFERENCES

1. Ciba Foundation Chest Symposium. Terminology, definitions and classification of chronic pulmonary emphysema and related conditions. Thorax 1959; 14:286–299.
2. American Thoracic Society. Chronic bronchitis, asthma and pulmonary emphysema: a statement by the committee on diagnostic standards for non-tuberculous respiratory diseases. Am Rev Respir Dis 1962; 85:762–768.
3. Ryan G, Latimer KM, Dolovich J, Hargreave FE. Bronchial responsiveness to histamine: relationship to diurnal variation to peak flow rate, improvement after bronchodilator, and airway calibre. Thorax 1982; 37:423–429.
4. Bahous J, Cartier A, Malo JL. Monitoring of peak expiratory flow rates in subjects with mild airway hyperexcitability. Bull Eur Physiopathol Respir 1985; 21:25–30.
5. Benson MK. Bronchial responsiveness to inhaled histamine and isoprenaline in patients with airway obstruction. Thorax 1978; 33:211–213.
6. Pepys J. Types of allergic reaction. Clin Allergy 1973; 3:491–509.
7. Sakula A. Sir John Floyer's A Treatise of the Asthma. Thorax 1984; 39: 248–254.
8. Laënnec RTH. *Traité de l'Auscultation médiate et des maladies des poumons et du coeur*. Paris, tome 2, 1826 pp 92.
9. Alexander HL, Paddock R. Bronchial asthma: response to pilocarpin and epinephrin. Arch Intern Med 1921; 27:184–191.
10. Dautrebande L, Philippot E. Crise d'asthme expérimental par aérosols de carbaminoylcholine chez l'homme traitée par dispersat de phénylaminopropane. La Presse Médicale 1941; 49:942–946.
11. Curry JJ. The action of histamine on the respiratory tract in normal and asthmatic subjects. J Clin Invest 1946; 25:785–791.
12. Tiffeneau R, Beauvallet M. Epreuve de bronchoconstriction et de bronchodilatation par aérosols. Emploi pour le dépistage, la mesure et le contrôle des insuffisances respiratoires chroniques. Bulletin de l'Académie de Médecine (Paris) 1945; 129:165–168.
13. De Vries K, Booij-Noord H, Goei JT, Grobler NJ, Sluiter HJ, Tammeling

GJ, Orie NGM. Hyperreactivity of the bronchial tree to drugs, chemical and physical agents. In: *Bronchitis II*. Orie NGM, Sluiter HJ, eds. Assen, Royal OVan Gorcum, 1964, pp 167-180.
14. Chai H, Farr RS, Froehlich LA, Mathison DA, McLean A, Rosenthal RR, Sheffer AL, Spector SL, Townley RG. Standardization of bronchial inhalation challenge procedures. J Allergy Clin Immunol 1975;56:323-327.
15. Cockcroft DW, Killian DN, Mellon JJA, Hargreave FE. Bronchial reactivity to inhaled histamine: a method and clinical survey. Clin Allergy 1977; 7:235-243.
16. Orehek J, Gayrard P. Les tests de provocation bronchique non spécifiques dans l'asthme. Bull Eur Physiopathol Respir 1976; 12:565-598.
17. Boushey HA, Holtzman MJ, Sheller JR, Nadel JA. Bronchial hyperreactivity. Am Rev Respir 1980; 121:389-413.
18. Hargreave FE, Ryan G, Thomson NC, O'Byrne PM, Latimer K, Juniper EF, Dolovich J. Bronchial responsiveness to histamine and methacholine in asthma: measurement and clinical significance. J Allergy Clin Immunol 1981;68:347-355.
19. SEPCR Working Group. Eiser NM, Kerrebijn KF, Quanjer PH. Guidelines for standardization of bronchial challenges with (nonspecific) bronchoconstricting agents. Bull Eur Physiopathol Respir 1983; 19:495-514.
20. Chen WY, Horton DJ. Heat and water loss from the airways and exercise-induced asthma. Respiration 1977;34:305-313.
21. Deal EC, McFadden ER, Ingram RH, Jaeger JJ. Hyperpnea and heat flux: initial reaction sequence in exercise-induced asthma. J Appl Physiol 1979; 46:476-483.
22. Hahn A, Anderson SD, Morton AR, Black JL, Fiftch KD. A reinterpretation of the effect of temperature and water content of the inspired air in exercise-induced asthma. Am Rev Respir Dis 1984; 130:575-579.
23. Scharf SM, Heimer D, Walters M. Bronchial challenge with room temperature isocapnic hyperventilation. Chest 1985; 88:586-593.
24. Tessier P, Cartier A, L'Archevêque J, Ghezzo H, Martin RR, Malo JL. Within- and between-day reproducibility of isocapnic cold air challenges in subjects with asthma. J Allergy Clin Immunol 1986; 78:379-387.
25. Deal EC Jr, McFadden ER Jr, Ingram RH Jr, Breslin F, Jaeger JJ. Airway responsiveness to cold air and hyperpnea in normal subjects and in those with hay fever and asthma. Am Rev Respir Dis 1980; 121:621-628.
26. Welty C, Weiss ST, Tager IB, Munoz A, Becker C, Speizer FE, Ingram RH Jr. The relationship of airways responsiveness to cold air, cigarette smoking, and atopy to respiratory symptoms and pulmonary function in adults. Am Rev Respir Dis 1984; 130:198-203.
27. Allegra L, Bianco S. Non-specific broncho-reactivity obtained with an ultrasonic aerosol of distilled water. Eur J Respir Dis 1980; 61:41-49.
28. Schoeffel RE, Anderson SD, Altounyan REC. Bronchial hyperreactivity in response to inhalation of ultrasonically nebulised solutions of distilled water and saline. Br Med J 1981; 283:1285-1287.
29. Barbee RA. The epidemiology of asthma. Monogr Allergy 1987;21:21-41.

30. Malo JL, Lockhart A. Hyper-excitabilité bronchique non allergénique. Médecine-Sciences 1987; 9:522–529.
31. Malo JL, Pineau L, Cartier A, Martin RR. Reference values of the provocation concentrations of methacholine that cause 6% and 20% changes in forced expiratory volume in one second in a normal population. Am Rev Respir Dis 1983; 28:8–11.
32. Bahous J, Cartier A, Ouimet G, Pineau L, Malo JL. Non-allergic bronchial hyperexcitability in chronic bronchitis. Am Rev Respir Dis 1984; 129: 216–220.
33. Hogg JC. The pathology of asthma. In: *Bronchial Asthma: Mechanisms and Therapeutics*. Weiss EB, Segal MS, Stein M, eds. Boston, Little, Brown and Co., 1985, pp 209–217.
34. Hargreave FE, Dolovich J, O'Byrne PM, Ramsdale EH, Daniel EE. The origin of airway hyperresponsiveness. J Allergy Clin Immunol 1986; 78: 825–832.
35. Macklem PT. Bronchial hyporesponsiveness. Chest 1985; 87:158S.
36. Souhrada JF, Dickey DC. Effect of antigen challenge on sensitized guinea pig trachea. Respir Physiol 1976; 27:241–251.
37. Stephens NL. Airway smooth muscle. Am Rev Respir Dis 1987; 135:960–975.
38. Woolcock AJ, Salome CM, Yan K. The shape of the dose–response curve to histamine in asthmatic and normal subjects. Am Rev Respir Dis 1984; 130:71–75.
39. Hogg JC. Bronchial mucosal permeability and its relationship to airways hyperreactivity. J Allergy Clin Immunol 1981; 67:421–425.
40. Hogg JC, Hulbert WC, Armour C, Paré PD. The effect of mucosal inflammation on airways reactivity. In: *Asthma: Physiology, Immunopharmacology, and Treatment*. Kay B, Austen KM, Lichtenstein LM, eds. London, Academic Press, 1984, pp 327–338.
41. Nadel JA, Barnes PJ, Holtzman MJ. Autonomic factors in hyperreactivity of airway smooth muscle. In: *Handbook of Physiology. Section 3. The Respiratory System. Vol III. Mechanics of Breathing*. Fishman AP, Macklem PT, Mead J, Geiger SR, eds. Baltimore, Williams and Wilkins, 1986, pp 693–702.
42. Szentivanyi A. The beta-adrenergic theory of the atopic abnormality in bronchial asthma. J Allergy 1968; 42:203–232.
43. Barnes PJ. Neural control of human airways in health and disease. Am Rev Respir Dis 1986; 134:1289–1314.
44. Thomson NC, Daniel EE, Hargreave FE. Role of smooth muscle alpha-1 receptors in nonspecific bronchial responsiveness in asthma. Am Rev Respir Dis 1982; 126:521–525.
45. Jenkins C, Breslin ABX, Marlin GE. The role of alpha and beta adrenoceptors in airway hyperresponsiveness to histamine. J Allergy Clin Immunol 1985; 75:364–372.
46. Richardson J, Béland J. Nonadrenergic inhibitory nervous system in human airways. J Appl Physiol 1976; 41:764–771.

47. Michoud MC, Amyot R, Jeanneret-GrosJean A, Couture J. Reflex decrease of histamine-induced bronchoconstriction after laryngeal stimulation in humans. Am Rev Respir Dis 1987; 136:618–622.
48. Barnes PJ. Asthma as an axon reflex. Lancet 1986; I:242–245.
49. Chung KH. Role of inflammation in the hyperreactivity of the airways in asthma. Thorax 1986; 41:657–662.
50. Fabbri LM, Aizawa H, Alpert SEm, Walters EH, O'Byrne PM, Gold BD, Nadel JA, Holtzman MJ. Airway hyperresponsiveness and changes in cell counts in bronchoalveolar lavage after ozone exposure in dogs. Am Rev Respir Dis 1984; 129:288–291.
51. Fabbri LM, Boschetto P, Zocca E, Milani G, Pivirotto F, Plebani M, Burlina A, Licata B, Mapp CE. Bronchoalveolar neutrophilia during late asthmatic reactions induced by toluene diisocyanate. Am Rev Respir Dis 1987; 136:36–42.
52. Cartier A, Thomson NC, Frith PA, Roberts R, Hargreave FE. Allergen-induced increase in bronchial responsiveness to histamine: relationship to the late asthmatic response and change in airway caliber. J Allergy Clin Immunol 1982; 70:170–177.
53. Michoud MC, Lelorier J, Amyot R. Factors modulating the interindividual variability of airway responsiveness to histamine. The influence of H1 and H2 receptors. Bull Eur Physiopathol Respir 1981; 17:807–821.
54. Sheppard D, Epstein J, Skoogh BE, Bethel RA, Nadel JA, Boushey HA. Variable inhibition of histamine-induced bronchoconstriction by atropine in subjects with asthma. J Allergy Clin Immunol 1984; 73:82–87.
55. Beaupré A, Malo JL. Comparison of the results of two methods of histamine bronchial challenges with the Wright nebulizer and the dosimeter. Clin Allergy 1979; 9:575–583.
56. Ryan G, Dolovich MB, Obminski G, Cockcroft DW, Juniper E, Hargreave FE, Newhouse MT. Standardization of inhalation provocation tests: influence of nebulizer output, particle size, and method of inhalation. J Allergy Clin Immunol 1981; 67:156–161.
57. Duiverman EJ, Neijens NJ, Van der Snee-van Smaalen, Kerrebijn KF. Comparison of forced oscillometry and forced expirations for measuring dose-related responses to inhaled methacholine in asthmatic children. Bull Eur Physiopathol Respir 1986; 22:433–436.
58. Lebecque OP, Spier S, Lapierre JG, Lamarre A, Zinman R, Coates AL. Histamine challenge test in children using forced oscillation to measure total respiratory resistance. Chest 1987; 92:313–318.
59. Michoud MC, Ghezzo H, Amyot R. A comparison of pulmonary function tests used for bronchial challenges. Bull Eur Physiopathol Respir 1982; 18:609–621.
60. Orehek J, Gayrard P, Smith AP, Grimaud C, Charpin J. Airway response to carbachol in normal and asthmatic subjects. Am Rev Respir Dis 1977; 115:937–943.
61. Malo JL, Cartier A, Pineau L, Gagnon G, Martin RR. Slope of the dose-response curve to inhaled histamine and methacholine and PC 20 in sub-

jects with symptoms of airway hyperexcitability and in normal subjects. Am Rev Respir Dis 1985; 132:644–647.

62. Cockcroft DW, Murdock KY, Mink JT. Determination of histamine PC 20. Comparison of linear and logarithmic interpolation. Chest 1983; 84:505–506.
63. Cartier A, Malo JL, Bégin P, Sestier M, Martin RR. Time course of the bronchoconstriction induced by inhaled histamine and methacholine. J Appl Physiol 1983; 54:821–826.
64. Juniper EF, Frith PA, Dunnett C, Cockcroft DW, Hargreave FE. Reproducibility and comparison of responses to inhaled histamine and methacholine. Thorax 1978; 33:705–710.
65. Dehaut P, Rachiele A, Martin RR, Malo JL. Histamine dose–response curves in asthma: reproducibility and sensitivity of different indices to assess response. Thorax 1983; 38:516–522.
66. Orehek J, Nicoli MM, Delpierre S, Beaupré A. Influence of the previous deep inspiration on the spirometric measurement of provoked bronchoconstriction in asthma. Am Rev Respir Dis 1981; 123:269–272.
67. Gayrard P, Orehek J, Grimaud C, Charpin J. Mechanisms of the bronchoconstrictor effects of deep inspiration in asthmatic patients. Thorax 1979; 34:234–240.
68. Ryan G, Dolovich MB, Roberts RS, Frith PA, Juniper EF, Hargreave FE, Newhouse MT. Standardization of inhalation provocation tests: two techniques of aerosol generation and inhalation compared. Am Rev Respir Dis 1981; 123:195–199.
69. Cockcroft DW, Berscheid BA, Murdock KY. Unimodal distribution of bronchial responsiveness to inhaled histamine in a random population. Chest 1983; 83:751–754.
70. Woolcock AJ, Peat JK, Salome CM, Yan K, Anderson SD, Schoeffel RE, McCowage G, Killalea T. Prevalence of bronchial hyperresponsiveness and asthma in a rural adult population. Thorax 1987; 42:361–368.
71. Burney PGJ, Britton JR, Chinn S, Tattersfield A, Papacosta AO, Kelson MC, Anderson F, Corfield DR. Descriptive epidemiology of bronchial reactivity in an adult population: results from a community study. Thorax 1987; 42:38–44.
72. Stanescu DC, Frans A. Bronchial asthma without increased airway reactivity. Eur J Respir Dis 1982; 63:5–12.
73. Taylor RG, Joyce H, Gross E, Holland F, Pride NB. Bronchial reactivity to inhaled histamine and annual rate of decline in FEV 1 in male smokers and ex-smokers. Thorax 1985; 40:9–16.
74. Rachiele A, Malo JL, Cartier A, Ghezzo H, Martin RR. Circadian variations of airway hyperexcitability to histamine in asthmatic subjects. Bull Eur Physiopathol Respir 1983; 19:465–469.
75. De Vries K, Goei JT, Booij-Noord H, Orie NGM. Changes during 24 hours in the lung function and histamine hyperreactivity of the bronchial tree in asthmatic and bronchitis patients. Int Arch Allergy 1962; 20:93–101.

76. Manning PJ, Jones GL, O'Byrne PM. Tachyphylaxis to inhaled histamine in asthmatic subjects. J Appl Physiol 1987; 63:1572-1577.
77. Ruffin RE, Alpers JH, Crockcett AJ, Hamilton R. Repeated histamine inhalation test in asthmatic patients. J Allergy Clin Immunol 1981; 67:285-289.
78. Lemire I, Cartier A, Malo JL, Pineau L, Ghezzo H, Martin RR. Effect of sodium cromoglycate on histamine inhalation tests. J Allergy Clin Immunol 1984; 73:234-239.
79. Cartier A, Lemire I, L'Archevêque J, Ghezzo H, Martin RR, Malo JL. Theophylline partially inhibits bronchoconstriction due to inhaled histamine in asthmatic subjects. J Allergy Clin Immunol 1986; 77:570-575.
80. Malo JL, Filiatrault S, Martin RR. Bronchial responsiveness to inhaled methacholine in young asymptomatic smokers. J Appl Physiol 1982; 52:1464-1470.
81. Casale TB, Rhodes BJ, Donnelly AL, Weiler JM. Airway responses to methacholine in asymptomatic nonatopic cigarette smokers. J Appl Physiol 1987; 62:1888-1892.
82. Eggleston PA, Fish JE. Upper airway disease and bronchial hyperreactivity. Clin Rev Allergy 1984; 2:429-441.
83. Bahous J, Cartier A, Pineau L, Bernard C, Martin RR, Malo JL. Pulmonary function tests and airway responsiveness to methacholine in chronic bronchiectasis of the adult. Bull Eur Physiopathol Respir 1984; 20:375-380.
84. Pison C, Malo JL, Rouleau JL, Malo J. Effects of acute and chronic left ventricular failure on bronchial responsiveness to methacholine (abstr). Am Rev Respir Dis 1988; 137:292.
85. Cabanes L, Weber S, Matran R, Regnard J, Delauture D, Degeorges M, Lockhart A. Bronchial hyperresponsiveness to methacholine in patients with impaired left-ventricular function (abstr). Am Rev Respir Dis 1988; 137:291.
86. Ryan G, Latimer KM, Juniper EF, Roberts RS, Hargreave FE. Effect of beclomethasone dipropionate on bronchial responsiveness to histamine in controlled nonsteroid-dependent asthma. J Allergy Clin Immunol 1985; 75:25-30.
87. Kraan J, Koeter GH, Mark TWVD, Sluiter HJ, de Vries K. Changes in bronchial hyperreactivity induced by 4 weeks of treatment with antiasthmatic drugs in patients with allergic asthma: a comparison between budesonide and terbutaline. J Allergy Clin Immunol 1985; 76:628-636.
88. Holtzman MJ, Cunningham JH, Sheller JR, Irsigler GB, Nadel JA, Boushey HA. Effect of ozone on bronchial reactivity in atopic and nonatopic subjects. Am Rev Respir Dis 1979; 120:1059-1067.
89. Empey DW, Laitinen LA, Jacobs L, Gold WM, Nadel JA. Mechanisms of bronchohyperreactivity in normal subjects after upper respiratory tract infections. Am Rev Respir Dis 1976; 113:131-139.
90. Jenkins CR, Breslin ABX. Upper respiratory tract infections and airway reactivity in normal and asthmatic subjects. Am Rev Respir Dis 1984; 130:879-883.

91. Tessier P, Cartier A, Ghezzo H, Martin RR, Malo JL. Bronchoconstriction due to exercise combined with cold air inhalation does not generally influence bronchial responsiveness to inhaled histamine in asthmatic subjects. Eur Respir J 1988; 1:133–138.
92. Mattoli S, Foresi A, Corbo GM, Valente S, Patalano F, Ciappi G. Increase in bronchial responsiveness to methacholine and late asthmatic response after the inhalation of ultrasonically nebulized distilled water. Chest 1986; 70:726–732.
93. Sotomayor H, Badier M, Vervloet D, Orehek J. Seasonal increase of carbachol airway responsiveness in patients allergic to grass pollen. Am Rev Respir Dis 1984; 130:56–58.
94. Cartier A, Malo JL, Forest F, Lafrance M, Pineau L, St-Aubin JJ, Dubois JY. Occupational asthma in snow crab-processing workers. J Allergy Clin Immunol 1984; 74:261–269.
95. Tiffeneau R. Hypersensibilité cholinergo-histaminique pulmonaire de l'asthmatique. Acta Allergol Suppl 1958; 5:187–221.
96. Cockcroft DW, Ruffin RE, Frith PA, Cartier A, Juniper EF, Dolovich J, Hargreave FE. Determinants of allergen-induced asthma: dose of allergen, circulating IgE antibody concentration, and bronchial responsiveness to inhaled histamine. Am Rev Respir Dis 1979; 120:1053–1058.
97. Cockcroft DW, Murdock KY, Kirby J, Hargreave F. Prediction of airway responsiveness to allergen from skin sensitivity to allergen and airway responsiveness to histamine. Am Rev Respir Dis 1987; 135:264–267.
98. Adelroth C, Hargreave FE, Ramsdale EH. Do physicians need objective measurements to diagnose asthma? Am Rev Respir Dis 1986; 134:704–707.
99. Desjardins A, De Luca S, Cartier A, L'Archevêque J, Ghezzo H, Malo JL. Non specific bronchial hyperresponsiveness to inhaled histamine and hyperventilation of cold dry air in individuals with respiratory symptoms of uncertain etiology. Am Rev Respir Dis 1988; 137:1020–1025.
100. Enarson DA, Chan-Yeung M, Tabona M, Jus J, Vedal S, Lam S. Predictors of bronchial hyperexcitability in grainhandlers. Chest 1985; 87:452–455.
101. Dales RE, Erns P, Hanley JA, Battista RN, Becklake MR. Prediction of airway reactivity from responses to a standardized respiratory symptom questionnaire. Am Rev Respir Dis 1987; 135:817–821.
102. Rijcken B, Schouten JP, Weiss ST, Speizer FE, Van der Lende R. The relationship of nonspecific bronchial responsiveness to respiratory symptoms in a random population sample. Am Rev Respir Dis 1987; 136: 62–68.
103. Pratter MR, Hingston DM, Irwin RS. Diagnosis of bronchial asthma by clinical evaluation: an unreliable method. Chest 1983; 84:42–47.
104. Dales RE, Nunes F, Partyka D, Ernst P. Clinical prediction of airways hyperresponsiveness. Chest 1988; 93:984–986.
105. Juniper EF, Frith PA, Hargreave FE. Airway responsiveness to histamine and methacholine: relationship to minimum treatment to control symptoms of asthma. Thorax 1981; 36:575–579.

106. Malo JL, Cartier A. Investigation of occupational asthma due to low molecular weight agents. In: *Highlights in Asthmology*. Michel F, Bousquet J, Godard P, eds. Berlin, Springer-Verlag, 1987, pp 345-350.
107. Chan-Yeung M. Evaluation of impairment/disability in patients with occupational asthma. Am Rev Respir Dis 1987; 135:950-951.
108. Herxheimer H. Hyperventilation asthma. Lancet 1946; 1:83-87.
109. Godfrey S. Exercise-induced asthma. Clinical, physiological, and therapeutic implications. J Allergy Clin Immunol 1975; 56:1-17.
110. Edmunds AT, Tooley M, Godfrey S. The refractory period after exercise-induced asthma: its duration and relation to the severity of exercise. Am Rev Respir Dis 1978; 117:247-254.
111. Anderson SD, Schoeffel RE. Standardization of exercise testing in the asthmatic patient: a challenge in itself. In: *Airway Responsiveness-Measurement and Interpretation*. Hargreave FE, Woolcock AJ, eds. Burlington, Astra Pharmaceuticals 1985, pp 51-59.
112. Eggleston PA, Rosenthal RR, Anderson SA, Anderton R, Bierman CW, Bleecker ER, Chai H, Cropp GJA, Johnson JD, Konig P, Morse J, Smith LJ, Summers RJ, Trautlein JJ. Guidelines for the methodology of exercise challenge testing of asthmatics. J Allergy Clin Immunol 1979; 64: 642-645.
113. Eggleston PA. Methods of exercise challenge. J Allergy Clin Immunol 1984; 73:666-669.
114. Hargreave FE, Dolovich J, Boulet LP. Inhalation provocation tests. Sem Respir Med 1983; 4:224-236.
115. Lockhart A, Régnard J, Dessanges JF, Florentin D, Lurie A. Exercise- and hyperventilation-induced asthma. Bull Eur Physiopathol Respir 1985; 21:399-409.
116. O'Byrne PM, Jones G. The effect of indomethacin on exercise-induced bronchoconstriction and refractoriness after exercise. Am Rev Respir Dis 1986; 134:69-72.
117. Anderton RC, Cuff MT, Frith PA, Cockcroft DW, Morse JLC, Jones NL, Hargreave FE. Bronchial responsiveness to inhaled histamine and exercise. J Allergy Clin Immunol 1979; 63:315-320.
118. Mellis CM, Kattan M, Keens TG, Levison H. Comparative study of histamine and exercise challenges in asthmatic children. Am Rev Respir Dis 1978; 117:911-915.
119. Henriksen JM. Reproducibility of exercise-induced asthma in children. Allergy 1986; 41:225-231.
120. Menkes HA. Airways reactivity and the need for a simple test. Am Rev Respir Dis 1980; 121:619-620.
121. Kivity S, Souhrada JF. A new diagnostic test to assess airway reactivity in asthmatics. Bull Eur Physiopathol Respir 1981; 17:243-254.
122. Eschenbacher WL, Sheppard D. Respiratory heat loss is not the sole stimulus for bronchoconstriction induced by isocapnic hyperpnea with dry air. Am Rev Respir Dis 1985; 131:894-901.

123. Smith CM, Anderson SD. Hyperosmolarity as the stimulus to asthma induced by hyperventilation? J Allergy Clin Immunol 1986;77:729–736.
124. Noviski N, Bar-Yishay E, Gur I, Godfrey S. Exercise intensity determines and climatic conditions modify the severity of exercise-induced asthma. Am Rev Respir Dis 1987;136:592–594.
125. Phillips YY, Jaeger JJ, Laube BL, Rosenthal RR. Eucapnic voluntary hyperventilation of compressed gas mixture. A simple system for bronchial challenge by respiratory heat loss. Am Rev Respir Dis 1985; 131:31–35.
126. O'Byrne PM, Ryan G, Morris M, McCormack D, Jones NL, Morse JLC, Hargreave FE. Asthma induced by cold air and its relation to nonspecific bronchial responsiveness to methacholine. Am Rev Respir Dis 1982; 125:281–285.
127. Malo JL, Cartier A, L'Archevêque J, Ghezzo H, Martin RR. Kinetics of the recovery from bronchial obstruction due to hyperventilation of cold air in asthmatic subjects. Eur Respir J (in press).
128. Tessier P, Ghezzo H, L'Archevêque J, Cartier A, Malo JL. Shape of the dose–response curve to cold air inhalation in normal and asthmatic subjects. Am Rev Respir Dis 1987;136:1418–1423.
129. Malo JL, Cartier A, L'Archevêque J, Ghezzo H, Martin RR. Cold air inhalation has a cumulative bronchospastic effect when inhaled in consecutive doses for progressively increasing degrees of ventilation. Am Rev Respir Dis 1986;134:990–993.
130. Weiss JW, Rossing TH, McFadden ER, Ingram RH. Relationship between bronchial responsiveness to hyperventilation with cold and methacholine in asthma. J Allergy Clin Immunol 1983;72:140–144.
131. Ramsdale EH, Morris MM, Roberts RS, Hargreave FE. Bronchial responsiveness to methacholine in chronic bronchitis: relationship to airflow obstruction and cold air responsiveness. Thorax 1984;39:912–918.
132. Latimer KM, O'Byrne PM, Morris MM, Roberts R, Hargreave FE. Bronchoconstriction stimulated by airway cooling. Am Rev Respir Dis 1983;128:440–443.
133. O'Byrne PM, Thomson NC, Morris M, Roberts RS, Daniel EE, Hargreave FE. The protective effect of inhaled chlorpheniramine and atropine on bronchoconstriction stimulated by airway cooling. Am Rev Respir Dis 1983;128:611–617.
134. Merland N, Cartier A, L'Archevêque J, Ghezzo H, Malo JL. Theophylline minimally inhibits bronchoconstriction induced by dry cold air inhalation of asthmatic subjects. Am Rev Respir Dis 1988; 137:1304–1308.
135. Ahrens RC, Bonham AC, Maxwell GA, Weinberger MM. A method for comparing the peak intensity and duration of action of aerosolized bronchodilators using bronchoprovocation with methacholine. Am Rev Respir Dis 1984;129:903–906.
136. Anderson SD, Schoeffel RE, Finney M. Evaluation of ultrasonically nebulised solutions for provocation testing in patients with asthma. Thorax 1983;38:284–291.

137. Boulet LP, Legris C, Thibaullt L, Turcotte H. Comparative bronchial responses to hyperosmolar saline and methacholine in asthma. Thorax 1983;42:953-958.
138. Woolcock AJ, Yan K, Salome CM. Effect of therapy on bronchial hyperresponsiveness in the long-term management of asthma. Clin Allergy 1988;18:165-176.

5

Atopy and Asthma

DONALD W. COCKCROFT

University Hospital
Saskatoon, Saskatchewan, Canada

INTRODUCTION

The relationship between atopy or sensitivity to inhaled allergens and asthma has long been known, dating back to before the term "atopy" was coined early in this century. The precise role and importance of inhalant (and other) allergens in the pathogenesis of asthma, or of symptoms in asthmatics, has not been clear, and has been a source of much controversy. Extreme views have ranged from that of a respiratory physiologist stating "I don't believe in allergy!" to that of a clinical ecologist who believes that all asthma and rhinitis, and in fact many other common human ailments, are "allergic" (atopic or otherwise) in nature. The more prevalent view has been to regard atopic inhalant allergens as one of a number of triggering factors known to provoke bronchospasm in subjects with asthma (i.e., pre-existing airway hyperresponsiveness). More recent views expressed in a comprehensive 1985 North American asthma textbook state that atopic allergy (among some other asthma triggers) is responsible for producing disease in subjects with airway responsiveness, is known to influence airway responsiveness, and "tends to enhance asthma severity" (1). The possibility that atopy, or more appropriately, chronic/recurrent atopic allergic airways inflammation might lead to transient and persistent airway hyperresponsiveness and thus be one ***cause*** of asthma has, until recently, been given little consideration.

Advances in knowledge in the past decade have changed our concepts regarding the pathogenesis of airway hyperresponsiveness and asthma. A number of asthma triggers have been identified to actually worsen asthma by leading to transient enhancement of airway hyperresponsiveness. These triggers include inhalant allergen exposure, occupational low-molecular weight sensitizing agent exposure, viral/mycoplasma respiratory tract infections, oxidizing gas (ozone, nitrogen dioxide) exposure, and possibly others (2,3). The common feature shared by these triggers is their association with airways inflammation. Such "inducing" triggers of airway responsiveness can be differentiated from the purely bronchospastic "inciting" triggers such as exercise, cold air, emotional stress, pharmacologic triggers, and inhaled irritants (2,3). These inciting triggers produce airways smooth muscle contraction which depends chiefly on the level of underlying airway hyperresponsiveness, without significantly modulating airway responsiveness itself; thus, responses to these bronchospastic triggers can be regarded as manifestations of the underlying disease rather than causative factors.

The recent recognition of allergic airways inflammation as a cause of both transient and possibly persistent airway hyperresponsiveness has led to increased appreciation of the importance of atopy in the pathogenesis of asthma. Evidence for atopy as a major (perhaps *the* major) cause of airway hyperresponsiveness and asthma will be presented in this review of atopy and asthma.

ATOPY

The term atopy, like asthma, is a commonly used term which does not have a universally acceptable definition. It was initially applied to a group of clinical disorders which included infantile/childhood eczema, conjunctivitis, rhinitis, and asthma, and in which historical evidence of inhalant allergen sensitivity was commonly evident. With the recognition of skin test sensitivity and reaginic antibody, more recently identified as IgE, it is obvious that a sizable number of asthma and rhinitis sufferers lack this immunologic sensitivity. A reasonably acceptable definition has been proposed by Pepys: "The essential feature of atopy is that form of immunological reactivity of the subject in which IgE antibody is ***readily*** produced in response to ***ordinary exposure*** to the common allergens of the subject's environment" (4).

The mechanism and pathogenesis of atopy are not entirely clear. Atopy probably is not simply the ability to produce IgE in increased amounts. The difference between atopic and nonatopic individuals may lie at the level of mucosal surfaces and probably relates to allergen transport and/or handling rather than IgE production per se (5). It appears that with "nonordinary exposure," that is, "injection" of allergen, IgE antibodies will develop readily even in nonatopic individuals (4,5).

The common allergens referred to in the definition are airborne protein-containing particles. Identified allergens are soluble globular proteins in the molecular weight range 3000-70,000 (predominantly in the 20-40,000 range) (6). The sources of these protein or protein-containing molecules in the atmosphere are many, and new sources are continually being identified. The major common allergens have been grouped into four categories: pollen, fungal spores, animal proteins, and house dust (7,8). The pollens responsible for sensitization are primarily those of wind-pollenated plants and include trees, grasses, and weeds. The seasonal variation depends on geographical/climatic conditions, but is usually spring, summer, and fall for trees, grasses, and weeds, respectively. Atmospheric fungal spores, produced by decaying vegetation, are significant causes of late summer and fall symptoms and also possibly spring symptoms in areas of late snow melting. Important animal allergens are chiefly those from mammalian species (cats, dogs, horses, etc.) and from avian species. Allergens contained within house dust are probably the most important cause of sensitization. There are many identified and possibly unidentified allergens which may be contained within house dust. House dust mites (***Dermatophagoides farinae, D. pteronyssinus***) are likely the single most common sensitizing allergen in the world. House dust may also contain insect allergens (cockroach), and mammalian allergens (particularly cat) among others. In addition, protein-containing allergens from virtually any phylum of the plant or animal kingdom can trigger atopic Type 1 sensitization. Many of these are commonly but not exclusively encountered in occupational settings. An incomplete list would include exotic birds and mammals (animal handlers, veterinarians, pet store owners, and laboratory workers), arthropods (shrimp, lobster, crab), insects (inhaled allergens in beekeepers, from silkworms, etc.), molluscs (clam, oyster workers), bacteria (***B. subtilus*** enzymes in detergents), and numerous plant allergens (psyllium used in laxatives, tobacco leaf, cocoa bean, coffee bean, castor bean, grain dust, etc.). In rare circumstances, atopic sensitivity can be so great that molecular exposure to the odors of cooking foods, particularly fish or eggs, can provoke symptoms.

IgE-mediated reactions to allergens which are either ingested or injected can also provoke asthma. Usually this occurs as part of a systemic anaphylactic reaction, however, occasionally symptomatic asthma is the major complaint. Ingested allergens include foods and drugs (usually a drug-protein haptene), while injected allergens include drugs, therapeutic allergen injections, and insect stings or bites. Although uncommon, these allergens may be causes of genuinely sudden life-threatening asthma and should be borne in mind in such cases. Subjects with such reactions may not necessarily be "atopic." IgE-mediated responses possibly to drugs (9), and almost certainly to insect stings (10), are no more frequent in otherwise atopic individuals than in nonatopic individuals; food hypersensitivity is somewhat more common in atopic than nonatopic individuals; whereas therapeutic allergen injections (excepting insect venom) should be exclusively limited to atopic individuals. Aside from the brief mention here for the sake of completion, ingested and injected allergens will not be discussed further.

There is a marked familial tendency toward atopy (11). It is almost certainly under major genetic control, however, the genetics for the inheritance of atopy are not known. Genetic studies are hampered by a number of facts, including the commonness of the condition, the lack of understanding of the pathophysiologic abnormality, and the continuous spectrum between atopy and nonatopy with a less than clearly identified "cutoff." Hypotheses have included autosomal-recessive inheritance with variable penetrance, and multiple gene or polygenic inheritance. The picture is further complicated by the observation that environment itself can have an important influence on at least the expression of, and perhaps even the presence of atopy. Such things as month of birth, concomitant infections, and age of first presentation to a given allergen may be relevant in development of sensitivity.

Based on the above definition, atopy is best defined by positive wheal and flare responses on prick skin testing to a battery of indigenous allergens (4). The prevalence of atopy in most populations ranges from 30 to slightly in excess of 50% in some areas where house dust mite sensitivity is particularly common (12-14). There are suggestions that the prevalence of both atopy and atopic diseases may have increased dramatically over the past 100 or so years (15), however no objective data are available. An alternate explanation, for at least part of the increased prevalence, is increased recognition of a common and perhaps previously ignored medical condition, as well as the fact that "allergy" has become a very fashionable disease of the twentieth century. Some studies in more primitive peoples, which have become "civilized" in the past few decades, strongly suggest that alterations and modernization of lifestyle might cause significant increases in the prevalence of atopy and atopic disease (16). In a typical North American population, the prevalence of atopy is approximately one-third, with about half of these having some atopic symptoms (rhinitis or conjunctivitis), and about half of these symptomatic individuals having some symptoms to suggest asthma (17). Thus, approximately 1 in 3 subjects will be atopic based on skin test, approximately 1 in 6 will also have some allergic rhinitis, and approximately 1 in 12 will have allergic asthma.

ALLERGEN INHALATION IN THE LABORATORY

Over the past 35 years, we have learned a great deal about the patterns and pathogenesis of allergen-induced asthmatic responses by utilizing allergen provocation tests in the laboratory (18). Such tests are generally performed by the inhalation of nebulized aerosols of aqueous allergen extracts. Compared to natural allergen exposure, inhalation challenges produce a relatively brief relatively high exposure of particles which may be smaller than those naturally encountered. These challenges, therefore, do not precisely mimic naturally occurring exposures.

The responses to inhaled allergen can be divided into early (within the first minutes to one hour) largely bronchospastic responses, and late (beyond two or three hours) which are, at least in part, due to airway inflammation.

The early asthmatic response is an episode of airflow obstruction which occurs almost immediately following allergen challenge, is maximal between 10 and 30 minutes after allergen exposure, and resolves spontaneously between 1 and 2 hours (Fig. 1a). The early asthmatic response is likely mainly bronchospastic, however some mucosal edema and mucous hypersecretion may also occur. The early asthmatic response is determined by the amount of mediators released from mast cells (dependent on allergen dose and specific IgE level) and the level of airway responsiveness (19). Smooth muscle contraction is likely due to the direct effects of mediators which are released or synthesized de novo from mast cells following the interaction between allergen and IgE fixed to mast cells. The importance of various mast cell-derived mediators has not been precisely clarified. One elegant in vitro study suggests the requirement for histamine and both cyclo-oxygenase products and lipoxygenase products of arachidonic acid metabolism as being necessary together to produce the early response (20). This study further suggested that histamine might be responsible for the early part of the contraction and the leukotrienes for the late part of the early asthmatic response.

The pharmacology of the early asthmatic response is as follows. Inhaled beta-adrenoreceptor agonists provide the best inhibition of the early asthmatic response (21-25). This may be because of its effect on smooth muscle but also could be due to inhibition of mast cell mediator release (26,27). The other bronchodilators, both methyl xanthines (28-31) and anticholinergic (24,32-35), provide significant but relatively minor protection against allergen-induced early asthmatic responses. Sodium cromoglycate provides very good inhibition of the early asthmatic response though not generally so complete as that provided by beta agonists (21,22,25,36-38). Single dose and short course corticosteroids do not inhibit the early response (21,22,25,37-40). Longer periods of corticosteroids inhibit at least partially the early asthmatic response by as yet unclear mechanisms (39,40). One possibility is steroid-induced improvement in nonallergic airway responsiveness (41), which is known to be an important determinant of the early asthmatic response (19); this possibility has not been investigated. H_1 receptor blockers provide partial inhibition of the early asthmatic response (21,22,42,43); some observations suggest that the early component of the early response is preferentially inhibited (43). Ketotifen, an H_1 blocker with possibly some antiallergic properties, has produced variable results regarding inhibition of the early asthmatic response (44,45). The effect of other specific mediator antagonists or mediator synthetase antagonists alone or in

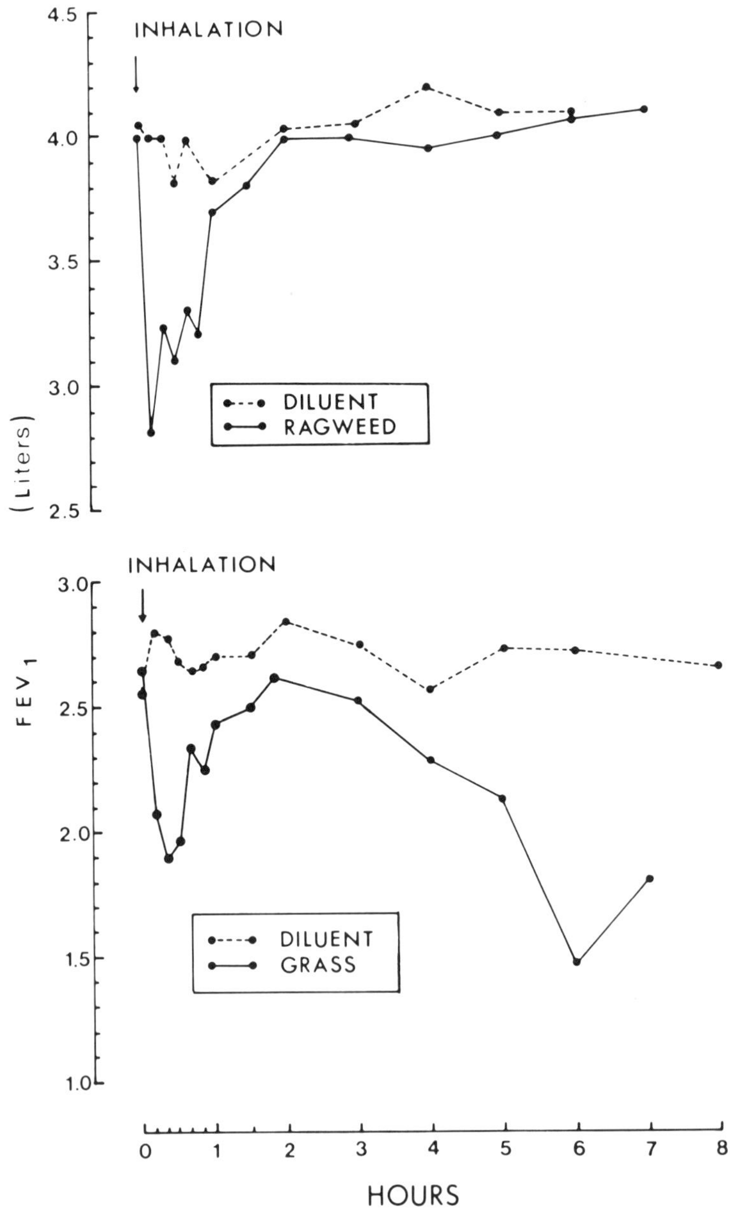

FIGURE 1 Controlled allergen challenges showing early asthmatic response (top panel) and dual asthmatic response (bottom panel). FEV_1 (%Δ) on vertical axis is graphed vs. time (h) on horizontal axis. From Ref. 85.

combination in human asthma remains to be confirmed. Nonsteroidal anti-inflammatory agents do not influence the early asthmatic response (46-48).

The late asthmatic response, first clearly described by Blackley in 1873 following accidental exposure to whole pollen in the laboratory (49), has now been more clearly described as an episode of airflow obstruction occurring generally between 3 and 8 hours after allergen exposure (Fig. 1b) (18,50,51). Mild to moderate late responses are largely reversible by beta-adrenergic agonists (52, 53). There is the impression, however, that beta agonists may be required more frequently than usual to maintain normal airway caliber during a late response. Larger late responses, of greater than 30 or 40% FEV_1 fall, are at least partially refractory to beta agonists (54); this led to the speculation earlier that a component of the late response was due to edema or inflammation within the airways. The late response following inhaled allergen occasionally lasts for up to 12 hours, rarely longer.

Allergen-induced increase in airway responsiveness is the second major feature of the late response induced by allergen. Airway responsiveness to histamine or methacholine (or exercise/cold air, etc.) was first identified following natural allergen exposure almost 25 years ago by Altounyan (55), and was first identified in the laboratory in 1977 (Fig. 2) (56). Airway responsiveness appears to increase between 2 and 3 hours after allergen exposure (57-59), is maximal between 7 hours and several days after exposure (56,60) and may last for a few days to a week or 10 days, sometimes longer (60). The increased airway responsiveness is closely associated with both the appearance and magnitude of the late asthmatic response (60). Increased airway responsiveness may occur with late responses which are very small (56,60). Increased airway responsiveness can occur occasionally in the absence of a late response, particularly in an individual who has received a dose of allergen which is just below the threshold required for a late response (59). It appears that subjects with normal or mildly increased airway responsiveness have a smaller late response relative to the magnitude of increase in airway responsiveness. By contrast, subjects with greater airway hyperresponsiveness, as expected from other studies, appear to develop more bronchospasm (greater late response) relative to the increased responsiveness. Increased airway responsiveness is associated with increased asthma symptoms particularly at night and on exposure to bronchospastic triggering factors (exercise, cold air, smoke, dust, etc.) (56,60). The increased responsiveness persists beyond any measurable changes in airway caliber (60).

Recurrent episodes of nocturnal bronchospasm has been reported as a separate allergic response (61). It is likely that recurrent nocturnal asthma represents enhanced diurnal variation of airway caliber secondary to the increased airway responsiveness (62).

The mechanism(s) underlying the late asthmatic response are a subject of much interest and study but are as yet far from clearly understood. A "second

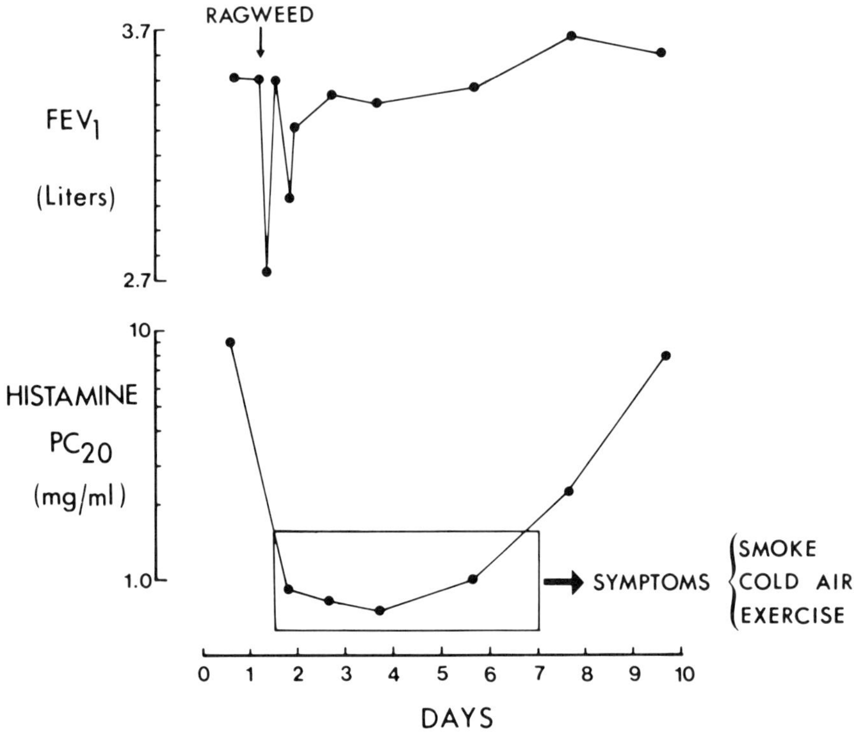

FIGURE 2 Allergen induced increase in airway responsiveness to inhaled histamine. The FEV_1 (%Δ) in top and histamine PC_{20} (mg/ml) on bottom is graphed vs. time (days), following a single brief inhalation of ragweed pollen allergen. From Ref. 85.

wave" of mediators released either from mast cells or other effector cells has been identified (63) and may be responsible in part for the bronchospastic component of the last asthmatic response. There is also increasing circumstantial evidence for the importance of cellular inflammation in the genesis of late responses. The evidence includes the following: (a) The level of airway responsiveness correlates well with inflammatory cells (eosinophils, metachromatic cells) recovered from bronchoalveolar lavage (64,65). Therefore, measurement of airway responsiveness may be a useful in vivo assessment of the presence of airways inflammation. (b) Inhibition of the late response with corticosteroids (21,22,25,37-40) is supportive of one late response being an inflammatory event. (c) Bronchoalveolar lavage studies in humans have shown that cellular inflammation, particularly eosinophils, is present in late but not isolated early asthmatic responders (66,67). (d) Animal studies have more clearly identified the importance of cellular inflammation in allergen-induced responses. Animals depleted of granulocytes do not develop late responses or increased airway responsiveness following allergen provocation (68,69).

A number of mediators have the potential to recruit inflammatory cells. These include neutrophil chemotactic factor (70,71), eosinophil chemotactic factor (71), leukotriene B_4 (72), and platelet activating factor (73). The precise means whereby inflammatory cells, predominantly eosinophils in allergen-induced late responses, increase airway responsiveness is also not clear. A number of studies have suggested that increased airway responsiveness induced by a variety of inflammatory triggers can be attenuated by cyclo-oxygenase inhibitor and/or thromboxane synthetase inhibitors (48,74-76), suggesting the possibility of the importance of thromboxane or thromboxane-like mediators, however, such studies are only preliminary.

The pharmacologic modulation of the late asthmatic response is less well documented than of the early response. Inhaled beta agonists in doses sufficient to reduce mast cell mediator release, do not prevent the late asthmatic response (21-23,25), nor do they prevent the increased airway responsiveness (25). Beta agonists, however, do largely reverse the late response when only mild or moderate in severity (52,53), and continuous use of a beta agonist would be expected to largely mask the late response, again without altering airway responsiveness. Theophylline preparations have only recently been studied in the late response. Theophylline reduces the magnitude of the late response from 25-50% (29-31). All studies performed have maintained therapeutic theophylline levels throughout the duration of the study, therefore it is not clear whether inhibition of the late response is occurring because of inhibition of the inflammatory response or by virtue of bronchoactive effects. Nevertheless, it appears that despite reduction in the late response, allergen-induced increase in airway responsiveness is not inhibited by theophylline (30,31). Anticholinergic drugs do not inhibit the late asthmatic responses (35), nor do they likely inhibit increased airway responsiveness. An anticholinergic bronchodilator will at least partially reverse the airflow obstruction seen during the late asthmatic response (52). Sodium cromoglycate administered before but not after allergen exposure will inhibit the late response (21,22,25,36-38) and increased airway responsiveness (25). Corticosteroids will also inhibit both the late asthmatic response (21,22,25,37-40) and the increased airway responsiveness (25). The effects of other drugs are less certain. Antihistamines do not appear to affect the late asthmatic response. The influence of ketotifen on the late response is uncertain; although there is one favorable report (45), further studies are required. Non-steroidal anti-inflammatory agents have been reported by some (47), but not by others (48) to inhibit the late response. Indomethacin appears to ameliorate the increased responsiveness seen following allergen exposure (48).

NATURAL ALLERGEN EXPOSURE

Difficulties in identifying the timing, duration, and dose of exposure to inhaled allergens under natural conditions leads to difficulties in appreciating the equivalents of the early and late allergen-induced responses following natural allergen exposure. This may be further complicated by multiple sensitivities and concomitant exposures which are often seen in atopic asthmatics. For these reasons, occupational asthma caused by sensitization to low-molecular weight chemicals, may provide a better model for understanding the course of natural sensitizing agent exposure. This is because occupational sensitization generally involves a single agent (or family of agents), exposure commences relatively late in life, the timing and duration of exposure are generally known, and at least a qualitative estimate of dose may be available.

The clinical equivalent of the early asthmatic response is often missing because of failure to recognize allergen exposure. This is particularly true with pollen, fungal spores, and house dust allergens. Furthermore, such allergen exposures may be accompanied by nonallergic triggers of bronchospasm (e.g., exercise plus grass pollen exposure when "mowing the lawn," exercise plus irritant effect plus allergen exposures in a dusty grain elevator, etc.). Thus the clinical appreciation of early asthmatic response is, for practical purposes, limited to those that occur following exposure to animals or exposure to an unusual allergen (often occupational). Acute immediate asthmatic symptoms are frequently reported in patients highly sensitized to animals, particularly cats and horses but also dogs, lab animals, and others. These historical reponses are more likely to be seen in subjects with milder asthma, often those requiring very little medications. Subjects with more continuous asthma, either perennial or seasonal, often do not provide a history to suggest early asthmatic responses. The reasons for this include: (a) failure to appreciate the timing of allergen exposure, (b) complete ablation of early asthmatic responses by frequent use of inhaled beta agonists, (c) absence of early asthmatic responses after exposure, as is seen commonly with occupational exposures and occasionally (in the lab) following allergen exposures, and (d) failure to differentiate an early response from responses produced by other bronchospastic (possibly concomitant) triggers. Furthermore, the possibility exists that intermittent or chronic low-grade allergen exposures, in a subject who is not highly allergic, might not provoke severe enough mediator release to produce an early asthmatic response yet may be responsible for gradual onset chronic late responses. This failure to document the early asthmatic response may have led to controversy and underappreciation of the importance of atopic allergen exposure in the pathogenesis of asthma. A cited but unpublished study noted that only 8% of 500 asthmatic admissions over a 10 year period were felt to be (presumably historically) attributable to allergen exposure (77), although undoubtedly a greater proportion of these patients were atopic. Furthermore, in the same practice about 50% of outpatients had some evidence (again presumably historically) of some symptoms due to allergens, largely animal danders or molds, and generally occurring mildly asthmatic individuals. This appreciation of some allergen-induced (early) asthmatic responses in milder but not more severe or hospitalized asthmatics is consistent with the concepts expressed above.

Late asthmatic responses are likely much more important in the pathogenesis of asthma. They are even more difficult to identify historically or clinically than are early responses, in part, because of the same difficulties noted above, added to which is the fact that the delayed and prolonged symptoms may direct the asthmatic away from the true cause. Nevertheless, in a small number of asthmatics a history of the late response and increased airway responsiveness can be obtained. Once again, the primary prerequisite is ability to identify fairly precisely the time and duration of allergen exposure and therefore again these episodes can be more often related to animal exposure or occupational allergen exposure. Occasionally, patients will report that following exposure to an animal, usually acute symptoms will develop, followed by asthma which worsens several hours later, often in the middle of the night. The same patients might note that a single exposure to an allergen may provoke symptoms of several days duration. Such histories are unusual, and, again, in our experience are more common in those who otherwise have generally mild asthma. Occasionally patients will notice a general worsening and improving of their asthma concomitant with, but lagging behind, exposure and nonexposure to an animal. On a larger time-scale, the seasonal worsening of asthma in subjects with pollen sensitivity, again lagging in onset and resolution often by several weeks behind the pollen count, is a well recognized feature of the seasonal allergic asthmatic. This probably represents the natural equivalent of allergen-induced increase in airway responsiveness.

There are few objective data available surrounding natural allergen exposure. The original excellent description of the relationship of asthma and rhinitis to pollen exposure and of a classic late asthmatic response was performed over 100 years ago using exposure to whole pollen, although in high doses (49). The observations, however, were purely clinical. Perhaps the most important objective data on natural exposure to allergens follows upon the 25-year-old observation of Altounyan, who noted seasonal increases in airway responsiveness to inhaled histamine in asthmatics sensitive to grass pollen (55,78). These studies have since been confirmed in other centers and other countries. Increased responsiveness to either histamine or to a cholinergic analog has been demonstrated in the ragweed pollen season in Canada (79), the grass pollen season in France (80), and the birch pollen season in Scandinavia (81). The reverse approach has also confirmed the existence of allergen-induced increases in airway responsiveness under natural conditions. A number of studies involving environmental control in house dust-sensitive asthmatics have confirmed that reduction in allergen exposure can be associated with improvements, frequently marked, in nonallergic airway responsiveness (82-84). We have similarly noted, anecdotally, improvement in airway responsiveness without changes in airways caliber, following removal of an animal from the home. These studies thus provide good evidence that natural exposure to allergen(s) can substantially increase airways responsiveness, and the reduction of such exposure can improve airways responsiveness. Based on the relationship of airways responsiveness to airways inflammation, as well as observations and speculations from laboratory data, these increases in airway responsiveness probably are related to atopic allergen-

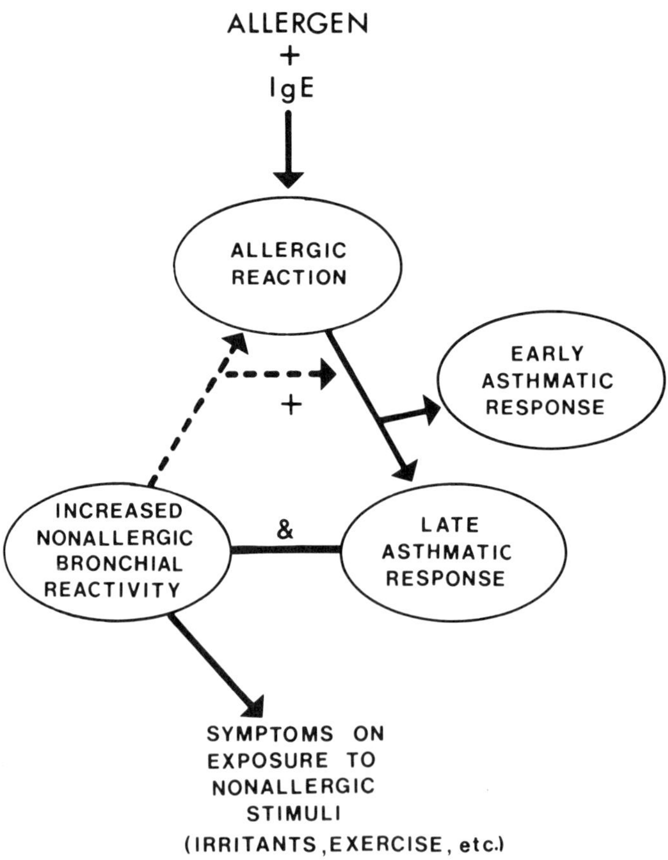

FIGURE 3 Vicious cycle hypothesis for the development and maintenance of airway hyperresponsiveness in atopic allergic asthma. From Ref. 85.

induced airways inflammation. This hypothesis however has not been rigorously tested in seasonal allergic asthmatics.

The small number of studies available would tend to confirm the studies in the laboratory regarding the pharmacology of natural allergen-induced increases in airway responsiveness. Seasonal studies have demonstrated that corticosteroids (80) and sodium cromoglycate (78,81) will prevent or reverse the seasonal increases in airway responsiveness, whereas bronchodilators (generally used in the control groups of the same studies) do not appear to prevent this.

Transient allergen-induced increases in airways inflammation and airway hyperresponsiveness have been hypothesized to be of major importance in the pathogenesis of both seasonal and perennial allergic asthma (85) (Fig. 3). A recent population study has suggested that the majority of purely seasonal allergic asthmatics may have only the transient component of allergen-induced airway hyperresponsiveness (17). However, in some seasonal asthmatics and likely all perennial allergic asthmatics, there exists a component of airway hyperresponsiveness which appears to be resistant to environmental control or corticosteroids. In such subjects, one component of their airway hyperresponsiveness appears to be transient and potentially reversible, whereas another component appears to be persistent and potentially nonreversible. Evidence is accumulating to support the hypothesis that the persistent (as well as the transient) component of airway hyperresponsiveness might be caused by allergic airways inflammation.

ALLERGENS AS A CAUSE OF PERSISTENT AIRWAY HYPERRESPONSIVENESS

The possibility that atopy, or chronic/recurrent allergic airways inflammation might be the cause of persistent airway hyperresponsiveness, and therefore the ***cause*** of asthma follows logically upon the observations that allergen exposure can lead to transient airway hyperresponsiveness (55-60,78-81), and that atopy is strongly associated with asthma (4). Prospective studies are difficult to perform because of the early onset of atopy, particularly in more severe allergic asthmatics. Retrospective (historical) assessment is difficult because of the early age of onset, multiple sensitivities, and inability to quantitate timing and dose of allergen exposure. However, occupational asthma, induced by low-molecular weight sensitizing chemicals, may serve as a useful model. There is strong retrospective evidence, which suggests that continued exposure to an occupational sensitizing agent, once sensitization has developed, may lead to permanent airway hyperresponsiveness and permanent asthma (86-88). There is reason to speculate that repeated allergen exposure, even if subclinical, might be an important cause of persistent airway responsiveness.

Within the past 4 years, five separate groups in three countries have studied random populations varying in size from 105 to almost 2500 (14,89-93). Airway responsiveness to inhaled histamine was measured by one of two frequently used methods (94,95), and atopy was defined in a similar fashion based on both number and size of positive prick skin tests to a standardized battery of 3 to 14 common allergens. Although the definitions of atopy and airway hyperresponsiveness varied slightly between studies, all five studies came to the same conclusion; in a total of over 5600 random subjects, there was a strong correlation between the degree of atopy and the prevalence of airway hyperresponsiveness. The four largest studies are summarized in Figure 4. The prevalence of airway hyperresponsiveness varied from about 5% to 10% in the nonatopic populations to between 30% and 50% in the most highly atopic populations. The relationship is greater in young populations but persists in older groups (89,92). Interestingly, this relationship appears to persist even when the symptomatic asthmatics are removed from the analysis (96). These studies provide evidence of both a quanitative and a qualitative relationship between atopy and airway hyperresponsiveness (and thus between atopy and asthma), however, such cross-sectional studies cannot prove causation. The most satisfactory explanation for these findings would be that either atopy, or recurrent/chronic atopic allergic airways inflammation, leads to persistent airway responsiveness (14,93). There is also evidence in animals that airway hyperresponsiveness can result from sensitization (97) or be passively transferred (98). An alternate possibility is that some additional factor, either genetic or otherwise, may predispose to both atopy and airway hyperresponsiveness. In this regard, a genetic linkage between two inherited traits has been suggested (90). This is based largely on the assumption that clinically significant airway hyperresponsiveness is a predominantly genetically determined characteristic. The evidence to support this is weak. The identification of atopy, an important genetically determined trait, as a possible major determinant of airway hyperresponsiveness stresses that future studies must be carefully designed so that possible genetic influences in airway hyperresponsiveness can be separated from atopy. Much of the reported inheritance pattern for airway hyperresponsiveness might in fact be due to atopy. The final possible explanation for the relationship, included here only for the sake of completion, is the unlikely possibility that airway hyperresponsiveness might predispose to the development of atopy.

There are no prospective data available in humans. The documented large increase in the prevalence of atopy and asthma in the natives of Papua, New Guinea upon importation of blankets, presumably caused by new exposure to house dust mites, supports this hypothesis (16).

There is a great deal of evidence to support the hypothesis that recurrent allergen-induced airways inflammation might lead to persistent airway hyperresponsiveness and thus be a *cause* of asthma. Nevertheless, these studies do not

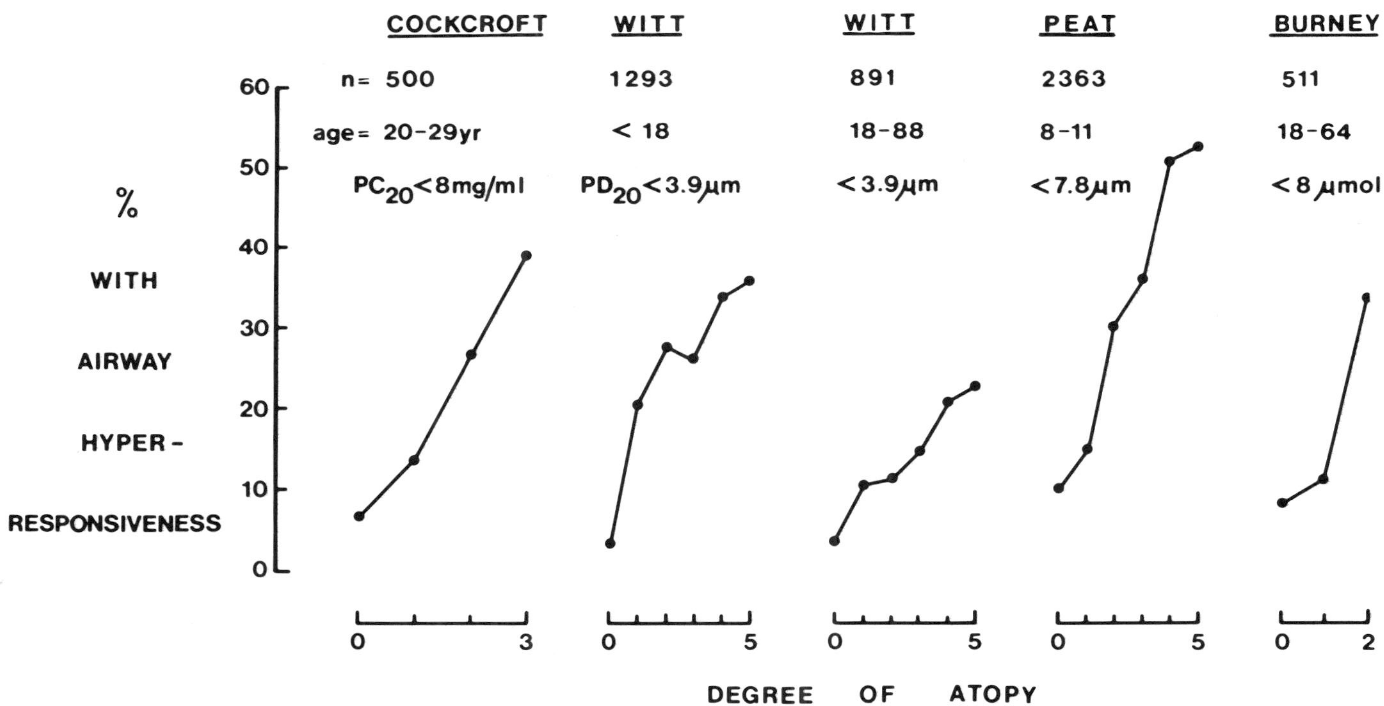

FIGURE 4 Relationship between degree of atopy and prevalence of airway hyperresponsiveness from 4 studies (14,89,91,92, 93). The degree of atopy from nonatopic (0) to increasing degree of atopy (higher numbers) using similar criteria from a prick skin test battery is on the horizontal axis and the prevalence (%) of airway hyperresponsiveness (defined on legend using PC_{20} (94) in panel 1 and PD_{20} (95) in panels 2–5) on the horizontal axis. From Ref. 93.

prove the case conclusively. The hypothesis, however, should be testable (with difficulty) by using long-term longitudinal prospective studies.

CLINICAL RELEVANCE

Appreciation that airway hyperresponsiveness and asthma can be caused transiently and possibly permanently by allergen-induced airways inflammation has greatly improved our understanding of the pathogenesis of allergic asthma. Such increased knowledge is clinically important with regards to both the diagnosis and management of asthma.

Diagnostically, this relates to assessment of atopic triggering factors in asthma. It is important to understand that one or more allergens may be responsible for causing asthma (or an asthma exacerbation) without causing any immediate chest symptoms that can be clearly related to exposure. This is often the case with low to moderate degree of atopic sensitivity to an animal in the home, in occupational allergy, and in seasonal allergy. History remains the major instrument for the identification of possibly relevant allergens. The history should be directed toward identifying allergens or potential allergens in the asthmatic's environment not only in the home, but also at school, work, and during recreational activities. Although historical evidence of sensitization (acute symptoms upon exposure) may be lacking in the chest, there may be other clues to sensitization. Acute conjunctivitis or rhinitis may be present following allergen exposure in the absence of noticeable acute chest symptoms in an asthmatic. This may be a particular problem if the allergen is transferred by hand to the eye following allergen handling (e.g., an animal). The development of urticaria following licking or scratching (cats, lobsters) may also be a clue to sensitivity. It is, however, not possible to exclude completely atopic sensitization in asthmatics no matter how nonallergic the history sounds. Perhaps the most useful historical clue in this regard is the age of onset of asthma; atopic allergic asthma generally has its onset within the first 2 or 2.5 decades of life whereas adult onset asthma is much more likely to be nonatopic (99). Nevertheless, it is wise to assess the atopic status of all asthmatics using a battery of relevant indigenous antigens (dust, mite, feathers, animals, fungal spores, and pollen) accompanied by any special allergens that might be indicated based on the patient's environment (unusual mammals, birds, or plant products).

Although management of asthma will be covered elsewhere, brief mention of the obvious therapeutic corollaries will be made here. Treatment strategies which will either prevent or reverse allergen-induced increases in airway responsiveness (i.e., airways inflammation) should be preferred over those strategies which do not. The only therapeutic strategies which have been clearly identified to play such a role are environmental control, sodium cromoglycate, and both inhaled and oral corticosteroids. Bronchodilators alone or in combination appear unlikely to prevent or reverse these allergen-induced inflammatory sequelae. In addition to the obvious short-term benefit, these same anti-inflammatory therapeutic strategies might on theoretical grounds have a long-term prophylactic benefit. If recurrent allergic airways inflammation does indeed lead to permanent airway hyperresponsiveness, then early environmental control and/or early use of anti-inflammatory medications might either prevent the development of persistent asthma or at least favorably modulate its severity. Like the underlying hypothesis, this hypothesis also should be possible to test (again with difficulty) with large and long-term longitudinal prospective studies.

ACKNOWLEDGMENTS

The author would like to thank Brenda Gore and Jacquie Bramley for their assistance in preparing this manuscript.

REFERENCES

1. Weiss ST, Speizer FE. The epidemiology of asthma: risk factors and natural history. In: *Bronchial Asthma: Mechanisms and Therapeutics*. Weiss EB, Segal MS, Stein M, eds. Boston, Little Brown and Co., 1985, pp 14–23.
2. Dolovich J, Hargreave FE. The asthma syndrome: inciters, inducers, and host characteristics. Thorax 1981; 36:641–644.
3. Cockcroft DW. Airway hyperresponsiveness: Therapeutic implications. Ann Allergy 1987; 59:405–414.
4. Pepys J. Atopy. In: *Clinical Aspects of Immunology*. Gell PGH, Coombs RRA, Lachman PJ, eds. Oxford, Blackwell Scientific Publications, 1975, pp 877–902.
5. Leskowitz S, Salvaggio JE, Schwartz HJ. An hypothesis for the development of atopic allergy in man. Clin Allergy 1972; 2:237–246.
6. King TP. Immunochemical properties of antigens that cause atopic diseases in man. In: *Bronchial Asthma: Mechanisms and Therapeutics*. Weiss EB, Segal MS, Stein M, eds. Boston, Little Brown and Co., 1985, pp 52–56.
7. Solomon WR. Aerobiology and inhalant allergens. I Pollens & Fungi. In: *Allergy, Principles and Practice*. Middleton Jr E, Reed CE, Ellis EF, eds. St. Louis, CV Mosby, 1978, pp 899–945.
8. Mathews KP. Aerobiology and inhalant allergens. II Other Inhaled Allergens. In: *Allergy, Principles and Practice*. Middleton Jr E, Reed CE, Ellis EF, eds. St. Louis, CV Mosby, 1978, pp 945–956.
9. Austen KF. Diseases of immediate type hypersensitivity. In: *Harrison's Principles of Internal Medicine*. Isselbacher KJ, Adams RD, Braunwald E, Petersdorf RG, Wilson JD, eds. New York, McGraw Hill, 1980, pp 342–347.
10. Settipane GA, Newstead GJ, Boyd GK. Frequency of hymenoptera allergy in atopic and normal populations. J Allergy 1972; 50:146–150.

11. Cohen C. Genetic aspects of allergy. Med Clin N Am 1974;58:25–42.
12. Woolcock AJ, Colman MH, Jones MW. Atopy and bronchial reactivity in Australian and Melanesian populations. Clin Allergy 1978;8:155–164.
13. Brown WG, Halonen MJ, Kaltenborn WT, Barbee RA. The relationship of respiratory allergy, skin test reactivity, and serum IgE in a community population sample. J Allergy Clin Immunol 1979; 63:328–335.
14. Cockcroft DW, Murdock KY, Berscheid BA. Relationship between atopy and bronchial responsiveness to histamine in a random population. Ann Allergy 1984;53:26–29.
15. Emanuel MB. Hay fever, a post industrial revolution epidemic. Clin Allergy 1988;18:295–304.
16. Dowse GK, Turner KJ, Stewart GA, Alpers MP, Woolcock AJ. The association between *Dermatophagoides* mites and the increasing prevalence of asthma in village communities within the Papua New Guinea highlands. J Allergy Clin Immunol 1985;75:75–83.
17. Cockcroft DW, Berscheid BA, Murdock KY, Gore BP. Sensitivity and specificity of histamine PC20 measurements in a random population. J Allergy Clin Immunol 1985; 75:142.
18. Pepys J, Hutchcroft BJ. Bronchial provocation tests in etiologic diagnosis and analysis of asthma. Am Rev Respir Dis 1975; 112:829–859.
19. Cockcroft DW, Murdock KY, Kirby J, Hargreave F. Prediction of airway responsiveness to allergen from skin sensitivity to allergen and airway responsiveness to histamine. Am Rev Respir Dis 1987; 135:264–267.
20. Schellenberg RR, Duff MJ, Foster A. Human bronchial responses to anti-IgE *in vitro*. Clin Invest Med 1985;8:A41.
21. Booij-Noord H, deVries K, Sluiter HJ, Orie NGM. Late bronchial obstructive reaction to experimental inhalation of house dust extract. Clin Allergy 1972;2:43–61.
22. Orie NGM, Van Lookeren Campagne JG, Knol K, Booij-Noord H, deVries K. Late reactions in bronchial asthma. In: *Intal in Bronchial Asthma*. Pepys J, Yamamura I, eds. Proceedings of the 8th International Congress of Allergology, Tokyo 1974, pp 17–29.
23. Hegardt B, Pauwels R, Van Der Straeten M. Inhibitory effect of KWD 2131, terbutaline, and DSCG on the immediate and late allergen-induced bronchoconstriction. Allergy 1981;36:115–122.
24. Ruffin RE, Cockcroft DW, Hargreave FE. A comparison of the protective effect of Sch1000 and fenoterol on allergen-induced asthma. J Allergy Clin Immunol 1978;61:42–47.
25. Cockcroft DW, Murdock KY. Comparative effects of inhaled salbutamol, sodium cromoglycate and beclomethasone dipropionate on allergen-induced early asthmatic responses, late asthmatic responses and increased bronchial responsiveness to histamine. J Allergy Clin Immunol 1987; 79:734–740.
26. Church MK, Young KD. The characteristics of inhibition of histamine release from human lung fragments by sodium cromoglycate, salbutamol, and chlorpromazine. Br J Pharmacol 1983;78:671–679.

27. Howarth PH, Durham SR, Lee TH, Kay B, Church MK, Holgate ST. Influence of albuterol, cromolyn sodium, and ipratropium bromide on the airway and circulating mediator responses to allergen bronchial provocation in asthma. Am Rev Respir Dis 1985; 132:986-992.
28. Nissim JE, Bleecker ER, Norman PS, Menkes H, Permutt S, Rosenthal RR. Failure of aminophylline pretreatment to prevent antigen-induced bronchospasm. J Allergy Clin Immunol 1980; 65:180.
29. Pauwels R, Van Der Straeten M. Drugs that modify mast-cell function: their mode of action. In: *The Mast-Cell, Its Role in Health and Disease*. Pepys J, Edward AM, eds. London, Pitman Medical, 1979.
30. Cockcroft DW, Murdock KY, Gore BP, O'Byrne PM, Manning P. Theophylline does not inhibit allergen-induced increase in airway responsiveness to methacholine. J Allergy Clin Immunol 1989; 83:913-920.
31. Crescioli S, Spinazzi D, Paleari M, Pozzan M, Mapp CE, Fabbri LM. Theophylline inhibits early and late asthmatic reactions induced by allergens in atopic subjects with asthma. Am Rev Respir Dis 1985; 137 Suppl: 35 (Abstract).
32. Yu DYC, Galant SP, Gold WM. Inhibition of antigen-induced bronchoconstriction by atropine in asthmatic patients. J Appl Physiol 1972; 32: 823-828.
33. Orehek J, Gayrard P, Grimaud Ch, Charpin J. Bronchoconstriction provoquee par inhalation d'allergene dans l'asthme: effet antagoniste d'un anticholinergique de synthese. Bull Eur Physiopathol Respir 1975; 11: 193-201.
34. Fish JE, Rosenthal RR, Summer WR, Menkes H, Norman PS, Permutt S. The effect of atropine on acute antigen-mediated airway constriction in subjects with allergic asthma. Am Rev Respir Dis 1977; 115:371-379.
35. Cockcroft DW, Ruffin RE, Hargreave FE. Effect of Sch 1000 in allergen-induced asthma. Clin Allergy 1978; 8:361-372.
36. Pepys J, Chan M, Hargreave FE, McCarthy DS. Inhibitory effects of disodium cromoglycate on allergen-inhalation tests. Lancet 1968; ii:134-137.
37. Booij-Noord H, Orie NGM, deVries K. Immediate and late bronchial obstructive reactions to inhalation of house dust and protective effects of disodium cromoglycate and prednisolone. J Allergy Clin Immunol 1971; 48:344-354.
38. Pepys J, Davies RJ, Breslin ABX, Hendricks DJ, Hutchcroft BJ. The effects of inhaled beclomethasone dipropionate (Becotide) and sodium cromoglycate on asthmatic reactions to provocation tests. Clin Allergy 1974; 4: 13-24.
39. Van Der Star JG, Berg WC, Steenhuis EJ, deVries K. Invloed van beclometason-dipropionaat per aerosol op de obstructieve reactie in de bronchien na huisstofinhalatie. Ned T Geneesk 1976; 120:1928-1932.
40. Burge PS, Efthimiou J, Turner-Warwick M, Nelmes PTJ. Double-blind trials of inhaled beclomethasone diproprionate and fluocortin butyl ester in allergen-induced immediate and late reactions. Clin Allergy 1982; 12:523-531.

41. Dutoit JI, Salome CM, Woolcock AJ. Inhaled corticosteroids reduce the severity of bronchial hyperresponsiveness in asthma but oral theophylline does not. Am Rev Respir Dis 1987; 136:1174-1178.
42. Phillips MJ, Ollier S, Gould CAL, Davies RJ. Effect of antihistamines and antiallergic drugs on responses to allergen and histamine provocation tests in asthma. Thorax 1984; 39:345-351.
43. Holgate ST, Emanuel MB, Howarth PH. Astemizole and other H_1-antihistaminic drug treatment of asthma. J Allergy Clin Immunol 1985; 76: 375-380.
44. Esau S, Del Carpio J, Martin JG. A comparison of the effects of ketotifen and clemastine on cutaneous and airway reactivity to histamine and allergen in atopic asthmatic subjects. J Allergy Clin Immunol 1984; 74:270-274.
45. Adachi M, Kobayashi H, Aoki N, Iijima M, Kokubu F, Furuya A, Takahashi T. A comparison of the inhibitory effects of ketotifen and disodium cromoglycate on bronchial responses to house dust, with special reference to the late asthmatic response. Pharmatherapeutica 4 1984; 36-42.
46. Fish JE, Ankin MG, Adkinson NF Jr, Peterman VI. Indomethacin modification of immediate-type immunologic airway responses in allergic asthmatic and nonasthmatic subjects. Am Rev Respir Dis 1981; 123:609-614.
47. Fairfax AJ. Inhibition of the late asthmatic response to house dust mite by non-steroidal anti-inflammatory drugs. Prostagland Leukotrienes Med 1982; 8:239-248.
48. Kirby JG, Hargreave FE, Cockcroft DW, O'Byrne PM. Indomethacin inhibits allergen-induced airway hyperresponsiveness but not allergen-induced asthmatic responses. J Appl Physiol 1989; 66:578-583.
49. Blackley CH. In: *Experimental Researches on the Cause and Nature of Catarrhus aestivus (Hay-Fever or Hay-Asthma)*. London, Balliere Tindall & Cox, 1873; reprinted by Dawson's of Pall Mall, London 1959, p 80.
50. Herxheimer H. The late bronchial reaction in induced asthma. Int Arch Allergy Appl Immunol 1952; 3:323-333.
51. Robertson DG, Kerigan AT, Hargreave FE, Chalmers R, Dolovich J. Late asthmatic responses induced by ragweed pollen allergen. J Allergy Clin Immunol 1974; 54:244-254.
52. Dorsch W, Baur X, Emslander HP, Fruhman G. Zu pathogenese und therapie der allergeninduzierten veizogerten bronchialobstruktion. Prax Klin Pneumol 1980; 34:461-468.
53. Cockcroft DW. Pharmacologic modulation of late phase responses: Beta-adrenergic agonists. In: *Late Phase Allergic Reactions*. Dorsch W, ed. Boca Raton, CRC Press, 1988. (In press)
54. McCarthy DS, Pepys J. Allergic bronchopulmonary aspergillosis. Clinical Immunology: (2) Skin nasal and bronchial tests. Clin Allergy 1971; 1:415-432.
55. Altounyan REC. Variation of drug action on airway obstruction in man. Thorax 1964; 19:406-415.

56. Cockcroft DW, Ruffin RE, Dolovich J, Hargreave FE. Allergen-induced increase in nonallergic bronchial reactivity. Clin Allergy 1977; 7:503-513.
57. Cockcroft DW, Murdock KY. Changes in bronchial responsiveness to histamine at intervals after allergen challenge. Thorax 1987; 42:302-308.
58. Hargreave FE, Dolovich J, O'Byrne PM, Ramsdale EH, Daniel EE. The origin of airway hyperresponsiveness. J Allergy Clin Immunol 1986; 78: 825-832.
59. Cockcroft DW. Allergen-induced airway hyperresponsiveness: Link with the late asthmatic response. In: *New Developments in Mechanisms and Treatment of Bronchial Obstruction*. Dijkman JH, van Herwaarden CLA, Hilvering CHR, Kerrebijn KF (eds), The Netherlands, Astra Pharmaceuticals, 1988, pp 65-76.
60. Cartier A, Thomson NC, Frith PA, Roberts R, Hargreave FE. Allergen-induced increase in bronchial responsiveness to histamine: relationship to the late asthmatic response and change in airway caliber. J Allergy Clin Immunol 1982; 70:170-177.
61. Newman Taylor AJ, Davies RJ, Hendrick DJ, Pepys J. Recurrent nocturnal asthmatic reactions to bronchial provocation tests. Clin Allergy 1979; 9:213-219.
62. Cockcroft DW, Hoeppner VH, Werner GD. Recurrent nocturnal asthma after bronchoprovocation with Western Red Cedar sawdust: association with acute increase in nonallergic bronchial responsiveness. Clin Allergy 1984; 14:61-68.
63. Durham SR, Lee TH, Cromwell O, Shaw RJ, Merrett T, Merrett J, Cooper P, Kay AB. Immunologic studies in allergen-induced late-phase asthmatic reactions. J Allergy Clin Immunol 1984; 74:49-60.
64. Kirby JC, Hargreave FE, Gleich GJ, O'Byrne PM. Bronchoalveolar cell profiles of asthmatic and non-asthmatic subjects. Am Rev Respir Dis 1987; 136:379-383.
65. Wardlaw AT, Dunnette S, Gleich GJ, Collins JV, Kay AB. Eosinophils and mast cells in subjects with mild asthma: Relationship to bronchial hyperreactivity. Am Rev Respir Dis 1988; 137:62-69.
66. de Monchy JGR, Kauffman HF, Venge P, Koeter GH, Jansen HM, Sleuter HJ, de Vries K. Bronchoalveolar eosinophilia during allergen-induced late asthmatic reactions. Am Rev Respir Dis 1985; 131:373-376.
67. Metzger WJ, Richerson WB, Worden K, Monick M, Hunninghake GW. Bronchoalveolar lavage of allergic asthmatic patients following allergen bronchoprovocation. Chest 1986; 89:477-83.
68. Murphy KR, Irvin CG, Glezen LS, Marsh WR, Larsen GL. The effect of polymorphonuclear leukocyte depletion in the late asthmatic response and changes in airways reactivity. Am Rev Respir Dis 1985; 131:A6.
69. Chung KF, Becker AB, Lazarus SC, Frick OL, Nadel JA, Gold WM. Antigen-induced hyperresponsiveness and pulmonary inflammation in allergic dogs. J Appl Physiol 1985; 58:1347-1353.
70. Kay AB, Lee TH. Neutrophil chemotactic factor of anaphylaxis. J Allergy Clin Immunol 1982; 70:317-320.

71. Metzger WJ, Richerson HB, Wasserman SI. Generation and partial characterization of eosinophil chemotactic activity and neutrophil chemotactic activity during early and late phase asthmatic response. J Allergy Clin Immunol 1986; 78:282-290.
72. Ford-Hutchinson AW, Bray MA, Doig MV, Shipley ME, Smith MJH. Leukotriene B_4, a potent chemokinetic and aggregating substance released from polymorphonuclear leukocytes. Nature (London) 1980; 286:264-265.
73. Basran GS, Page CP, Paul W, Morley J. Platelet-activating factor: a possible mediator of the dual response to allergen? Clin Allergy 1984; 14:75-79.
74. Aizawa H, Chung KF, Leikauf GD, Ueki I, Bethel RA, O'Byrne AM, Hirose T, Nadel JA. Significance of thromboxane generation in ozone-induced airway hyperresponsiveness in dogs. J Appl Physiol 1985; 59:1918-1923.
75. Chung KF, Aizawa H, Becker AB, Frick O, Gold WM, Nadel JA. Inhibition of antigen-induced airway hyperresponsiveness by a thromboxane synthetase inhibitor (OKY-046) in allergic dogs. Am Rev Respir Dis 1986; 134:258-261.
76. Chung KF, Aizawa H, Leikauf GD, Ueki IF, Evans TN, Nadel JA. Airway hyperresponsiveness induced by platelet activating factor: Role of thromboxane generation. J Pharmacol Exp Ther 1987; 236:580-584.
77. Reed CE, Ouellette JJ: Cited in: Lichtenstein LM. An evaluation of the role of immunotherapy in asthma. Am Rev Respir Dis 1978; 117:191-197.
78. Altounyan REC. Changes in histamine and atropine responsiveness as a guide to diagnosis and evaluation of therapy in obstructive airways disease. In: *Disodium Cromoglycate in Allergic Airways Disease*. Pepys J, Franklands AW, eds. London, Butterworths, 1970, pp 47-53.
79. Boulet LP, Cartier A, Thomson NC, Roberts RS, Dolovich J, Hargreave FE. Asthma and increases in nonallergic bronchial responsiveness from seasonal pollen exposure. J Allergy Clin Immunol 1983; 71:399-406.
80. Sotomayor H, Badier M, Vervloet D, Orehek J. Seasonal increase of carbachol airway responsiveness in patients allergic to grass pollen. Am Rev Respir Dis 1984; 130:56-58.
81. Lowhagen O, Rak S. Modification of bronchial hyperreactivity after treatment with sodium cromoglycate during pollen season. J Allergy Clin Immunol 1985; 75:460-467.
82. Zuidema PS. Cited in: Kerrebijn KF: Endogenous factors in childhood CNSLD. In: *Bronchitis III*. Orie NGM, van der Lende R, eds. Assen, Royal van Gorcum, 1970, pp 38-48.
83. Platts-Mills TAE, Mitchell EB, Nock P, Tovey ER, Moszoro H, Wilkins SR. Reduction of bronchial hyperreactivity during prolonged allergen avoidance. Lancet 1982; 2:675-678.
84. Murray AB, Ferguson AC. Dust-free bedrooms in the treatment of asthmatic children with house dust or house dust mite allergy: a controlled trial. Pediatrics 1983; 71:418-422.
85. Cockcroft DW. Mechanism of perennial allergic asthma. Lancet 1983; 2:253-256.
86. Cockcroft DW. Acquired persistent increase in nonspecific bronchial reac-

tivity associated with isocyanate exposure. Ann Allergy 1982; 48:93-95.
87. Chan-Yeung M, Lam S, Koener S. Clinical features and natural history of occupational asthma due to Western Red Cedar (Thuja plicata). Am J Med 1982;72:411-415.
88. Mapp CE, Corona PC, de Marzo N, Fabbri L. Persistent asthma due to isocyanates. Am Rev Respir Dis 1988; 137:1326-1329.
89. Witt C, Stuckey MS, Woolcock AJ, Dawkins RC. Positive allergy prick skin tests associated with bronchial histamine responsiveness in an unselected population. J Allergy Clin Immunol 1986;77:698-702.
90. Cookson WOCM, Musk AW, Ryan G. Associations between asthma history, atopy, and non-specific bronchial responsiveness in young adults. Clin Allergy 1984; 16:425-432.
91. Peat JK, Britton WJ, Salome CM, Woolcock AJ. Bronchial hyperresponsiveness in two populations of Australian school children: III Effect of exposure to environmental allergens. Clin Allergy 1987; 17:291-300.
92. Burney PFJ, Britton JR, Chinn S, Tattersfield AE, Papacosta AO, Kelson MC, Anderson F, Corfield DR. Descriptive epidemiology of bronchial reactivity in an adult population: results from a community study. Thorax 1987;42:38-44.
93. Cockcroft DW, Hargreave FE. Relationship between atopy and airway responsiveness. In: *Bronchitis IV*. van der Lende R, Sluiter HJ, eds. Assen, van Gorcum, 1988, pp 23-32.
94. Cockcroft DW, Killian DN, Mellon JJA, Hargreave FE. Bronchial reactivity to inhaled histamine: a method and clinical survey. Clin Allergy 1977; 7:235-243.
95. Yan K, Salome C, Woolcock AJ. Rapid method for measurement of bronchial responsiveness. Thorax 1983;38:760-765.
96. Woolcock AJ. Bronchial hyperresponsiveness: Reply. Clin Allergy 1988; 18:312 (correspondence).
97. Vane JR. Mediators of the anaphylactic reaction. In: *Identification of Asthma*. Ciba Foundation Symposium Study Group No. 38, Porter R, Birch J, eds. London, Churchill Livingston, 1971.
98. Fink JN, Schlueter DP. Passive transfer of methacholine sensitivity. J Allergy 1969;43:167-168.
99. Scadding JG. Definitions and clinical categories of asthma. In: *Asthma*. Clark TJH, Godfrey S, eds. London, Chapman and Hall, 1983; pp 1-11.

6

Occupational Asthma

LEONARDO M. FABBRI, CRISTINA E. MAPP,
MARINA SAETTA, and LUIGI ALLEGRA

Interuniversity Center on Cellular and Molecular Mechanisms of Lung Injury
Universities of Brescia, Ferrara, Milan, Padova, and Parma, Italy

INTRODUCTION

Occupational asthma is a disease characterized by variable airflow limitation and airway hyperresponsiveness caused by agents present in the work place (1). If one accepts this definition, the long-lasting variable airflow limitation and airway hyperresponsiveness caused by acute exposure to irritant gases (2,3) may also be classified as occupational asthma, whereas occupational lung diseases such as byssinosis (4,5) or hypersensitivity pneumonitis (6), which may indeed manifest with variable airflow limitation, should not be considered occupational asthma because they are not usually associated with airway hyperresponsiveness.

The widespread use of new chemical agents leads to greater frequency of asthma in exposed subjects, and occupational asthma may well exceed pneumoconiosis as the most important cause of occupational lung diseases (1,7).

DIAGNOSIS OF OCCUPATIONAL ASTHMA

The diagnosis of occupational asthma is based on (a) the history, (b) the demonstration of variable airflow limitation (by recording the peak expiratory flow rate over a period of time while the subject is at work and while the subject is on leave) and (3) the results of inhalation challenges with nonspecific agents (e.g., histamine or methacholine) and/or with specific sensitizing agents present in the workplace. Sensitized subjects may develop asthmatic symptoms within minutes or over several hours after exposure to the sensitizing agent in their place of work. Thus, one should suspect occupational asthma even when asthma symptoms develop hours after cessation of exposure to the causative agent. Most subjects with a history of occupational asthma have airway hyperresponsiveness to histamine or methacholine, but some develop airway hyperresponsiveness only during or shortly after exposure to the sensitizing agent (8,9). Thus, in a subject with history of work-related asthma, the diagnosis of occupational asthma should not be disregarded if airway responsiveness is within normal limits. Serial measurements of airway responsiveness and periodic recording of peak expiratory flow rates showing variability of peak expiratory flow on return to work and normalization when away from work may indeed confirm objectively a diagnosis of occupational asthma (8,10-12).

Inhalation challenges with recognized sensitizing agents should be performed *only* in specialized hospitals by experienced personnel, and resuscitation facilities should be available in the place where challenges are carried out. There is anedoctal evidence of at least one death after an inhalation challenge with isocyanates, and almost every investigator with experience in the field could report severe asthmatic reactions even after exposure to very low concentrations of the sensitizing agent. After challenge with sensitizing agents in the laboratory, sensitized subjects develop immediate and/or late asthmatic reactions, and the determinants and mechanisms of the different pattern of reactions are poorly understood (10,11,13).

MECHANISMS OF SENSITIZATION TO OCCUPATIONAL AGENTS

The pathogenesis of variable airflow limitation and airway hyperresponsiveness induced by agents present in the workplace is largely unknown. Some sensi-

FIGURE 1 Forced expiratory volume in 1 sec (FEV_1) before and after exposure to toluene diisocyanate (TDI) in two groups of subjects. The horizontal axes indicate time in hours, and the vertical axes indicate FEV_1 in liters. The graph reports the reaction to the screening TDI inhalation challenge (open circles) and to the TDI inhalation challenges performed on the day of bronchoalveolar lavage (closed circles), either after no treatment (left panel) or after treatment with prednisone (right panel). Subjects who received no treatment developed a late or dual asthmatic reaction of time-course and intensity similar to control challenge. By contrast, subjects who received prednisone did not develop dual or late asthmatic reaction (reproduced with permission from Ref. 38).

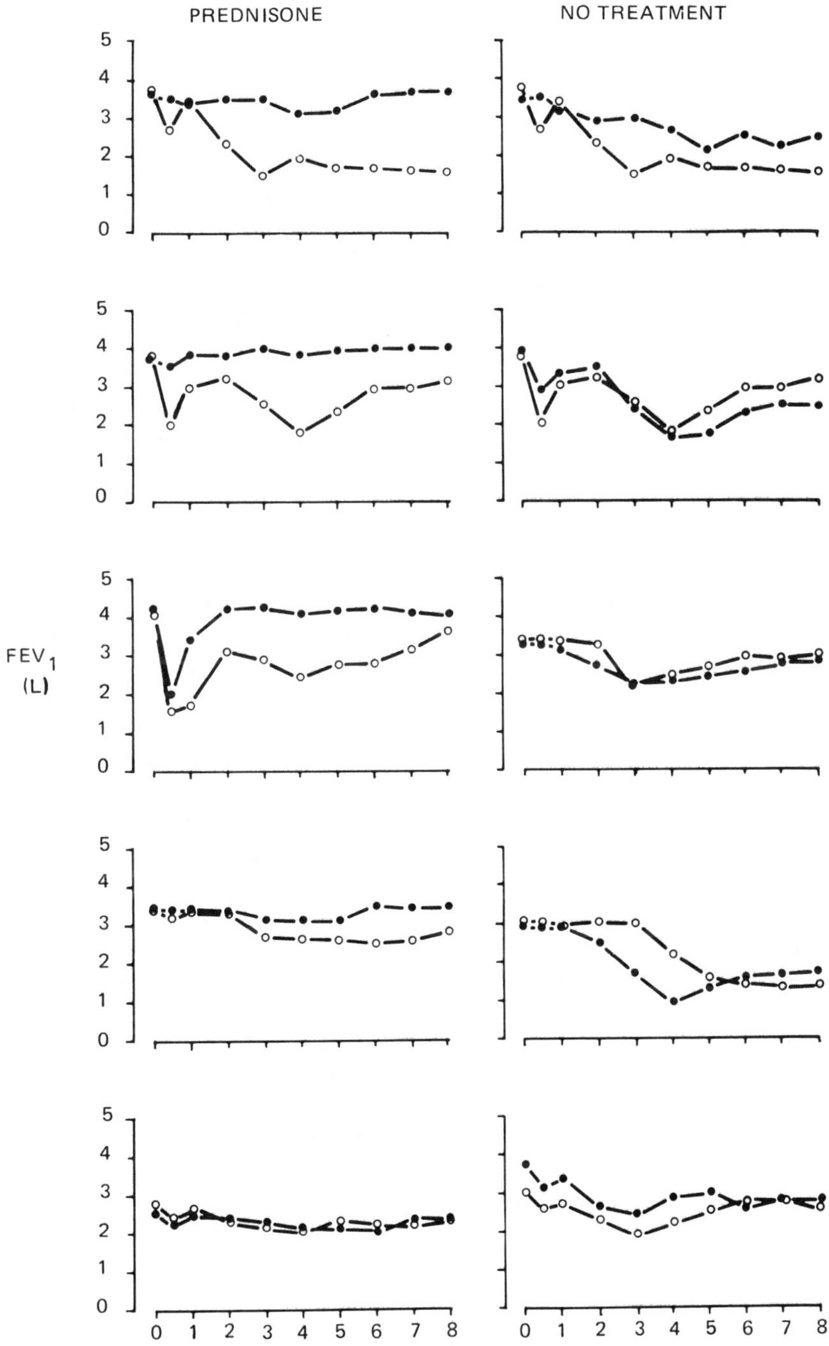

PREDNISONE
NO TREATMENT
FEV1
(L)
HOURS AFTER TDI

tizing agents, mainly high-molecular weight compounds (e.g., animal products, grain dust, flours, detergents, vegetables), but also low-molecular weight compounds (e.g., plicatic acid present in red cedar) can stimulate the production of specific antibodies in exposed subjects (10). Although specific antibodies may interact with sensitizing agents and trigger the release of mediators responsible for the development of airway hyperresponsiveness and of asthma attacks, several subjects have been demonstrated to have antibodies but not asthma, and do not develop asthma attacks even after exposure to the sensitizing agents. These observations suggest that the antibodies may represent a response to exposure but not necessarily the mechanism of development of airway hyperresponsiveness or asthma. Alternative theories regarding the beta-blocking effect (14), the stimulating effect of some inciters (15) on lung irritant receptors, or the effect on airway smooth muscle of some agents (16) have not been firmly established.

Unfortunately the characteristics that distinguish the subjects who become sensitized compared with subjects with similar exposure who remain healthy are unknown. Atopy may be a risk factor in some subjects, particularly those sensitized to high-molecular weight compounds (10); whereas smoking habits, genetic predisposition, gender, or even airway hyperresponsiveness do not represent significant risk factors (1,10,17). There is some evidence that the process of sensitization may be associated with acute exposure to the sensitizing agent (18,19), or with viral infections of the upper airways (20), causing a syndrome similar to the reactive airways diseases induced by acute exposure to irritant gases (2). In both cases the common effects are long lasting variable airflow limitation and airway hyperresponsiveness, but the sensitization process is associated with a specific hyperresponsiveness to a sensitizing agent. In fact, sensitized subjects develop bronchoconstriction after exposure to concentrations of the sensitizing agent that do not cause bronchoconstriction in unsensitized subjects. Although exposure to spills (e.g., isocyanates; 21) and viral infections of the upper airway (22) are likely to be associated with acute airway inflammation, the reversible airflow limitation and long lasting airway hyperresponsiveness of sensitized subjects may not be associated with inflamed airways when these subjects recover from an acute exposure (23,24). In addition to long lasting airway hyperresponsiveness acquired during the process of sensitization, sensitized subjects may develop transient increases of airway responsiveness during exacerbations of asthma and particularly after exposure to the sensitizing agent that results in a dual or late asthmatic reaction (11,13, 25,26) (Figs. 1,2).

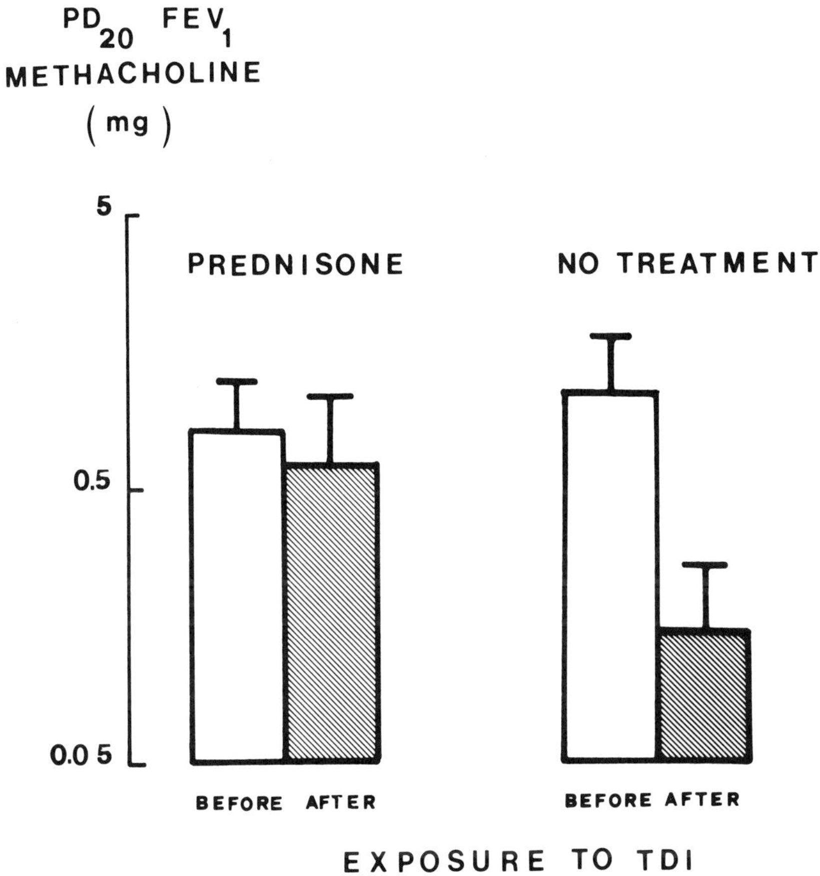

FIGURE 2 PD_{20} FEV_1 methacholine before (open column) and 8 h after (striped column) exposure to TDI in two groups of subjects. Subjects who received no treatment had an increased airway responsiveness to methacholine associated with the late or dual asthmatic reaction, whereas subjects who received prednisone did not develop a significant increase of airway responsiveness. Interestingly airway responsiveness before exposure to TDI was not modified by prednisone treatment, suggesting that baseline long-lasting bronchial responsiveness is steroid unsensitive, thus possibly not related to airway inflammation (reproduced with permission from Ref. 38).

ASTHMATIC REACTIONS, TRANSIENT INCREASE OF NONSPECIFIC AIRWAY RESPONSIVENESS, AND AIRWAY INFLAMMATION INDUCED BY OCCUPATIONAL SENSITIZERS

While the pathogenesis of the long lasting airway hyperresponsiveness associated with the process of sensitization remains almost completely unexplained, the pathogenesis of the transient increase of airway responsiveness associated with late asthmatic reactions is reasonably clear. Several pieces of evidence suggest that it is caused by an acute inflammatory reaction of the airways characterized by epithelial damage, polymorphonuclear leukocyte infiltration of the airway mucosa and release of inflammatory mediators (23-27).

Early Asthmatic Reactions

Early asthmatic reactions are in part due to smooth muscle contraction because they quickly reverse either spontaneously or after bronchodilator therapy (11). However, there is increasing evidence that early asthmatic reactions induced by allergens are associated with extravasation of proteins (28,29), suggesting increased microvascular leakage, and release of inflammatory mediators (30-32), and, at least in experimental animals, with dramatic changes of flow in bronchial arteries (33). Thus, it may well be that early asthmatic reactions are determined not only by airway smooth muscle contraction, but also by mucosal edema, as it appears by looking through the bronchoscope during local instillation of allergens (34). Indeed, the association of increased blood flow, increased protein leakage from the microvasculature, and release of inflammatory mediators closely resemble the features of the exudative phase of an acute inflammatory process. Unfortunately bronchoalveolar lavage during or immediately after an early asthmatic reaction induced by occupational sensitizing agents has not been performed, thus we do not know whether these agents cause the same effects of allergens. Bronchoalveolar lavage obtained at 8 hours after early asthmatic reactions induced by isocyanates or plicatic acid do not contain an increased albumin concentration (24), suggesting that extravasation of proteins does not occur; however these experiments need to be repeated immediately after an early reaction to exclude that it indeed occurs but is transient.

Late Asthmatic Reactions

Late asthmatic reactions induced by occupational sensitizing agents are not inhibited by bronchodilators (11,35), but only by anti-inflammatory steroids (11,36-39) and are associated with an increased number of leukocytes in bronchoalveolar lavage, mainly eosinophils after plicatic acid (the sensitizing agent contained in red cedar) (23), or mainly neutrophils after isocyanates

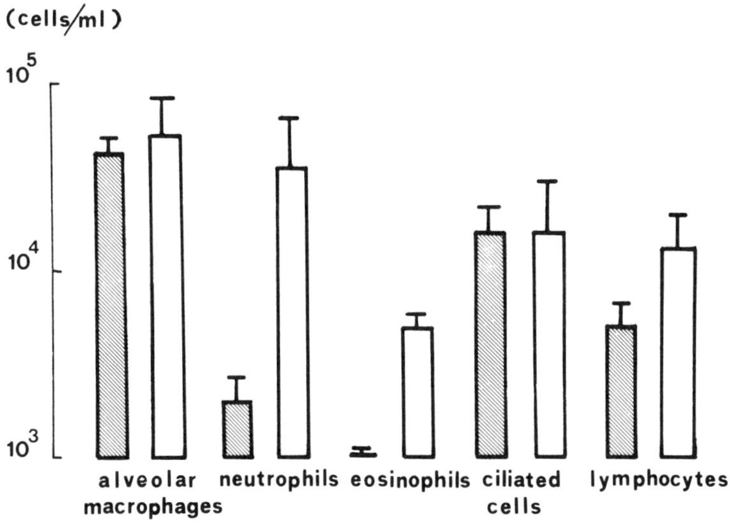

FIGURE 3 Cell counts in bronchoalveolar lavage fluid obtained 8 h after exposure to TDI in the two groups of subjects examined. Neutrophils and eosinophils were significantly increased in subjects who received no treatment (open column) and developed a late asthmatic reaction after exposure to TDI, compared with subjects who were treated with prednisone (striped column) and did not develop a late asthmatic reaction after exposure to TDI (reproduced with permission from Ref. 38).

(24,40) (Fig. 3) or cobalt (41). The bronchoalveolar leukocytosis is associated with increased concentration of albumin in the supernatant (Fig. 4) (23,24). Steroids inhibit late asthmatic reactions and the associated increase in bronchial responsiveness to methacholine (Figs. 1, 2) while preventing the migration of neutrophils and eosinophils and the extravasation of albumin in the air spaces (38) (Figs. 3, 4). These actions further support the hypothesis that, like allergen-induced late asthmatic reactions (25), late asthmatic reactions induced by occupational agents (e.g., TDI) may be caused by the combination of bronchoconstriction and airway inflammation.

Late asthmatic reactions induced by allergens are associated with an increased number of neutrophils and eosinophils in bronchoalveolar lavage (28,29,42), with an increased neutrophil chemotactic activity and eosinophilia in the circulation (32) and are inhibited by steroids (43). The increased number of neutrophils and eosinophils observed during late asthmatic reactions induced by occupational sensitizing agents, and the absence of such increase in subjects who did not develop late asthmatic reactions when treated with steroids suggest that

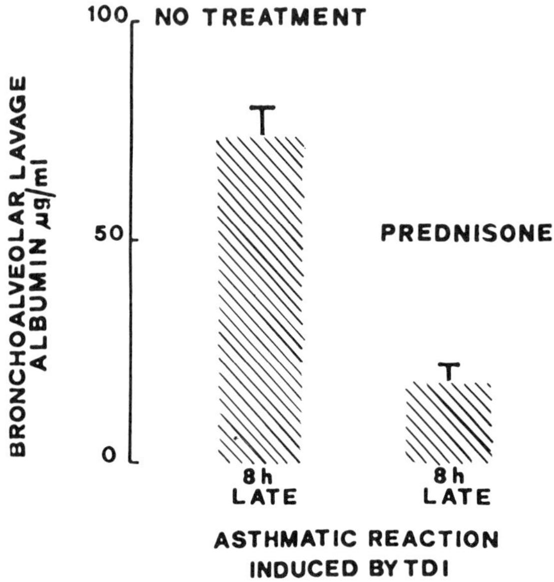

FIGURE 4 Albumin concentration in bronchoalveolar lavage fluid obtained 8 h after exposure to TDI in two groups of subjects. Albumin concentration was significantly increased in subjects who received no treatment and developed a late asthmatic reaction and increased bronchial responsiveness after exposure to TDI, compared with subjects who were treated with prednisone and who developed neither late asthmatic reaction nor increased bronchial responsiveness after exposure to TDI (modified from Ref. 38).

polymorphonuclear leukocyte infiltration may be required for the development of late asthmatic reactions and increased responsiveness induced by exposure to the sensitizing agent. Ongoing studies aim to identify the chemical structure and source of the chemotactic factors that attract neutrophils and/or eosinophils in the air spaces and the chemical structure of the mediators released from these cells that increase bronchial responsiveness. Although the concentration of LTB_4 in bronchoalveolar lavage fluid is increased during late asthmatic reactions induced by toluene diisocyanate, we still do not know whether its increase is the cause or the effect of neutrophil influx into the airspaces.

Subjects sensitized to TDI show both a steroid-sensitive and a nonsteroid-sensitive component of airway hyperresponsiveness. The former may be due to airway inflammation while the latter is due to unknown mechanisms (36-39). Both the late asthmatic reaction and the increase in bronchial responsiveness induced by TDI are inhibited by oral and inhaled steroids (36-39) (Figs. 1, 2) which, at the same time, prevent the inflammatory reaction that accompanies them (38) (Figs. 3, 4). However, steroids do not modify the airway hyperresponsiveness that precedes exposure to the sensitizing agent (Fig. 2), and which is not associated with airway inflammation (24). Interestingly, in some subjects with late asthmatic reactions, airway hyperresponsiveness to methacholine develops only after exposure to TDI at the time when the airways are inflamed (8): in these subjects, airway hyperresponsiveness appears to be caused entirely by airway inflammation.

Epithelial damage has been associated with airway inflammation and might cause bronchoconstriction and airway hyperresponsiveness by exposing or sensitizing vagal sensory receptors (44) triggering vagal or axon reflexes (45), or increasing mucosal permeability (46). However, the number of ciliated epithelial cells in bronchoalveolar lavage fluid is increased during a late asthmatic reaction induced by plicatic acid (24), but not after isocyanates (25), suggesting that epithelial damage may be involved in late asthmatic responses induced by red cedar, but not in late asthmatic reactions and in the associated airway hyperresponsiveness induced by isocyanates. Albumin concentration increases during late asthmatic reactions induced by plicatic acid and isocyanates. In the latter, such increase is prevented by steroids (38). These results suggest that the increased vascular permeability associated with the inflammatory reaction is inhibited by steroids, but the importance of the increased vascular permeability for the late asthmatic reaction remains to be determined (47). Inflammatory mediators released by neutrophils and/or eosinophils during the late asthmatic reaction induced by occupational sensitizing agents may cause bronchoconstriction, edema, and hypersecretion (48) either acting directly on smooth muscle, vasa, and glands, or indirectly via axon reflexes (44).

The mediators responsible for or involved in the late asthmatic reactions induced by occupational sensitizing agents are unknown. Late asthmatic reactions induced by TDI are inhibited by steroids but not by indomethacin, a specific inhibitor of cyclooxygenase (37). Since the main biochemical effect of steroids is the inhibition of phospholipase A and, consequently, the inhibition of release of arachidonic acid and other phospholipid metabolites from cell membranes (49,50), these results suggest that either lipoxygenase metabolites of arachidonic acid or other membrane phospholipid derivatives inhibited by steroids, but not cyclooxygenase metabolites of arachidonic acid, may be involved in the late asthmatic reactions induced by TDI in sensitized subjects. Interestingly, although indomethacin has no effect in late asthmatic reactions induced by allergens, indomethacin inhibits the airway hyperresponsiveness to histamine that follows the late asthmatic reactions (51), suggesting that the airway hyperresponsiveness induced by allergens, in contrast with the airway hyperresponsiveness induced by TDI, may be mediated by cyclooxygenase arachidonate metabolites.

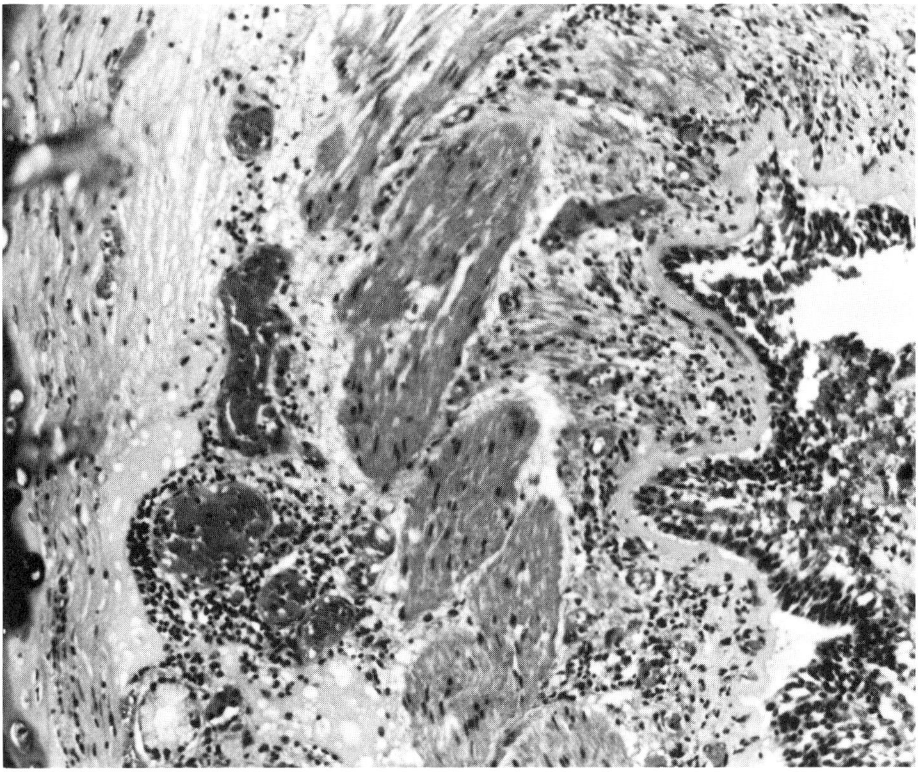

(a)

FIGURE 5 (a) Photomicrograph showing morphologic features of the airways: mucous plug partially occluding the lumen, desquamation of epithelium, thickening of the basement membrane, hypertrophy and disarray of smooth muscle, inflammatory infiltrate and edema of the bronchial wall. Magnification X25; stain: hematoxylin-eosin. (b) photomicrograph showing morphologic features of the lung parenchyma: alveolar wall destruction with fragments of septa floating in the alveolar spaces. Magnification: X125; stain: hematoxylin-eosin.

PATHOLOGY OF OCCUPATIONAL ASTHMA

The pathology of death from asthma caused by exposure to occupational agents include airway and lung inflammation. We have recently reported an asthma death caused by exposure to isocyanates at work in a subject previously demonstrated to be sensitized to toluene diisocyanate (52). Lung pathology included

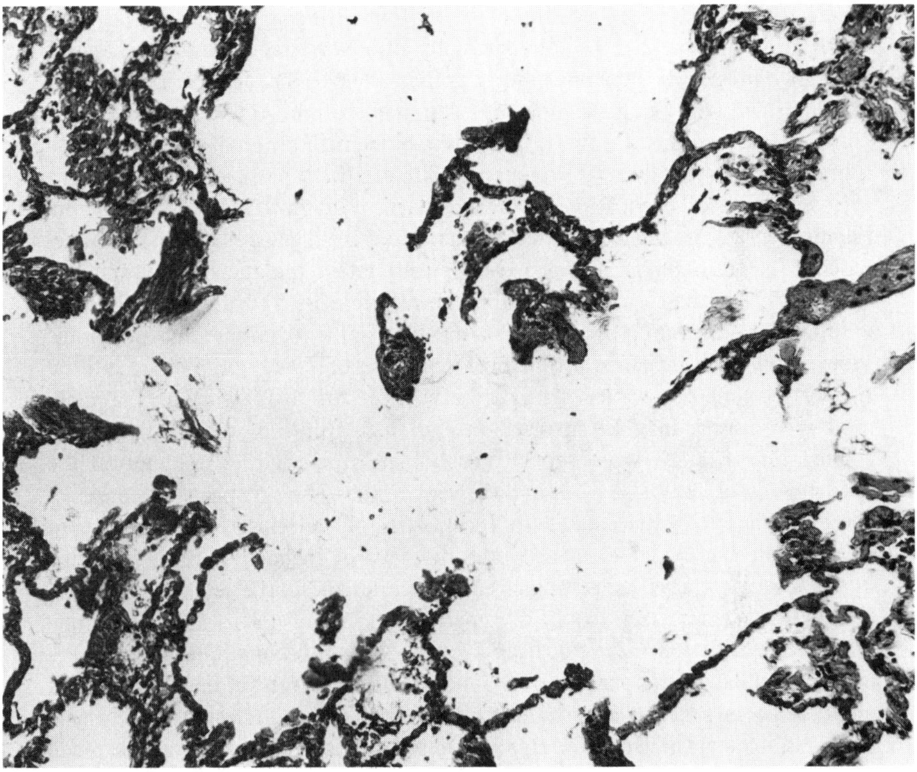

(b)

some previously discussed characteristic features of fatal asthma, but also some pathological findings which were different. Macroscopically, lungs were overinflated and did not collapse on opening of the pleural cavities. Airways were plugged with mucus containing abundant exudate. Microscopy showed morphological abnormalities of both airways (Fig. 5, panel a) and lung parenchyma (Fig. 5, panel b). In the airways, we observed extensive epithelial desquamation, edema of the bronchial wall, diffuse infiltration of inflammatory cells including eosinophils and neutrophils, and marked thickening of the basement membrane in addition to extensive plugging of the bronchioles. Mucous glands were hyperplastic and bronchial smooth muscle was hypertrophic and disarrayed with loss of the usual regular intersections of fibers that criss-cross unevenly and form whirls (Fig. 5, panel a). While hypertrophy of airway smooth muscle is almost invariably present in previous reports on nonoccupational asthma, the disarray of smooth muscle fibers has not been described before. Among the pathologic features observed in the airways, the eosinophilic infiltration of the mucosa and submucosa was particularly pronounced. Subjects with persistent stable asthma after cessation of occupational exposure have been shown to have chronic inflammation of the airway mucosa, characterized by slight infiltration of eosinophils (53). Eosinophilia is also present during late asthmatic reaction induced by plicatic acid and during late asthmatic reactions by TDI (24,25). Although eosinophilic infiltration is present in the lungs of both atopic and nonatopic subjects who die in status asthmaticus (54), the observed eosinophilic infiltration of the lung of a subject who died after exposure to TDI suggests that common mechanisms may be involved in the final events of different types of asthma. Surprisingly, we observed morphologic abnormalities not only at the bronchial level, but also within the alveolar walls (Fig. 5, panel b): areas of acute emphysema alternated with focal areas of atelectasis. The presence of acute emphysema is confirmed by the presence of fragments of septa floating in the alveolar spaces, suggesting alveolar wall destruction. These areas of focal destruction were adjacent to areas of perfectly intact alveolar walls. Interestingly, these focal lesions have not been described in nonoccupational asthma, and are very similar to the parenchymal abnormalities observed in the early stage of emphysema in a group of smokers in whom the classic indices of emphysema were still normal (55,56). Alveolar wall destructions may decrease elastic recoil and, because the elastic loads against which bronchial smooth muscle contracts is an important determinant of the degree of airway narrowing, alveolar wall destruction may decrease the elastic load against which airway smooth muscle contracts which, together with airway edema, may facilitate airway narrowing (57).

ACKNOWLEDGMENTS

Supported by Grants No. 87.00266.56 and 87.01476.04 from the National Research Council, by the Italian Ministry of Education, by the European Community for Coal and Steel, and by Regione Veneto.

REFERENCES

1. Fabbri LM, Salvaggio JE (Eds). Occupational asthma. Folia Allergol Immunol Clin 1985;32:1–65.
2. Brooks SM, Weiss MA, Bernstein IL. Reactive airways dysfunction syndrome (RADS). Persistent asthma syndrome after high level irritant exposures. Chest 1985;86:376–384.

3. Chan-Yeung M. Occupational asthma update. Chest 1988; 93:407–411.
4. Schilling RSF. Byssinosis in cotton and other textile workers. Lancet 1956; 2:261–265, 319–325.
5. Mundie TG, Ainsworth SK. Etiopathogenetic mechanisms of bronchoconstriction in byssinosis. Am Rev Respir Dis 1986; 133:1181–1185.
6. Cotes JE, Steel J. Extrinsic Allergic Alveolitis. In: *Work Related Lung Disorders*. Blackwell Scientific Publications, Oxford, 1987, p 320.
7. Venables KM. Epidemiology and the prevention of occupational asthma. Br J Industr Med 1987; 44:73–75.
8. Hargreave FE, Ramsdale EH, Pugsly SO. Occupational asthma without bronchial hyperresponsiveness. Am Rev Respir Dis 1984; 130:513–515.
9. Mapp CE, Dal Vecchio L, Boschetto P, De Marzo N, Fabbri LM. Toluene diisocianate-induced asthma without airway hyperresponsiveness. Eur J Respir Dis 1986; 68:89–95.
10. Chan-Yeung M, Lam S. Occupational asthma. Am Rev Respir Dis 1986; 133:686–703.
11. Pepys J, Hutchroft BJ. Bronchial provocation tests in etiologic diagnosis and analysis of asthma. Am Rev Respir Dis 1975; 112:829–859.
12. Burge PS, O'Brien IM, Harries MG. Peak flow rate records in the diagnosis of occupational asthma due to colophony. Thorax 1979; 34:308–316.
13. Mapp CE, Di Giacomo R, Broseghini C, et al. Late, but not early, asthmatic reactions induced by toluene diisocyanate (TDI) are associated with increased airway responsiveness. Eur J Respir Dis 1986; 68:276–284.
14. Butcher BT. Mechanism of isocyanate-induced asthma. Eur J Respir Dis 1982; 63 (suppl 123):82–86.
15. Dolovich J, Hargreave FE. The asthma syndrome: incitizers, inducers and host characteristics. Thorax 1981; 36:641–643.
16. Mckay RT, Brooks SM. Hyperreactive airway smooth muscle responsiveness after inhalation of toluene diisocyanate vapors. Am Rev Respir Dis 1984; 129:296–300.
17. Mapp CE, Boschetto P, Dal Vecchio L, Maestrelli P, Fabbri LM. Occupational asthma due to isocyanates. Eur J Respir Dis 1988; 1:273–279.
18. Diem JE, Jones RN, Hendrick DJ, et al. Five-year longitudinal study of workers employed in a new toluene diisocyanate manufacturing plant. Am Rev Respir Dis 1982; 126:493–498.
19. Brooks SM. The evaluation of occupational airways disease in the laboratory and workplace. J Allergy Clin Immunol 1982; 70:56–66.
20. Chester EH, Martinez-Catinchi FL, Schwartz HJ, et al. Patterns of airway reactivity to asthma produced by exposure to toluene diisocyanate. Chest 1979; 75 (suppl):229–231.
21. NIOSH Criteria for a Recommended standard. Occupational exposure to Diisocyanates. U.S. Department of Health, Education, and Welfare. Washington DC, Publication No. 78-215, 1978.
22. Walsh JJ, Dietlein LF, Low GB, Burch GB, Mogabgab WJ. Bronchotracheal response in human influenza. Arch Intern Med 1961; 108:376–380.
23. Lam S, LeRiche J, Phillips D, Chan-Yeung M. Cellular and protein changes

in bronchoalveolar lavage fluid after late asthmatic reactions in patients with red cedar asthma. J Allergy Clin Immunol 1987; 80:44-50.

24. Fabbri LM, Boschetto P, Zocca E, Milani GF, Pivirotto F, Burlina A, Plebani M, Licata B, Mapp CE. Bronchoalveolar neutrophilia during late asthmatic reactions induced by toluene diisocyanate (TDI). Am Rev Respir Dis 1987; 136:36-42.
25. O'Byrne PM, Dolovich J, Hargreave FE. Late asthmatic responses. Am Rev Respir Dis 1987; 136:740-751.
26. Mapp CE, Boschetto P, Zocca E, Milani GF, Pivirotto F, Tegazzin V, Fabbri LM. Pathogenesis of late asthmatic reactions induced by exposure to isocyanates. Bull Eur Physiopathol Respir 1987; 23:583-586.
27. Zocca E, Boschetto P, Mapp CE, Milani GF, Pivirotto F, Fabbri LM. LTB4-like substance in bronchoalveolar lavage supernatant released during asthmatic reactions induced by toluene-diisocyanate in sensitized subjects. Twenty third Annual Meeting of the S.E.P.C.R., Athens, June 20-24th, 1988.
28. Metzger WJ, Richerson HB, Worden K, Monick M, Hunninghake GW. Bronchoalveolar lavage of allergic asthmatic patients following allergen bronchoprovocation. Chest 1986; 89:477-483.
29. Fick RB, Metzger WJ, Richerson HB, et al. Increased bronchovascular permeability after allergen exposure in sensitive asthmatics. J Appl Physiol 1987; 63:1147-1155.
30. Atkins PC, Norman ME, Zweiman B. Antigen-induced neutrophil chemotactic activity in man. Correlation with bronchospasm and inhibition by disodium cromoglycate. J Allergy Clin Immunol 1978; 62:149-155.
31. Murray JJ, Tonnel AB, Brash AR, et al. Release of prostaglandin D2 into human airways during acute antigen challenge. N Engl J Med 1986; 315: 800-804.
32. Kay AB, Wadlaw AJ, Moqbel R, Diana R, Buchanan DR, Cromwell O, Fitzharris P. Leukocytes and the asthma process. In: *Allergy and Inflammation*. Kay AB (ed.). Academic Press, London, 1987, pp 203-223.
33. Baier H, Long WM, Wanner A. Bronchial circulation in asthma. Respiration 1985; 48:199-208.
34. Metzger WJ, Zavala D, Richerson HB, Moseley P, Iwamota P, Monick M, Sjordsma K, Hunninghake GW. Local allergen challenge and bronchoalveolar lavage of allergic asthmatic lung. Description of the model and local airway inflammation. Am Rev Respir Dis 1987; 135:433-440.
35. Paggiaro PL, Bacci E, Talini D, Dente FL, Rossi D, Pulera N, Fabbri LM, Giuntini C. Atropine does not inhibit late asthmatic responses induced by toluene diisocyanate in sensitized subjects. Am Rev Respir Dis 1987; 136:1237-1241.
36. Fabbri LM, Chiesura-Corona P, Dal Vecchio L, Di Giacomo GR, Zocca E, De Marzo N, Maestrelli P, Mapp CE. Prednisone inhibits the late asthmatic reaction and the associated increase in bronchial responsiveness induced by toluene-diisocyanate in sensitized subjects. Am Rev Respir Dis 1985; 132:1010-1014.

37. Fabbri LM, Di Giacomo R, Dal Vecchio L, Zocca E, De Marzo N, Maestrelli P, Mapp CE. Prednisone, indomethacin and airway responsiveness in toluene diisocyanate sensitized subjects. Bull Eur Physiopathol Resp 1985;21:421-426.
38. Boschetto P, Fabbri LM, Zocca E, Milani GF, Pivirotto F, Dal Vecchio A, Plebani, Mapp CE. Prednisone inhibits late asthmatic reactions and airway inflammation induced by toluene diisocyanate in sensitized subjects. J Allergy Clin Immunol 1987;80:261-267.
39. De Marzo N, Fabbri LM, Crescioli S, Plebani M, Testi R, Mapp CE. Dose dependent inhibitory effect of inhaled beclomethasone on late asthmatic reactions and increased airway responsiveness to methacholine induced by toluene diisocyanate in sensitized subjects. Pul Pharmacol 1988; 1:15-20.
40. Mapp CE, Dal Vecchio L, Boschetto P, Fabbri LM. Combined asthma and alveolitis due to diphenylmethane diisocyanate (MDI) with demonstration of no crossed respiratory reactivity to toluene diisocyanate (TDI). Ann Allergy 1985;54:424-429.
41. Van Cutsem EJ, Ceuppens JL, Lacquet LM, Demetz M. Combined asthma and alveolitis induced by cobalt in a diamond polisher. Eur J Respir Dis 1987;70:54-61.
42. De Monchy JGR, Kauffman HF, Venge P, et al. Bronchoalveolar eosinophilia during allergen-induced late asthmatic reactions. Am Rev Respir Dis 1985;131:373-376.
43. Booy-Noord H, Orie NGM, De Vries K. Immediate and late bronchial obstructive reactions to inhalation of house dust and protective effect of disodium cromoglycate and prednisolone. J Allergy Clin Immunol 1971; 48:344-354.
44. Barnes PJ. Asthma as an axon reflex. Lancet 1986;i:242-245.
45. Nadel JA, Barnes PJ. Autonomic regulation of the airways. Annu Rev Med 1984;35:451-467.
46. Hogg JC. Bronchial mucosal permeability and its relationship to airways hyperreactivity. J Allergy Clin Immunol 1981;67:421-425.
47. Persson CGA, Erjefalt I. Airway microvascular permeability to large molecules. Bull Eur Physiopath Respir 1986;22:23-31.
48. Nadel JA, Holtzman MJ. Regulation of airway responsiveness and secretion: role of inflammation. In: *Asthma, Physiology, Pharmacology, and Treatment*. Kay AB, Austen KF, Lichtenstein LM, eds. Academic Press, Inc., London, 1985, pp 129-155.
49. Pauwels R. Mode of action of corticosteroids in asthma and rhinitis. Clin Allergy 1986;16:281-288.
50. Morris H. Mechanisms of action and therapeutic role of corticosteroids in asthma. J Allergy Clin Immunol 1985;75:1-13.
51. Kirby JG, Hargreave FE, O'Byrne PM. Indomethacin inhibits allergen-induced airway hyperresponsiveness but not allergen-induced asthmatic responses. Am Rev Respir Dis 1987;135:A312.
52. Fabbri LM, Danieli D, Crescioli S, Bevilacqua P, Meli S, Saetta M, Mapp

CE. Fatal asthma in a toluene diisocyanate sensitized subject. Am Rev Respir Dis 1988; 137:1494-1498.
53. Paggiaro PL, Paoletti P, Bacci E, et al. Eosinophils in bronchoalveolar lavage (BAL) of patients with toluene diisocyanate (TDI) asthma after cessation of work. Am Rev Respir Dis 1987; 135:A234.
54. Hogg JC. The pathology of asthma. In: *Bronchial Asthma*. Weiss SB, Barsan GC, Segal MS, Stein M, eds. Little, Brown, and Company, Boston, 1985, pp 209-217.
55. Saetta M, Shiner RJ, Angus GE, Kim WD, Wang NS, King M, Ghezzo N, Cosio MG. Destructive index: a measurement of lung parenchymal destruction in smokers. Am Rev Resp Dis 1985; 131:764-768.
56. Saetta M, Ghezzo H, Kim WD, et al. Loss of alveolar attachments in smokers. A morphometric correlate of lung function impairment. Am Rev Respir Dis 1985; 132:894-900.
57. Moreno RH, Hogg JC, Pare PD. Mechanics of airway narrowing. Am Rev Respir Dis 1986; 133:1171-1180.

7

Airway Inflammation and Asthma

PAUL M. O'BYRNE

McMaster University
Hamilton, Ontario, Canada

INTRODUCTION

Asthma is a disease known, from earliest antiquity (1), to be intermittent, sometimes severe, and occasionally fatal. Asthma symptoms occur because of variable airflow obstruction, sometimes precipitated by a stimulus known to provoke airflow obstruction, but more often with no obvious stimulus.

Over the past 40–50 years, the ability of the airways of asthmatic subjects to constrict when exposed to inhaled constrictor agonists or to naturally occurring stimuli, such as exercise, has been described (2,3) and extensively investigated. This is airway hyperresponsiveness, which means that asthmatic airways require much smaller concentrations of inhaled bronchoconstrictor mediators to induce the same degree of airway narrowing than nonasthmatic airways (4) (Fig. 1). Also, asthmatic airways can narrow to a greater extent than nonasthmatic airways (5).

Past studies examining the pathogenesis of airway hyperresponsiveness and symptomatic asthma have focused on inhaled stimuli which cause airway hyperresponsiveness, such as allergen or occupational sensitizing agents, and mediators released from cells in asthmatic airways, such as mast cells. Studies attempting to implicate specific mediators have been difficult to perform, because of the difficulties in measuring the mediators at their site of action in the airways, and have not been definitive, mostly because of lack of potent and specific mediator antagonists. Indeed, there is no convincing evidence that implicates any one

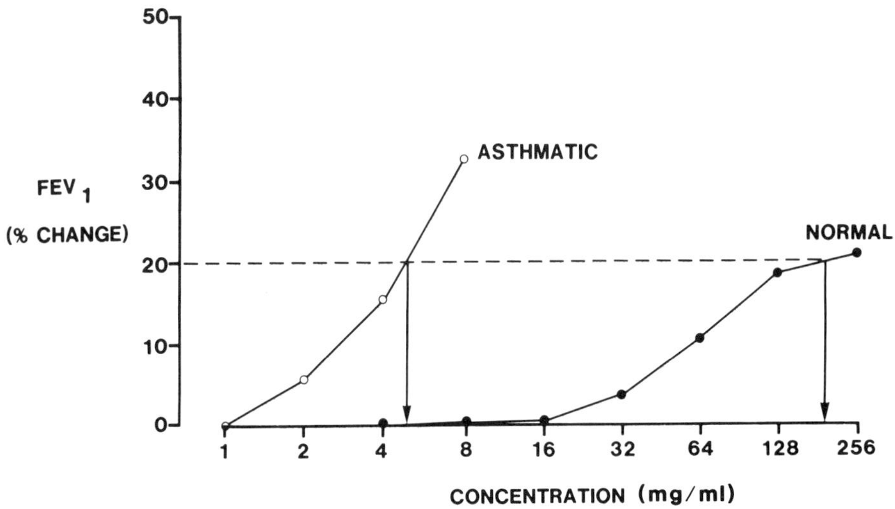

FIGURE 1 Dose–response curve to increasing concentrations of an inhaled bronchoconstrictor agonist. The response is measured as change in FEV_1 from baseline values in an asthmatic (open circles) and a normal (closed circles) subject. The response is expressed as the provocative concentration of agonist causing a 20% fall in FEV_1 (PC_{20}). The PC_{20} is lower in the asthmatic subject indicating airway hyperresponsiveness to the agonist. (Reproduced with permission from Ref. 4a.)

mediator in the pathogenesis of airway hyperresponsiveness or symptomatic asthma.

More recently, studies have also focused on the inflammatory cells which are present in stable asthmatic airways, as well as after inhaled stimuli. These studies have also examined the mediators which attract the cells into the airways and the state of activation of the cells.

The fact that severe airway inflammation was present in the airways of severe, fatal asthma is not new. Indeed, William Osler, described in the first edition of his book, *The Principals and Practice of Medicine*, "bronchial asthma . . . in many cases is a special form of inflammation of the smaller bronchioles" (6). A more complete description of airway inflammation and asthma was provided by Dunnill and colleagues (7) in the 1960s, again in patients dying of acute asthma.

More recently, however, the importance of airway inflammation in causing ongoing, even mild asthma or transient asthma after exposure to an inflammatory stimulus, has been recognized. This chapter is a review of the evidence that airway inflammation causes airway hyperresponsiveness and asthma and the impact that this improved understanding has had in treating asthma.

AIRWAY HYPERRESPONSIVENESS IN ASTHMA

Asthma is now defined as a disease which is characterized by both reversible airway narrowing and airway hyperresponsiveness (8). The release of constrictor mediators in airways and hyperresponsiveness to these mediators are both important in the clinical manifestations of asthma. The importance of airway hyperresponsiveness in asthma is more fully described in Chapter 5.

Airway hyperresponsiveness can be stable over several years in many asthmatic subjects (9). However, inhalation of a number of stimuli such as allergen (10-12), ozone (13), and low-molecular weight chemical sensitizers, such as toluene diisocyanate (TDI) (14,15), or plicatic acid from Western Red Ceder (16) can cause airway hyperresponsiveness in human subjects. This is associated with an increase in symptoms of asthma and an increase in the amount of treatment required to control symptoms (17). Therefore, in many asthmatics inhaled allergens or other stimuli are an important cause of asthma morbidity. Furthermore, Cockcroft (18) has suggested that in many patients with ongoing asthma, who are allergic to commonly encountered environmental allergens, such as house dust mite, their persisting symptoms are caused by regular allergen exposure. This hypothesis has been supported by several studies which have shown that allergen avoidance in patients with persisting asthma, can improve both airway hyperresponsiveness and asthma symptoms (19-21). This concept is more fully considered in Chapter 6.

AIRWAY INFLAMMATION AND HYPERRESPONSIVENESS IN ANIMALS

There is no animal model of human asthma. However, the stimuli known to cause airway hyperresponsiveness in humans also cause airway hyperresponsiveness in a number of animal species. This has allowed experimental studies to be carried out in animal models to investigate the pathogenesis of airway hyperresponsiveness, and has allowed hypotheses to be generated, some of which could be subsequently tested in human subjects.

Initial studies which suggested that some component(s) of acute airway inflammation is responsible for the development of transient airway hyperresponsiveness were performed in dogs after inhaled ozone (22) and allergen (23). Several other animal preparations of airway hyperresponsiveness have been described. These have been in rabbits after allergen (24); in guinea pigs after ozone (25), allergen (26), and toluene diisocyanate (TDI) (27); and in sheep after allergen (28). Each of these stimuli can cause acute airway inflammation, presumably through initiating the release of mediators chemotactic for inflammatory cells. The cells drawn into the airways subsequently release mediators which change airway responsiveness to bronchoconstrictor mediators. The precise role of individual inflammatory cells and mediators in initiating airway hyperresponsiveness is controversial and appears to vary between species and with the inciting stimulus.

INFLAMMATORY CELLS AND AIRWAY HYPERRESPONSIVENESS

Studies in dogs examining the pathogenesis of airway hyperresponsiveness demonstrated a temporal association between the development of airway hyperresponsiveness and the presence of neutrophils in the airways after inhalation of ozone (29). Inhaled ozone causes transient airway hyperresponsiveness, which is maximal several hours after exposure and which has completely recovered by one week (22). Biopsies of the central airways of dogs before and after inhaled ozone demonstrated that a large influx of neutrophils occurred after inhaled ozone, when the dogs had airway hyperresponsiveness and that both the influx of neutrophils and the airway hyperresponsiveness had resolved at one week (29). The influx of neutrophils was also demonstrated in bronchoalveolar lavage fluid from dogs after inhaled ozone (30). Other investigators have confirmed that neutrophils are present in the airways when airway hyperresponsiveness has developed in dogs (23) and rabbits after inhaling allergen (24).

These temporal associations, however, do not prove causality. To further test the hypothesis that neutrophils are important in the pathogenesis of airway hyperresponsiveness, dogs were depleted of circulating neutrophils using intravenous hydroxyurea and exposed to ozone (31). During the period of neutropenia, ozone inhalation did not lead to airway hyperresponsiveness. When the neutrophil counts had recovered, all dogs developed airway hyperresponsiveness after ozone.

Similar studies have been performed in rabbits sensitized to ***Alternaria tenuis***. The development of late responses and airway hyperresponsiveness after inhaled allergen is associated with the presence of polymorphonuclear leukocytes and mononuclear cells in the airways (24). In addition, leukocyte depletion abolished both of these responses. Lastly, repletion of cells by infusion of neutrophil-rich cell suspensions restored the ability to develop late responses and airway hyperresponsiveness (32).

The importance of neutrophils in the development of airway hyperresponsiveness appears to be species specific. For example, neutrophil depletion using cyclophosphamide does not inhibit airway hyperresponsiveness in guinea pigs after inhalation of ozone (33) or TDI (34). In sensitized guinea pigs, inhaled allergen causes influx of both neutrophils and eosinophils into airways (26).

However, only the presence of eosinophils appears to be necessary for the development of late responses.

A major problem, however, with all studies in which neutrophil depletion has been performed is the lack of specificity of the drug used to deplete neutrophils. Therefore, while the studies in dogs (31) suggested that neutrophils were involved in the development of airway hyperresponsiveness after ozone, and in rabbits (32) that polymorphonuclear leukocytes were involved in the development of airway hyperresponsiveness after allergen, they did not provide proof. To further clarify the ability of neutrophils to induce airway hyperresponsiveness, human neutrophils were isolated (>95% pure preparations) and stimulated with arachidonic acid and the calcium ionophore A23187. Inhalation of the supernatant fluid from the stimulated neutrophils caused airway hyperresponsiveness in dogs, while inhalation of arachidonic acid and A23187 alone did not. Also, inhaled supernatants from stimulated human neutrophils (35), but not eosinophils (36), caused airway hyperresponsiveness in allergic rabbits. These studies indicate that human neutrophils have the capacity to release mediators which cause airway hyperresponsiveness in dogs and rabbits.

To summarize the animal studies, all studies agree that some component(s) of an acute airway inflammatory response are important in the pathogenesis of airway hyperresponsiveness after inhaled stimuli such as allergen, ozone, and TDI. These studies have suggested, however, that the important effecter cell and possibly mediators for the development of airway hyperresponsiveness may vary between species, or possibly the stimulus used to cause airway hyperresponsiveness.

AIRWAY INFLAMMATION AND HYPERRESPONSIVENESS IN HUMANS

The association between the presence of inflammatory cells in the airways and airway hyperresponsiveness has also been investigated in human subjects. In these studies, numbers of cells and the cellular differential has been measured in bronchoalveolar lavage fluid before and after subjects have inhaled stimuli, known to cause airway hyperresponsiveness, such as ozone (37), the occupational sensitizing agents TDI (38), and western red cedar (39), and allergen (40,41). All of these studies have demonstrated an acute inflammatory response in the airways associated with the development of airway hyperresponsiveness. In addition, these studies have suggested that the stimulus which initiates airway hyperresponsiveness may determine the cellular response. For example, Stelzer et al. (37) demonstrated an isolated increase in neutrophils in bronchoalveolar lavage fluid in subjects with airway hyperresponsiveness after ozone. Also, a large increase in neutrophils and a smaller increase in eosinophils occurred in bronchoalveolar lavage fluid in subjects with airway hyperresponsiveness after toluene diisocyanate (38). By contrast, an increase in eosinophils but not neutrophils was demonstrated in lavage fluid after allergen inhalation in some studies (40) and in Western red cedar-induced asthma (39). In another study, however, both eosinophils and neutrophils are elevated after inhaled allergen (41), although measurements were made at a different time point. Therefore, while these studies have suggested that components of the airway inflammatory response cause airway hyperresponsiveness, the cellular responses may differ between stimuli or at different time points during the response.

AIRWAY INFLAMMATION AND STABLE ASTHMA

Several studies have provided information on cell populations in lavage fluid of stable asthmatics who have ongoing persisting airway hyperresponsiveness (42-45). These studies have all demonstrated the presence of inflammatory cells and have suggested that an increase in mast cells (42-45) and/or eosinophils (42,44, 45) exists in asthmatic airways.

Recent studies have related the numbers of mast cells and eosinophils with features of clinical relevance in asthma, such as measurements of airway hyperresponsiveness or spirometry. For example, one study performed bronchoalveolar lavage in one lung and a bronchial washing in the opposite lung in a group of mild, stable asthmatics with no clinical evidence of airway inflammation such as cough or sputum production, and a group of nonsmoking, nonasthmatic subjects (44). This study demonstrated a significant increase in the numbers of eosinophils and mast cells in both the lavage and washings of the asthmatics, consistent with other studies examining lavage fluid from asthmatics. In addition, there was close correlation between numbers of mast cells and the degree of airway hyperresponsiveness in the asthmatics in both lavage fluid ($r=-0.94$) (Fig. 2) and washings ($r=-0.85$), indicating that the more hyperresponsive subjects had the greatest number of mast cells. Also, eosinophil numbers in lavage fluid were correlated with the degree of airway hyperresponsiveness ($r=-0.71$) (Fig. 2). Similar correlations have been described by other investigators in asthmatic subjects (42,45).

In a more recent study, Kelly et al. (46) also showed correlations between the numbers of neutrophils and airway hyperresponsiveness. They also demonstrated that the activity of both the neutrophils and alveolar macrophages as indicated by luminol-enhanced chemiluminescence was increased in asthmatic subjects when compared with control subjects. Therefore, this study not only demonstrated the presence of inflammatory cells in asthmatic airways, but also that the cells are metabolically active, suggesting they play a role in ongoing asthma.

All of these studies have been consistent with the hypothesis that even in mild stable asthmatics, airway hyperresponsiveness is maintained as a conse-

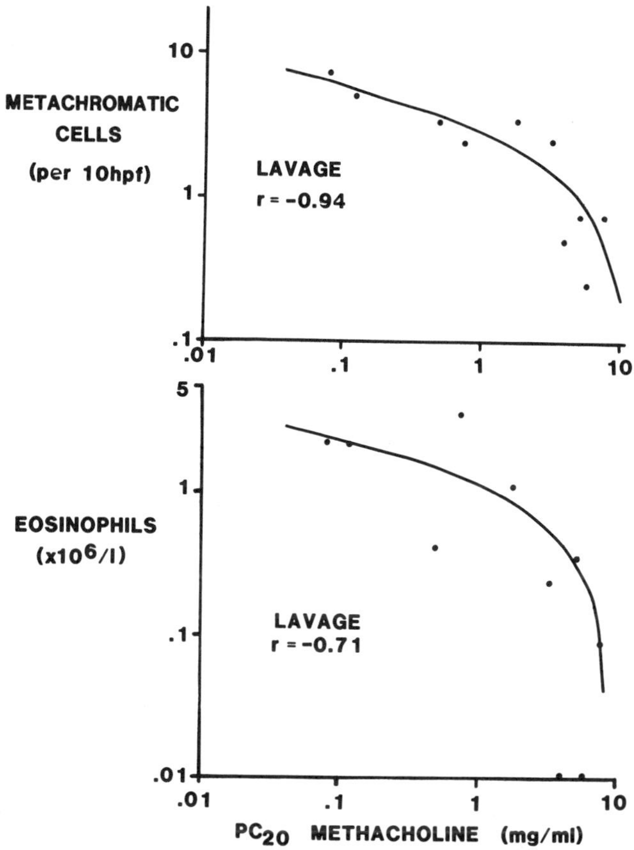

FIGURE 2 Correlation of the number of metachromatic cells (upper panel) and eosinophils (lower panel) and the degree of methacholine airway hyperresponsiveness in mild asthmatic subjects. The more airway hyperresponsiveness is present the more inflammatory cells in lavage fluid. (Modified with the authors permission from Ref. 44.)

quence of some component of the inflammatory response and that this response may involve mast cells, eosinophils, or neutrophils.

The close associations between the presence of inflammatory cells and the level of airway hyperresponsiveness in asthmatic subjects also suggests that measurements of airway hyperresponsiveness may be used as an, albeit indirect, indication of the presence and severity of airway inflammation in these subjects. This concept is useful in that no other noninvasive method exists to indicate the presence of airway inflammation in asthmatics, and improvements in airway hyperresponsiveness after appropriate treatment may reflect improvements in the degree of airway inflammation, although this remains to be proven.

INFLAMMATORY MEDIATORS AND AIRWAY HYPERRESPONSIVENESS

The importance of specific inflammatory mediators in the pathogenesis of airway hyperresponsiveness and asthma will be fully reviewed in Chapter 9.

Many mediators have been implicated in causing asthma. These mediators can be considered in three groups:

1. Mediators which cause transient bronchoconstriction, such as histamine or acetylcholine
2. Mediators which cause influx of inflammatory cells and possibly activation of cells in the airways, such as platelet activating factor or leukotriene B_4
3. Mediators which are released from inflammatory cells and which cause airway hyperresponsiveness [e.g., evidence for such mediators exists for thromboxane in dogs (47) and tachykinins in guinea pigs (48)]

The importance of thromboxane in causing airway hyperresponsiveness in dogs has come from studies where airway hyperresponsiveness occurred following inhalation of ozone (49), allergen (48), leukotriene B_4 (LTB_4) (50), and platelet-activating factor (PAF) (51). These studies have been done by both inhibition of the production of mediators, using specific synthetase inhibitors, and measurement of levels of mediators in lavage fluid at a time when airway hyperresponsiveness was present. Initially, indomethacin, an inhibitor of the cyclooxygenase pathway of arachidonate metabolism, was demonstrated to prevent airway hyperresponsiveness after ozone in dogs (52). This suggested that a prostaglandin or thromboxane was involved in the pathogenesis of airway hyperresponsiveness after this stimulus. Indomethacin has also been demonstrated to prevent airway hyperresponsiveness after C5a in rabbits (53) and after inhaled allergen in sheep (54).

Measurement of cyclooxygenase products in lavage fluid at a time airway hyperresponsiveness was present after inhaled LTB_4 in dogs, demonstrated an increase in thromboxane B_2 levels compared to controls (50). Inhibition of thromboxane synthesis using OKY-046, prevented both the rise in thromboxane in lavage and airway hyperresponsiveness after LTB_4 (50) and the increases in airway responsiveness after ozone (49), allergen (48), and PAF (51) in dogs. Lastly, pretreatment with the thromboxane mimetic U46619, can increase airway responsiveness (49). Therefore, thromboxane appears to be an important mediator for the development of airway hyperresponsiveness in dogs.

In contrast to these studies in dogs, in guinea pigs BW 755c, an inhibitor of both cyclooxygenase and lipoxygenase, but not indomethacin, prevented airway hyperresponsiveness after inhaled toluene diioscyanate (55). Thus, there appears to be species differences in the mediator(s) causing airway hyperresponsiveness. This has been further demonstrated by Thompson et al. (48), who demonstrated that tachykinins appear to be responsible for airway hyperresponsiveness caused by toluene diisocyanate in guinea pigs.

There is evidence which implicates prostaglandins or thromboxane in the pathogenesis of airway hyperresponsiveness after inhaled allergens in humans. A number of investigators (56,57) have demonstrated inhibition of the late response by inhibitors of cyclooxygenase, including indomethacin, implicating prostanoids in the pathogenesis of this response. However, Fabbri et al. (58) could not demonstrate any inhibition by indomethacin of the late response after inhaled toluene diisocyanate. A more recent study has examined the ability of indomethacin to inhibit the early and late asthmatic responses after inhaled allergen and also to inhibit the increases in airway responsiveness after allergen (59). Indomethacin did not inhibit the early or late asthmatic response, which suggests that prostanoids or thromboxane are not responsible for these responses. However, indomethacin did inhibit the increases in airway responsiveness after allergen. Therefore, these results are consistent with the hypothesis that prostanoids or thromboxane are involved in the development of airway hyperresponsiveness after stimuli such as allergen in human subjects.

IMPACT ON THE TREATMENT OF ASTHMA

The appreciation that airway inflammation plays a central role in the pathogenesis of not only acute exacerbations of asthma triggered by inflammatory stimuli, such as allergen or TDI, but also of ongoing persisting, even mild stable asthma, has changed the way which many clinicians treat patients with asthma. This is covered in greater detail in Chapter 12.

Drugs which are used to treat asthma can be considered in two broad categories, those which bronchodilate and provide rapid symptomatic relief, and those which influence the inflammatory response, which do not act rapidly but provide more long-term improvement in airway hyperresponsiveness and asthma symptoms. The most commonly used bronchodilating drugs are β_2-adrenoceptor agonists (60), theophyllines (61), and anticholinergics (62). The most effective anti-inflammatory drugs are glucocorticoids (63); others in this category include cromolyn (64) and nedocromil (65).

The major change in the treatment of asthma that has occurred in many (but by no means all) countries, has been to stress the importance of glucocorticoids, particularly inhaled, much earlier in the treatment of asthma, and to downplay the use of bronchodilating drugs as first-line treatment in most asthmatic subjects. This approach is supported by studies which have demonstrated improvements in airway hyperresponsiveness as well as symptoms of asthma after regular treatment with inhaled glucocorticoids, in patients with asthma which spans the range of severity from mild to severe (66,67). These improvements in airway hyperresponsiveness may also reflect a reduction in the degree of airway inflammation.

CONCLUSION

It is now widely accepted that some component(s) of an acute airway inflammatory response is responsible for the development of airway hyperresponsiveness after stimuli such as allergen and occupational sensitizing agents, leading to the development of symptomatic asthma. The sequence of events leading to airway hyperresponsiveness is partially understood in some animal species; however the importance of different inflammatory cells and mediators between species is still being debated. Studies in humans have supported the hypothesis that airway inflammation also results in stable airway hyperresponsiveness and asthma. However, a great deal more research is necessary to fully elucidate the interactions between the important cells and mediators involved. This improved understanding of the role of airway inflammation in asthma has also provided rationale for the earlier use of anti-inflammatory drugs, such as inhaled glucocorticoids, in the management of asthma.

REFERENCES

1. Adams F. The extent of the work of Aretaeus the Cappadocian. In: *The Proceedings of The Sydenham Society*, London, 1856.
2. Weiss S, Robb GP, Ellis LB. The systemic effects of histamine in man. Arch Intern Med 1932;49:360–396.
3. Curry JJ. Comparative action of acetyl-beta-methyl choline and histamine on the respiratory tract in normals, patients with hay fever and subjects with bronchial asthma. J Clin Invest 1947;26:430–438.
4. Hargreave FE, Ryan G, Thomson NC, O'Byrne PM, Latimer K, Juniper EF, Dolovich J. Bronchial responsiveness to histamine or methacholine in asthma: measurement and clinical significance. J Allergy Clin Immunol 1981;68:347–355.

4a. O'Byrne PM. Allergy and airway hyperresponsiveness. In: *The Allergic Basis of Asthma*. Kay AB (ed.). WB Saunders, London, 1988, pp 127–142.

5. Woolcock AJ, Salome CM, Yan K. The shape of the dose-response curve to histamine in asthmatic and normal subjects. Am Rev Respir Dis 1984; 130: 71–75.
6. Osler W. In: *The Principals and Practice of Medicine*. Appleton and Co., New York, 1892, p 497.
7. Dunnill MS, Massarell GR, Anderson JA. A comparison of the quantitive anatomy of the bronchi in normal subjects, in status asthmaticus, in chronic bronchitis and in emphysema. Thorax 1969; 24:176–179.

8. American Thoracic Society: definition of asthma. Am Rev Respir Dis 1962;134:704–707.
9. Juniper EF, Frith PA, Hargreave FE. Long term stability of bronchial responsiveness to histamine. Thorax 1982;37:288–291.
10. Cartier A, Thomson NC, Frith PA, Roberts R, Hargreave FE. Allergen-induced increase in bronchial responsiveness to histamine: relationship to the late asthmatic response and change in airway caliber. J Allergy Clin Immunol 1982;70:170–177.
11. Cockcroft DW, Ruffin RE, Dolovich J, Hargreave FE. Allergen-induced increase in non-allergic bronchial reactivity. Clinical Allergy 1977; 7:503–513.
12. Boulet LP, Cartier A, Thomson NC, Roberts RS, Dolovich J, Hargreave FE. Asthma and increases in nonallergic bronchial responsiveness from seasonal pollen exposure. J Allergy Clin Immunol 1983; 71:399–406.
13. Golden JA, Nadel JA, Boushey HA. Bronchial hyperirritability in healthy subjects after exposure to ozone. Am Rev Respir Dis 1978; 118:287–294.
14. Yeung M, Lam S, Tse KS. Measurement of airway responsiveness in occupational asthma. In: *Airway Responsiveness*. Hargreave FE, Woolcock AJ (eds.). Mississauga, Astra Pharmaceuticals 1985; 129–134.
15. Fabbri LM, Chiesura-Corona P, Dal Vecchio L, Di Giacomo GR, Zocca E, De Marzo N, Maestrelli P, Mapp CE. Prednisone inhibits late asthmatic reactions and the associated increase in airway responsiveness induced by toluene diisocyanate in sensitized subjects. Am Rev Respir Dis 1985; 132: 1010–1014.
16. Chan-Yeung M, Lam S, Koener S. Clinical features and natural history of occupational asthma due to Western Red Cedar (Thuja plicata). Am J Med 1982;72:411–415.
17. Juniper EF, Frith PA, Hargreave FE. Airway responsiveness to histamine and methacholine: relationship to minimum treatment to control symptoms of asthma. Thorax 1981;36:575–579.
18. Cockcroft DW. Mechanism of perennial allergic asthma. Lancet 1983; ii:253–256.
19. Platts-Mills TA, Mitchell EB, Nock P, Tovey ER, Moszor H, Wilkins S. Reduction of bronchial hyperreactivity during prolonged allergen avoidance. Lancet 1982; ii:675–678.
20. Murray AB, Ferguson AC. Dust-free bedrooms in the treatment of asthmatic children with house dust or house dust mite allergen: a controlled trial. Pediatrics 1983;71:418–422.
21. Dorward AJ, Colloff MJ, MacKay NS, McSharry C, Thomson NC. Effect of house dust mite avoidance measures on adult atopic asthma. Thorax 1988;43:98–102.
22. Holtzman MJ, Fabbri LM, Skoogh B.-E, O'Byrne PM, Walters EH, Aizawa H, Nadel JA. Time course of airway hyperresponsiveness induced by ozone in dogs. J Appl Physiol 1983;55(4):1232–1236.
23. Chung KF, Becker AB, Lazarus SC, Frick OL, Nadel JA, Gold WM.

Antigen-induced airway hyperresponsiveness and pulmonary inflammation in allergic dogs. J Appl Physiol 1985; 58:1347-1353.
24. Marsh WR, Irvin CG, Murphy KR, Behrens BL, Larsen GL. Increases in airway reactivity to histamine and inflammatory cells in bronchoalveolar lavage after the late asthmatic response in an animal model. Am Rev Resp Dis 1985; 131:875-879.
25. Murlas CG, Roum JH. Sequence of pathological changes in the airway mucosa of guinea pigs during ozone-induced bronchial hyperreactivity. Am Rev Respir Dis 1985; 131:875-879.
26. Hutson PA, Church MK, Clay TP, Miller P, Holgate ST. Early and late-phase bronchoconstriction after allergen challenge of nonanaesthetized guinea pigs. Am Rev Respir Dis 1988; 137:548-557.
27. Gordon T, Sheppard D, McDonald D, Distefano S, Scypinski L. Airway hyperresponsiveness and inflammation induced by toluene diisocyanate in guinea pigs. Am Rev Respir Dis 1985; 132:1106-1112.
28. Lanes S, Stevenson JS, Codias E, Hernandez A, Sielczak MW, Abraham WM. Effects of busesonide on late bronchial response and the associated airway hyperresponsiveness in allergic sheep. In: *Glucocorticoids, Inflammation and Bronchial Hyperreactivity*. Hogg JC, Ellul-Micallef R, Brattsand R, eds. Excerpta Med, New York, 1985, pp 38-50.
29. Holtzman MJ, Fabbri LM, O'Byrne PM, Gold BD, Aizawa H, Walters EH, Alpert SE, Nadel JA. Importance of airway inflammation for hyperresponsiveness induced by ozone. Am Rev Respir Dis 1983; 127:686-690.
30. Fabbri LM, Aizawa H, Alpert SE, Walters EH, O'Byrne PM, Gold BD, Nadel JA, Holtzman MJ. Airway hyperresponsiveness and changes in cell counts in bronchoalveolar lavage after ozone exposure in dogs. Am Rev Respir Dis 1984; 129:288-291.
31. O'Byrne PM, Walters EH, Gold BD, Aizawa HA, Fabbri LM, Alpert SE, Nadel JA, Holtzman MJ. Neutrophil depletion inhibits airway hyperresponsiveness induced by ozone exposure. Am Rev Respir Dis 1984; 130:2, 14-19.
32. Murphy KR, Wilson MC, Irvin CG, Glezen LS, Marsh WR, Haslett C, Henson PM, Larsen GL. The requirement for polymorphonuclear leukocytes in the asthmatic response and heightened airways reactivity in an asthmatic model. Am Rev Respir Dis 1986; 134:62-68.
33. Murlas C, Roum JH. Bronchial hyperreactivity occurs in steroid-treated guinea pigs depleted of leukocytes by cyclophospamide. J Appl Physiol 1985; 58:1630-1637.
34. Thompson JE, Scypinski LA, Gordon T, Sheppard D. Hydroxyurea inhibits airway hyperresponsiveness in guinea pigs by a granulocyte-independent mechanism. Am Rev Respir Dis 1986; 134:1213-1218.
35. Irvin C, Baltopoulos G, Honour J, Seccombe JF, Henson PM. Lipid mediators released by activated human neutrophils which increase airway reactivity. Am Rev Respir Dis 1986; 133:A175.
36. Uchida DA, Kimani G, Larsen GL, Irvin CG. Effects on airway function of supernatants from phagocytosing eosinophils. Am Rev Respir Dis 1987; 135:A178.

37. Stelzer J, Bigby BG, Stulbarg M, Holtzman MJ, Nadel JA, Ueki IF, Leifauf GD, Goetzl EJ, Boushey HA. Ozone-induced changes in bronchial reactivity to methacholine and airway inflammation in humans. J Appl Physiol 1986; 60:1321-1326.
38. Boschetto P, Zocca E, Milani GF, Licata B, Pivirotto F, Mapp CE, Fabbri LM. Bronchoalevolar neutrophilia during the late, but not early, asthmatic reactions induced by toluene diisocyanate (TDI). J Allergy Clin Immunol 1986;77:496A.
39. Lam S, Chan-Yeung M, Le Riche J, Kijek K, Phillip D. Cellular changes in bronchial lavage fluid following late asthmatic reactions in patients with red cedar asthma. Am Rev Respir Dis 1985;131:42A.
40. De Monchy JGR, Kauffman HF, Venge Per, Koeter GH, Jansen HM, Sluiter HJ, De Vries K. Bronchoalveolar eosinophilia during allergen-induced late asthmatic reaction. Am Rev Respir Dis 1985;131:373-376.
41. Metzger WJ, Zavala D, Richerson HB, Moseley P, Iwamota P, Monick M, Sjoerdsma K, Hunnunghake GW. Local allergen challenge and broncho-alveolar lavage of allergic asthmatic lungs. Am Rev Respir Dis 1987; 135: 433-440.
42. Flint KC, Leung KBP, Hudspith BN, Brostoff J, Pearce FL, Johnson NM. Bronchoalveolar mast cells in extrinsic asthma: a mechanism for the initiation of antigen specific bronchoconstriction. Br Med J 1985; 291:923-936.
43. Tomioka M, Ida S, Shindoh Y, Ishihara T, Takishima T. Mast cells in bronchoalveolar lumen of patients with bronchial asthma. Am Rev Respir Dis 1984;129:1000-1005.
44. Kirby J, Hargreave FE, Gleich GJ, O'Byrne PM. Bronchoalveolar cell profiles of asthmatic and nonasthmatic subjects. Am Rev Respir Dis 1987; 136:379-383.
45. Wardlaw AJ, Dunnette S, Gleich GJ, Collins JV, Kay AB. Eosinophils and mast cells in bronchoalveolar lavage in subjects with mild asthma. Am Rev Respir Dis 1988;137:62-69.
46. Kelly C, Ward C, Stenton CS, Bird G, Hendrick DJ, Walters EH. Number and activity of inflammatory cells in bronchoalveolar lavage fluid in asthma and their relation to airway responsiveness. Thorax 1988;43:684-692.
47. Thompson JE, Scypinski LA, Gordon T, Sheppard D. Tachykinins mediate the acute increase in airway caused by toluene diisocyanate responsiveness in guinea pigs. Am Rev Respir Dis 1987;136:43-49.
48. Chung KF, Aizawa H, Becker AB, Frick O, Gold WM, Nadel JA. Inhibition of antigen-induced airway hyperresponsiveness by a thromboxane synthetase inhibitor (OKY 046) in allergic dogs. Am Rev REspir Dis 1986; 134:258-261.
49. Aizawa H, Chung KF, Leikauf GD, Ueki I, Bethel RA, O'Byrne PM, Hirose T, Nadel JA. Significance of thromboxane generation in ozone-induced airway hyperresponsiveness in dogs. J Appl Physiol 1985;59:1918-1923.
50. O'Byrne PM, Leikauf GD, Aizawa H, Bethel RA, Ueki IF, Holtzman MJ, Nadel JA. Leukotriene B4-induced airway hyperresponsiveness in dogs. J Appl Physiol 1985;59:1941-1946.

51. Chung KF, Aizawa H, Leikauf GD, Ueki IF, Evens TW, Nadel JA. Airway hyperresponsiveness induced by platelet-activating factor: role of thromboxane generation. J Pharmacol Exp Ther 1986; 236:580-581.
52. O'Byrne PM, Walters EH, Aizawa H, Fabbri LM, Holtzman MJ, Nadel JA. Indomethacin inhibits the airway hyperresponsiveness but not the neutrophil influx induced by ozone in dogs. Am Rev Respir Dis 1984; 130:220-224.
53. Berend N, Armour CL, Black JL. Indomethacin inhibits C5a des arg-induced airway hyperresponsiveness in the rabbit. Am Rev Respir Dis 1985; 131:24A.
54. Lanes S, Stevenson JS, Codias E, Hernandez A, Sialczak MW, Wanner A, Abraham WM. Indomethacin and FPL 55321 inhibit antigen-induced airway hyperresponsiveness in sheep. J Appl Physiol 1986; 61:864-872.
55. Lee HK, Murlas C. Ozone-induced bronchial hyperreactivity in guinea pigs is abolished by BW 755c or FPL 55712 but not by indomethacin. Am Rev Respir Dis 1985; 132:1005-1009.
56. Shephard EG, Malan L, Macfarlane CM, Mouton W, Joubert JR. Lung function and plasma levels of thromboxane B2, 6-ketoprostaglandin F1a and B-thromboglobulin in antigen-induced asthma before and after indomethacin pretreatment. Br J Clin Pharmacol 1985; 19:459-470.
57. Fairfax AJ. Inhibition of the late asthmatic response to house dust mite by non-steroidal anti-inflammatory drugs. Prostaglandins Leukotrienes and Medicine 1982; 8:239-248.
58. Fabbri LM, Chiesura-Corona P, Dal Vecchio L, Di Giacomo GR, Zocca E, De Marzo N, Maestrelli P, Mapp CE. Prednisone inhibits late asthmatic reactions and the associated increase in airway responsiveness induced by toluene-diisocyanate in sensitized subjects. Am Rev Respir Dis 1985; 132:1010-1014.
59. Kirby JG, Hargreave FE, Cockcroft DW, O'Byrne PM. The effect of indomethacin on allergen-induced asthmatic responses. J Appl Physiol 1989; 66:578-583.
60. Newhouse MT, Dolovich MB. Control of asthma by aerosols. N Engl J Med 1986; 315:870-874.
61. Weinberger M. Theophylline for the treatment of asthma. J Pediatr 1978; 92:1-7.
62. Gross NJ, Skorodin MS. Anticholinergic antimuscurinic bronchodilators. Am Rev Respir Dis 1984; 129:856-870.
63. Morris HG. Mechanisms of glucocorticoid action in pulmonary disease. Chest 1985; 133S-141S.
64. Altounyan REC. Review of clinical activity and mode of action of sodium cromoglycate. Clin Allergy 1980; 10:481-489.
65. Holgate ST. Clinical evaluation of nedocromil sodium in asthma. Eur J Respir Dis 1986; 69:149-159.
66. Ryan G, Latimer KM, Juniper EF, Roberts RS, Hargreave FE. Effect of beclomethasone dipropionate on bronchial responsiveness to histamine

in controlled non-steroid-dependent asthma. J Allergy Clin Immunol 1985; 75:25–30.

67. Dutiot JI, Salome CM, Woolcock AJ. Inhaled corticosteroids reduce the severity of bronchial hyperresponsiveness in asthma but oral theophylline does not. Am Rev Respir Dis 1987; 136:1174–1178.

8

Inflammatory Mediators in Asthma

K. F. CHUNG

National Heart and Lung Institute
Brompton Hospital
London, England

INTRODUCTION

There is an increasing awareness of the pathophysiological significance of inflammatory mechanisms in asthma. Mucosal edema due to increased airway microvascular permeability, infiltration of the airway wall with eosinophils, neutrophils, and mononuclear cells, desquamation of the bronchial epithelium, and mucus secretion are some of the pathologic features of the asthmatic airway (1,2). Airway inflammation is a complex series of events which are likely to be triggered by inflammatory stimuli interacting with primary effector cells resident within the airways. Release of inflammatory mediators from these cells may in turn recruit and activate other effector cells or cell-independent systems, with generation of other mediators, thus augmenting the inflammatory process. Airway narrowing and hyperresponsiveness, which are both characteristic features of the airways of asthmatic subjects, are the likely results of the inflammatory process and the release of mediators (3).

A wealth of information is now available on the effect of many putative mediators of asthma on the airways (4). Improvements in biochemistry and pharmacology have led to better assays and to the development of specific

Supported by the Medical Research Council of Great Britain

pharmacologic antagonists for many mediators so that their role in asthma can be probed. Histamine was one of the first mediators to be implicated in asthma and, more recently, there has been interest in the cyclooxygenase and lipoxygenase products of arachidonic acid metabolism (5) and in platelet-activating factor (PAF) (6). Because of the possible involvement of noncholinergic neural mechanisms in asthma and of its interactions with inflammatory events, sensory neuropeptides released from airway nerves have been implicated in asthma (7). This review will be mostly devoted to these mediators, but the complexity of airway inflammation suggests that other classes of mediators are likely to be involved. Because of possible species differences, information obtained from studies in humans will be reviewed as far as possible.

ORIGIN AND SOURCE OF INFLAMMATORY MEDIATORS

Inflammatory mediators that have been implicated in asthma may be generated by resident cells within the airways and lungs, as well as by cells that have migrated into the airways from circulating blood (Fig. 1). Although the mast cell was initially the focus of most attention, it is now clear that airway epithelial cells, alveolar macrophages, and endothelial cells may be additional sources of inflammatory mediators, in addition to eosinophils which are attracted to the asthmatic airway (Table 1).

Histamine is a preformed mediator stored within cytoplasmic granules of mast cells and basophils, and is released into tissue surroundings immediately on stimulation. Other preformed mediators such as chemotactic factors for neutrophils and eosinophils, adenosine, and superoxide anions are also generated, in addition to granule-associated mediators such as heparin, neutral proteases, and superoxide dismutase (8).

TABLE 1 Profile of Mediators Released by Human Airway and Inflammatory Cells

Mast cell	Histamine, PGD_2, LTC_4, LTB_4, PAF, proteases
Macrophage	PGE_2, TxA_2, LTB_4, PAF, superoxide anions
Airway epithelium	15-HETE, PGE_2, 'relaxant factor'
Airway smooth muscle	PGE_2
Vascular endothelium	PGI_2, LTB_4, PAF
Eosinophils	15-HETE, LTC_4, PAF, cationic proteins, eosinophil, peroxidase
Neutrophils	TxA_2, HETE's, PAF, superoxide, proteases
Sensory neurones	Tachykinins (substance P, neurokinins)

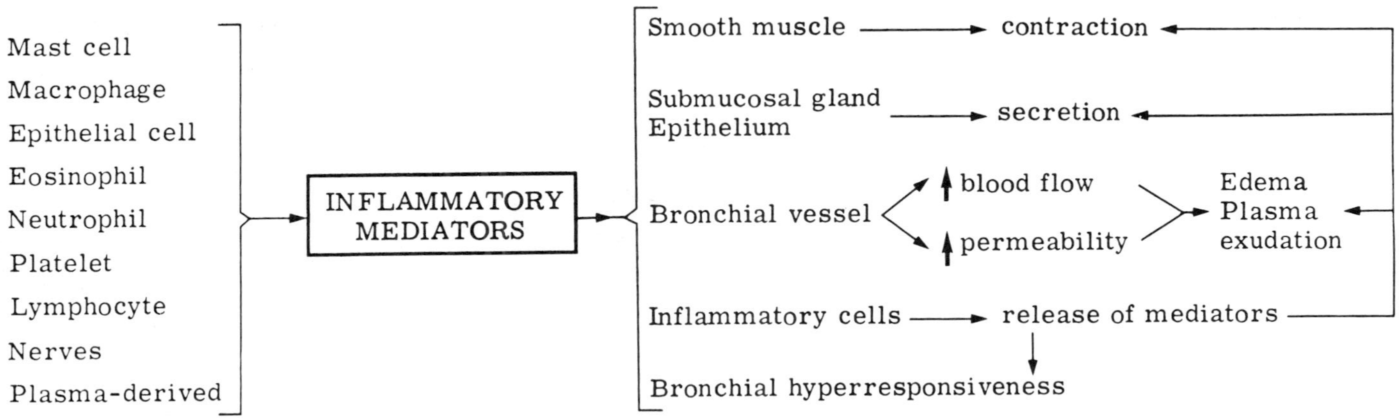

FIGURE 1 Cellular sources of inflammatory mediators and their effects on target cells in the airways.

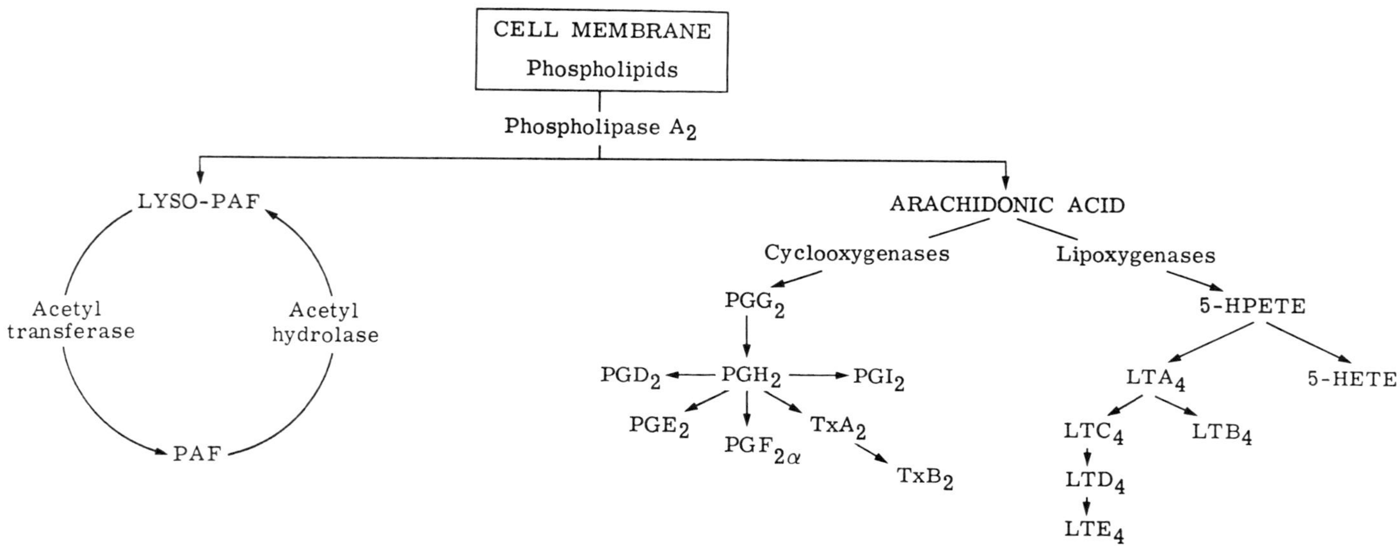

FIGURE 2 Pathways leading to the synthesis of prostaglandins (PG) and thromboxane (Tx), leukotrienes (LT), and platelet-activating factor (PAF) from cell membrane phospholipids. HPETE: hydroperoxyeicosatetraenoic acid; HETE: hydroeicosatetraenoic acid.

Cyclooxygenase and lipoxygenase derivatives of arachidonic acid metabolism are newly generated mediators synthesized following the release of arachidonic acid from cell membrane phospholipids by the enzyme phospholipase A_2. The metabolic pathways involved in the synthesis of the major cyclooxygenase and lipoxygenase products are shown on Figure 2 (9,10). PAF is formed from ether-linked phospholipids in the cell membrane through the generation of lyso-PAF; action of acetyltransferase enzyme converts lyso-PAF to PAF (11; Fig. 2).

Several cells types produce a spectrum of newly generated lipid mediators. IgE-mediated stimulation of purified human lung mast cells results in the generation of substantial amounts of prostaglandin D_2 (PGD_2) and leukotriene C_4 (LTC_4) with LTB_4 and PAF (12). Alveolar macrophages can also generate LTB_4 and PAF, and thromboxane A_2 (TxA_2) (13) and can be activated by IgE-dependent mechanisms (14). Of particular interest is the activity of human airway epithelial cells in releasing not only PGE_2 but also various 15-lipoxygenase products including 15-HETE (15). An epithelial-derived relaxing factor which inhibits smooth muscle contraction has also been described (16). Eosinophils are another source of LTC_4 and of PAF (17,18), and in addition secrete several granular constituents such as major basic protein, eosinophil cationic protein, and eosinophil peroxidase which are cytotoxic to airway epithelial cells (19). Alveolar macrophages and eosinophils can also release reactive oxygen species which can potentiate this effect. Vascular endothelial cells are an important site for the production of PAF (20) but similar to neutrophils and monocytes, only a small proportion of the synthesized PAF is released from the cell (21).

Many sensory neuropeptides including substance P (SP), neurokinin A (NKA), and calcitonin gene-related peptide (CGRP) have been localized in the respiratory tract (22). These peptides are synthesized in sensory neurones in the nodose and jugular ganglia and transported peripherally in sensory nerves. Activation of these airway afferent nerves leads to their release, with subsequent rapid inactivation by neutral endopeptidases (23).

Cell-independent effector systems include the complement and the kinin pathways. Complement activation may occur through either the classical or the alternative pathway to cause the generation of bioactive complement factors such as C3a and C5a (24). One of the better characterized mediators from the kinin pathway is bradykinin, which is generated from kininogens, which are $alpha_2$-globulins, by the action of kininogenases that may be released from mast cells and other inflammatory cells (25).

EFFECTS OF INFLAMMATORY MEDIATORS

Inflammatory mediators may have a variety of effects on several target cells within the airway and may thus mimic a wide range of abnormalities found in

TABLE 2 Effects of Inflammatory Mediators Implicated in Asthma

Mediator	Broncho-constriction	Airway secretion	Microvascular leakage	Chemo-taxis	Bronchial hyper-responsiveness
Histamine	+	+	+	+	–
Prostaglandins D_2, F_{2a}	++	+	?	?	+
Prostaglandin E_2	–	+	–	+	–
Thromboxane	++	?	–	±	+
Leukotriene B_4	–	–	±	++	±
Leukotrienes C_4, D_4, E_4	++	++	++	?	±
Platelet activating factor	++	+	++	++	++
Bradykinin	+	+	++	–	–
Substance P	+	++	++	±	–
Complement fragments	+	+	+	++	–

Key: ++ pronounced effect, + moderate effect, ± uncertain effect, ? information not available.

asthma (Fig. 1). They may lead to contraction of airway smooth muscle, either directly or indirectly, through the release other mediators or the activation of neural pathways. Some mediators have potent effects in increasing mucus secretion from submucosal glands and in causing microvascular leakage in the airways which results in airway edema and exudation of plasma into the airway lumen. Inflammatory mediators can attract and activate cells from the circulation, which in turn release other mediators. The detailed effects of several mediators of potential relevance to asthma with their possible contribution to the pathophysiology of asthma are described later but are summarized on Table 2.

Mediators produce their effects on target cells by the activation of specific cell surface receptors (26). Characterization and localization of these receptors have been made possible by the use of radioligand agonists or antagonists. Thus, SP receptors have been predominantly localized to airway smooth muscle of trachea down to terminal bronchioles, consistent with a potent direct contractile effect of SP on airway smooth muscle. Autoradiographic distribution of LTC_4 and LTD_4 binding sites has been obtained in guinea pig lung and trachea. High affinity binding sites for PAF have been demonstrated on inflammatory cells such as neutrophils, eosinophils, and on lung membranes using labelled PAF or PAF antagonists, but the localization of these receptors in the airways has not been determined. Classification of receptor subtypes for many of the inflammatory mediators including histamine (H-1 and H-2), the prostaglandins and thromboxane has been based on comparisons of the rank order of agonist potency.

The intracellular effects of inflammatory mediators and their relationship to functional effects are of interest both in airway smooth muscle and inflammatory cells. Activation of some receptors leads to inhibition of adenylate cyclase via an inhibitory guanine nucleotide protein, and for other receptors, breakdown of membrane phosphoinositides leads to the generation of inositol triphosphate which leads to the release of intracellular calcium (27). Whether inflammatory mediators can potentiate these intracellular mechanisms of airway smooth muscle or of other cells and possibly underlie the bronchial hyperresponsiveness of asthma is not known.

MEDIATOR INTERACTIONS

The release and generation of several inflammatory mediators may be enhanced in asthma. Bronchoalveolar lavage (BAL) fluid obtained from asthmatic subjects contain significantly more histamine than that from normal subjects (28,29), probably the result of increased releasability of histamine from airway mast cells (29). Alveolar macrophages obtained from BAL fluid of asthmatics produce more superoxide anions and PAF than that from normal subjects (30-32). Circulating eosinophils from symptomatic asthmatic subjects generate more chemiluminescence on stimulation in vitro by PAF and by a phorbol ester (33).

One potential mechanism for these enhanced responses is the priming effect of mediators. Thus, in vitro, PGD_2 is able to potentiate IgE-dependent release of histamine from basophils (34). Leukotriene generation from human eosinophils and neutrophils is potentiated by monokines released from mononuclear cells (35). Various cytokines such as interleukins 1 and 5 may enhance the response of eosinophils in vitro (36). The cellular mechanisms of this priming effect are not clear.

Mediator interactions may also occur at the level of the airway smooth muscle. The lipoxygenase products, 15-HETE and LTE_4 potentiate the response of airway smooth muscle to histamine in vitro (37,38); in addition, a thromboxane-mimetic drug (U46619) and SP potentiate the release of acetylcholine from cholinergic nerves in bronchial smooth muscle (39,40). In vivo, a transient increase in bronchial responses to histamine and methacholine has been observed with $PGF\text{-}_{2\alpha}$ and PGD_2 (41,42). More prolonged bronchial hyperresponsiveness has been reported with PAF, perhaps resulting from the induction of an inflammatory process (43). Potentiation of the microvascular leakage induced by histamine and bradykinin in the skin is also seen with vasodilators such as PGE_2 (44), but this interaction has not been demonstrated in the airways.

STUDY OF MEDIATORS IN ASTHMA

The possible involvement of mediators in asthma has been studied by measuring their release or by observing the effect of their antagonists or synthetic inhibitors either under baseline conditions or during challenge with stimuli such as allergen or exercise. Different mediators have been implicated during allergen-induced early and late phase responses, and bronchial hyperresponsiveness (45), suggesting heterogeneity of mediator involvement for several aspects of the airway response. Bronchial hyperresponsiveness induced by exposure to atmospheric pollutants such as ozone and to chemicals such as toluene diisocyanate have also been studied (3).

Measurement of Mediators

The precise quantity of mediators generated locally within airway tissue is not known and evidence for their release thus far has rested on the measurement of levels in circulating blood or in BAL. The amount of mediator recovered is dependent upon its concentration gradient from tissue levels, its diffusibility and its metabolic degradation by tissue and fluid enzymes. During an acute response such as inhalation of allergen, a rapid and transient release of histamine can be detected in the circulation and in BAL of sensitized dogs (46). Significant amounts of PGD_2 have also been detected in BAL of allergic asthmatics challenged with allergen (47). Ragweed-sensitive rhinitis patients PGD_2, LTC_4,

LTD_4, and LTE_4 as well as histamine and kinins into nasal washings after intranasal challenge with ragweed pollen (48,49). However, the profile of mediators released from intrapulmonary airways may not be similar to that observed from the nasal mucosa. Techniques for sampling specific portions of the lower airway may improve mediator recovery (50).

Recovery of mediators may be more difficult during the allergen late response, perhaps due to the slow release of mediators. Inflammatory cells may also potentiate the degradation of potent cyclooxygenase and lipoxygenase products. The peroxidase-H_2O_2-halide system produced by eosinophils and neutrophils may inactivate prostaglandins and leukotrienes (51,52). Nevertheless, increased recovery of LTE_4 has been observed in BAL fluid of stable asthmatic subjects (53), but LTD_4 is more difficult to detect in blood samples from patients with acute asthma (54). Rapid degradation of PAF by plasma acetylhydrolase present in biological fluids (54) and by alveolar epithelial cells (55) severely limit its recovery.

Mediator Antagonists and Inhibitors of Synthesis

Mediator antagonists or inhibitors of synthetic pathways are being increasingly used to elucidate the role of an individual mediator in asthma. The degree of specificity of the antagonist or inhibitor and the achievement of adequate tissue levels to block the effect of the endogenously generated mediator are important prerequisites for these studies and these may be difficult to obtain in human studies. Consequently, there is a relative paucity of such studies in humans. In addition, side effects from the antagonist may limit adequate dosing. Thus, the leukotriene antagonist, L-649,923, when administered orally was only mildly protective against bronchoconstriction induced by inhaled LTD_4 and was associated with gastrointestinal side effects (57). One possibility would be to administer antagonist drugs via the inhaled route to achieve high local airway concentrations. Inhibitors of synthetic pathway in addition to preventing the formation of a given mediator may divert the conversion of precursor substrates to other products. OKY-046, an inhibitor of thromboxane synthesis, has been shown to improve airway responsiveness to methacholine in asthma (58); however, this effect could have resulted from the shunting of prostaglandin endoperoxide to bronchodilator prostaglandins.

PUTATIVE ROLE OF SPECIFIC MEDIATORS IN ASTHMA

Histamine

Histamine is probably one of the most studied inflammatory mediators in asthma. Intravenous and inhaled histamine induces bronchospasm in asthmatics as well as in normal subjects at higher concentrations, an effect mediated through histamine H-1 receptors. The role of vagal reflexes in this response in human subjects has been variably reported as ranging from little effect of cholinergic blockade (59) to significant inhibition (60). It is possible that this response is dependent upon the duration and severity of the asthma. Histamine induces airway microvascular leakage in the proximal large airways of the guinea pig (61). When instilled on the human nasal mucosa, histamine causes an increase in the recovery of albumin and bradykinin, indicating an increase in both vascular and epithelial permeabilities (62). Histamine increases the secretion of mucus glycoproteins from human airways in vitro, an effect mediated by stimulation of H-2 receptors (63). Histamine has modest chemotactic activity for eosinophils in vitro (64).

Histamine is detectable in the circulation in humans with levels of 0.2 to 0.4 ng/ml, which are highest in the early hours of the morning and are elevated in stable asthmatic subjects (65). Modest rises have been reported in asthmatics during exercise- and allergen-induced bronchoconstriction (66,67). A secondary rise in plasma histamine but not in urinary excretion of histamine metabolites has also been reported during the late asthmatic response (68,69). It is possible that the rise in circulating basophils during exercise may account for the increase in histamine levels (70). Increased amounts of histamine have been recovered from an isolated airway segment after local exposure of the airways of asthmatic subjects to a hyperosmolar stimulus (50).

Chlorpeniramine, an H-1 histamine antagonist, has been studied extensively despite causing sedation when administered orally or intravenously and irritation when inhaled. It causes acute bronchodilation in asthmatic subjects (71). Inhaled clemastine, another potent H-1 antagonist, was as effective a bronchodilator as the beta-agonist, salbutamol, in asthmatic subjects (72), suggesting the presence of histamine 'tone' in asthmatic airways and supporting the concept of increased basal release of histamine in asthma. Inhaled clemastine also inhibits exercise- and antigen-induced bronchoconstriction (73,74). The more selective, nonsedative, and potent antihistamine, terfenadine, also cause bronchodilatation in asthmatic subjects with variable inhibitory effects against antigen-induced bronchoconstriction (75,76). Similarly, astemizole attenuates airway responses to exercise and to antigen in asthmatics (77). Clinical experience with antihistamines in asthma has not been encouraging (78,79), but the newer antihistamines, terfenadine and astemizole, remain to be tested clinically in asthma. Blockade of histamine H-2 receptors in asthmatic subjects does not alter baseline airway function or the acute response to allergen in asthmatic subjects (71).

Cyclooxygenase Products

PGD_2 and $F_{2\alpha}$ are potent bronchoconstrictor agents when administered by aerosol, and PGD_2 is 30 times more active than histamine (80,81). Ipratropium bromide partially inhibited PGD_2-induced constriction, suggesting the role of reflex cholinergic mechanisms (82). The effect of TxA_2 in humans is not known, but it is known to cause bronchoconstriction in animals (83). PGE_1 and E_2 are bronchodilators in asthmatic subjects (84), but bronchoconstrictor responses have also been reported (85), possibly caused by stimulation of airway afferent vagal C fibers. $PGF_{2\alpha}$ and PGD_2 can transiently enhance the airway response to histamine and methacholine (41,42). Potentiation of cholinergic neurotransmission by $PGF_{2\alpha}$ and TxA_2-mimetic (U46619) occurs in canine airways in vitro (39,43). $PGF_{2\alpha}$ and E_2 are potent inducers of cough (86). Inhaled $PGF_{2\alpha}$ increases airway secretions (87). Little is known about the potential of cyclo-oxygenase products to induce an inflammatory response in the airways. Injection of PGD_2 into human skin induces an immediate wheal and flare with a biphasic perivenular neutrophil infiltrate (88).

Raised levels of a $PGF_{2\alpha}$ metabolite and TXB_2 in plasma (89,90), and of PGD_2 in BAL (47) have been measured during antigen-induced bronchoconstriction in asthmatic subjects. Inhibition of the cyclo-oxygenase pathway with indomethacin has no effect on resting pulmonary function of normal and asthmatic subjects (91,92) although some asthmatics experience symptomatic worsening after taking aspirin or indomethacin (93). Indomethacin does not influence exercise-induced asthma, but prevents the tachyphylactic bronchoconstrictor response to successive bouts of exercise (94).

Indomethacin or aspirin has no effect on the early acute response induced by inhaled antigen in asthmatic subjects (90,91,95), despite inhibition of the early rise in plasma TxB_2 (90). Flurbiprofen, another inhibitor of the cyclo-oxygenase pathway, had a significant inhibitory effect in atopic nonasthmatic subjects challenged with allergen, an effect not potentiated by the concurrent administration of an H-1 antagonist (75). Whether these conflicting results represent differences between atopic asthmatics and nonasthmatics or differences in potency of cyclo-oxygenase inhibitors is not clear. The late response to antigen is inhibited by indomethacin, aspirin, or benaxoprofen (90,95), an effect which is accompanied by a fall in TxB_2 plasma levels and by a rise in PGI_2 levels (90). However, Kirby et al. (96) failed to inhibit antigen-induced late asthmatic responses with indomethacin in a double-blind, placebo-controlled trial, but they showed a significant reduction in the associated increase in bronchial responsiveness. These results are in accordance with the importance of cyclo-oxygenase products, particularly thromboxane A_2, for the development of airway hyperresponsiveness in dogs (97). In addition, inhibition of thromboxane synthetase by OKY-046 significantly improves bronchial hyperresponsiveness to methacholine in asthmatic subjects (58). The recent availability of thromboxane receptor antagonists will be most helpful in dissecting its contribution to asthmatic responses.

Lipoxygenase Products

LTC_4 and D_4 are approximately 1,000–5,000 times more potent than histamine in causing bronchoconstriction in normal and asthmatic subjects (98,99). LTE_4 is less potent than LTD_4, but has a longer duration of action (100). Asthmatic subjects are hyperresponsive to inhaled leukotrienes (100–102). In vitro, both LTC_4 and D_4 are potent stimulants of mucus release from human airways (103). LTC_4, D_4, and E_4 increase airway microvascular permeability in the guinea pig (104), possibly by a direct effect on postcapillary venular endothelial cells. The microvascular leakage induced by LTB_4 probably depends upon the emigration and interaction of neutrophils through the endothelial microvasculature (105).

LTB_4 is an extremely potent chemotactic and chemokinetic agent for neutrophils in vitro (106), but is less effective for eosinophils (107). When instilled locally into human airways in vivo, LTB_4 increases recovery of neutrophils in BAL (108). LTB_4 activates human neutrophils to cause the release of lysosomal enzymes (109) and of superoxide anions (110), and enhances the expression of surface complement receptors on human neutrophils and eosinophils (111). LTB_4 increases bronchial responsiveness to acetylcholine in dogs (112) but not in humans (113). LTE_4, but not LTD_4, transiently enhances the constrictor effect of histamine (99,114).

Dietary supplementation with eicosapentaenoic acid (fish oil) leads to decreased formation of lipoxygenase products by diversion to the less active eicosapentaenoic derivatives such as LTB_5, C_5, and D_5. However, no clinical benefit was observed in asthmatic subjects fed a fish oil diet (115).

Sulfidopeptide leukotrienes have been detected occasionally in the plasma of subjects with acute asthma (54), but LTE_4 has been recovered from BAL of asthmatic subjects (53). The 5-lipoxygenase inhibitors, AA-361 and REV 5901, had no effect on airway responsiveness (58) or on baseline lung function (116), respectively. In vitro, FPL 55712, a leukotriene antagonist, and Piriprost (U-60,257), an inhibitor of LTC_4 and LTD_4 synthesis, attenuates allergen-induced bronchial contraction of sensitized human airways (117,118). However, in vivo, Piriprost had no effect on allergen challenge in asthmatic subjects (119). Another LTD_4 receptor antagonist, L-649,923, had no significant effects on the early and late asthmatic response to antigen (120). However, it is not possible to ascertain whether this antagonist was effective at the doses used (57).

Platelet-Activating Factor (PAF)

Inhaled PAF causes a rapid onset of bronchoconstriction in humans, and is about 100-fold more potent than methacholine (43,121). This effect is rapidly tachyphylactic to further doses, preventing cumulative dose–response studies. Interestingly, asthmatic subjects who are hyperresponsive to methacholine, show similar bronchoconstrictor responses to PAF as normal subjects (121,122).

Because PAF does not contract human airway smooth muscle in vitro, its in vivo effects could be mediated by the recruitment and activation of circulating cells such as platelets (6). Part of the airway narrowing induced by PAF may be secondary to airway edema since PAF is one of the most potent inducers of airway microvascular leakage (61).

PAF activates a wide range of inflammatory cells in vitro including platelets, neutrophils, and monocytes. PAF is a most potent chemoattractant for eosinophils in vitro (107) and in vivo into the airways of guinea pigs (123). However, inhalation of PAF in humans and dogs only caused an increase in neutrophil recovery in BAL (124,125), but in the skin of atopic subjects, intradermal injection of PAF resulted in a selection accumulation of eosinophils (126). PAF activates eosinophils to cause the release of LTC_4 (127) and eosinophil peroxidase (128). Since PAF may also be generated by eosinophils (18) and eosinophil peroxidase may damage airway epithelium, the potential interactions between PAF and eosinophils may represent a self-potentiating mechanism for inflammatory responses within the asthmatic airway.

PAF induces bronchial hyperresponsiveness in normal human subjects (43, 121), an effect that may last for many weeks (43). Because of its rapid metabolism, this effect of PAF presumably results from secondary mechanisms such as the recruitment of inflammatory cells and perhaps the release of secondary mediators (6).

Using a bioassay technique, PAF has been detected in BAL of asthmatic subjects (129) and in the plasma of asthmatics during allergen-induced late responses (130). Potent PAF antagonists have recently been developed (131) and inhibit several effects of PAF of potential relevance to asthma such as eosinophil activation, bronchoconstriction, and increased airway microvascular permeability. In humans, the gingkolide mixture, BN52063, inhibits PAF- but not histamine-induced cutaneous responses (132); in addition, it inhibits the late phase cutaneous response to allergen in atopic subjects (133). When taken orally, it is only a modest antagonist of the bronchoconstrictor effects of inhaled PAF in humans (134). The protective effect of inhaled BN 52063 is not known. Other potent PAF antagonists such as the triazodiazepine WEB 2086 and the PAF analog CV 3398 are available and under current investigation. PAF antagonists inhibit allergen-induced bronchoconstriction and eosinophil infiltration of the airways in sensitized guinea pigs (123,135,136). In addition, BN 52021 has been reported to attenuate the late phase response and airway hyperresponsiveness induced by allergen in a sensitized rabbit model (137). Similar studies need to be carried out in asthmatic subjects.

Bradykinin

Inhaled bradykinin causes bronchoconstriction in asthmatics but not in normal subjects (138,139). Bradykinin is a potent stimulant of bronchial C fibers in dogs (140) and causes the release of sensory neuropeptides from capsaicin-sensitive nerves (141). The bronchoconstrictor effect of bradykinin may be mediated by these mechanisms as bradykinin does not contract human airways in vitro (139). Bradykinin increases airway microvascular permeability in the guinea pig (142). When applied to the human nasal mucosa, it causes a rise in albumin recovery in nasal washings (143).

Increased plasma kinins have been reported during asthma attacks (144) but the high values reported may represent spontaneous kinin generation in plasma. Allergen challenge of the nasal mucosa of allergic rhinitis subjects results in the recovery of bradykinin and lys-bradykinin in nasal washings (48), but similar measurements have not been made in the lower airways. However, increased kallikrein activity has been detected in BAL of stable asthmatic subjects, which may lead to increased generation of bradykinin within the airways (145). There are no bradykinin antagonists currently available for use in humans.

Sensory Neuropeptides

Tachykinins produce bronchoconstriction both in vitro and in vivo in animals (22). Although SP contracts human airways in vitro, infusion or inhalation of SP has no effect on lung function of normal and asthmatic subjects (146), perhaps due to the rapid enzymatic degradation of SP in the airway epithelium. On the other hand, inhaled NKA causes bronchoconstriction in asthmatic but not in normal subjects (147). SP is a potent inducer of airway microvascular leakage in guinea pig airways (142) and of submucosal gland secretion (148). Although SP may degranulate mast cells in human skin (149), there is no evidence that it does so in the airways. SP may be involved in the regulation of inflammatory responses (150).

There is no direct evidence for the involvement of sensory neuropeptides in asthma nor are there specific antagonists suitable for clinical use. Stimulation of sensory nerves by inflammatory mediators such as bradykinin may cause the release of sensory neuropeptides (141) to induce putative local axon reflexes in the airways (151). These reflexes may also be enhanced in the presence of epithelial damage and desquamation in asthma and have been proposed as a mechanism for amplifying and propagating inflammation in asthmatic airways, leading to enhanced bronchoconstriction and mucosal edema (144,151). Pretreatment of guinea pigs with capsaicin, which causes depletion of sensory neuropeptides, inhibits the edema of the nasal mucosa induced by cigarette smoke (152) and the bronchial hyperresponsiveness resulting from exposure to toluene diisocyanate (153). These results suggest that sensory neuropeptides are involved in the airway inflammatory response to exogenous irritants.

CONCLUSION

The large number of mediators that may be involved in asthma and their potential interactions make it unlikely that only one particular mediator can be responsible for all the pathophysiological manifestations of asthma. A network of mediators may contribute to a particular response of the asthmatic airway such as increased microvascular permeability or airway smooth muscle contraction, such that pharmacologic inhibition of one mediator may not be sufficient to achieve a complete effect. It is unlikely that all cells are activated by the same inflammatory stimulus with the release of all inflammatory mediators. Different profiles of mediators may be released from different cell types according to the stimulus, and this may form the basis for the heterogeneity of severity or presentation of the disease. For example, the self-limited bronchoconstriction induced by exercise may be due to a different spectrum of mediators from that induced by antigen challenge, particularly during the more prolonged late phase response or associated bronchial hyperresponsiveness. Although a great deal of information has now been gathered on the potential contribution of inflammatory mediators on the airways, relatively little is known about the effects resulting from interactions between mediators.

The involvement of many mediators in asthma suggest that inhibitors of individual inflammatory mediators will be less effective than general anti-inflammatory agents such as corticosteroids which act at several different sites to prevent mediator release and to suppress the effects of mediators. However, it is possible that there are initial steps in the inflammatory process that are of prime importance in the pathogenesis of asthma and that inhibition of the effect of the primary mediators involved may be beneficial. Eosinophil chemotaxis into the airways and its activation to release cationic proteins to damage airway epithelium may be such important events in the asthmatic airway, with the resulting damage to airway epithelium being the basis for bronchial hyperresponsiveness. Mediators involved in these early events may be more important to inhibit therapeutically than those acting later on airway target cells such as airway smooth muscle, vascular endothelium and airway nerves. It is also possible that combination of such mediator antagonists may be more effective in the treatment of asthma than when used individually.

ACKNOWLEDGMENTS

I thank Astrid Greenberry for her utmost care in the preparation of this manuscript.

REFERENCES

1. Dunnill MS. The pathology of asthma with special reference to changes in the bronchial mucosa. J Clin Pathol 1960; 13:27–33.
2. Laitinen LA, Heino M, Laitinen A, Kava T, Haahtela T. Damage of the airway epithelium and bronchial reactivity in patients with asthma. Am Rev Respir Dis 1985; 131:599–606.
3. Chung KF. Role of inflammation in the hyperreactivity of the airways in asthma. Thorax 1986; 41:657–662.
4. Barnes PJ, Chung KF, Page CP. Inflammatory mediators in asthma. Pharmacol Rev 1988; 40:49–84.
5. Lewis R, Robin J. Arachidonic acid derivatives as mediators of asthma. J Allergy Clin Immunol 1985; 76:259–264.
6. Barnes PJ, Chung KF, Page CP. Platelet-activating factor as a mediator of allergic disease. J Allergy Clin Immunol 1988; 81:919–934.
7. Barnes PJ. Neuropeptides in human airways: function and clinical implications. Am Rev Respir Dis 1987; 136:577–583.
8. Friedman NM, Kaliner M. The human lung mast cell and asthma. Am Rev Respir Dis 1987; 135:1157–1164.
9. Robinson C, Hardy C, Holgate S. Pulmonary synthesis, release and metabolism of prostaglandin. J Allergy Clin Immunol 1985; 76:265–271.
10. Lewis RA, Austen KF. The biologically active leukotrienes. J Clin Invest 1984; 73:889–897.
11. Snyder F. Chemical and biochemical aspects of platelet activating factor: A novel class of acetylated ether-linked choline phospholipids. Med Res Rev 1985; 5:107–140.
12. Peters SP, Schleimer RP, Naclerio RM, et al. The pathophysiology of human mast cells: in vitro and in vivo function. Am Rev Respir Dis 1987; 135:1196–1200.
13. Takemura R, Werb Z. Secretory products of macrophages and their physiological functions. Am J Physiol (H) 1984; 246:C1–9.
14. Tonnel AB, Joseph M, Gosset Ph, Fournier E, Capron A. Stimulation of alveolar macrophages in asthmatic patients after local provocation test. Lancet 1983; 2:1406–1408.
15. Hunter JA, Finkbeiner WE, Nadel JA, Goetzl EJ, Holtzman MJ. Predominant generation of 15-lipoxygenase metabolites of arachidonic acid by epithelial cells from human trachea. Proc Natl Acad Sci (USA) 1985; 82:4633–4637.
16. Barnes PJ, Cuss FMC, Palmer JBD. The effect of airway epithelium on smooth muscle contractility in bovine trachea. Br J Pharmacol 1985; 86:685–691.
17. Weller PF, Lee CW, Foster DW, Corey EJ, Austen KF, Lewis RA. Generation and metabolism of 5-lipoxygenase pathway leukotrienes by human eosinophils: predominant production of leukotriene C4. Proc Natl Acad Sci (USA) 1983; 80:7626–7630.
18. Lee TC, Lenihan DJ, Malone B, Roddy LL, Wasserman SI. Increased bio-

synthesis of platelet activating factor in activated human eosinophils. J Biol Chem 1984;259:5526–5530.
19. Frigas E, Gleich GJ. The eosinophil and the pathology of asthma. J Allergy Clin Immunol 1986;77:527–537.
20. Camussi G, Aglietta M, Malavasi F, Tetta C, Piacibello W, Sanavio F, Bussolino F. The release of platelet activating factor from human endothelial cells in culture. J Immunol 1983;131:2397–2403.
21. Lynch JM, Henson PM. The intracellular retention of newly-synthetized platelet-activating factor. J Immunol 1986;137:2653–2661.
22. Lundberg JM, Saria A, Lundblad L, Angaard A, Martling C-R, Theodorsson-Norheim E, Stjarne P, Hokfelt T. Bioactive peptides in capsaicin-sensitive C-fiber afferents of the airways: functional and pathophysiological implications. In: *The Airways: Neural Control in Health and Disease*. Kaliner MA, Barnes PJ, eds. New York, Marcel Dekker, 1987; pp 417–445.
23. Stimler-Gerard NP. Neutral endopeptidose-like enzyme controls the contractile activity of substance P in guinea pig lungs. J Clin Invest 1987;79:1819–1825.
24. Hugli TE, Marceau F, Lundberg C. Effects of complement fragments on pulmonary vascular smooth muscle. Am Rev Respir Dis 1987; 135:9–13.
25. Regoli D, Barabe J. Pharmacology of bradykinin and related kinins. Pharmacol Rev 1980;32:1–46.
26. Barnes PJ. Inflammatory mediator recepters and asthma. Am Rev Respir Dis 1987;135:S28–31.
27. Berridge MJ, Dawson RMC, Dawnes CP, Heslop JP, Irvine RF. Changes in the levels of inositol phosphates after agonist-dependent hydrolysis of membrane phosphoinositides. Biochem J 1983;212:473–482.
28. Tamioka M, Shiroh I, Shindoh Y, Ishihara T, Takishima T. Mast cells in the bronchoalveolar lumen of patients with bronchial asthma. Am Rev Respir Dis 1984;129:1000–1005.
29. Flint KC, Leung KBP, Hudspith BN, Brostoff J, Pearce FL, Johnson NM. Bronchoalveolar mast cells in extrinsic asthma: a mechanism for the initiation of antigen specific bronchoconstriction. Br Med J 1985; 291:923–926.
30. Godard P, Chaintreuil J, Damon M, Coupe M, Flandre O, Crastes de Paulet A, Michel FB. Functional assessment of alveolar macrophages: comparison of cells from asthmatics and normal subjects. J Allergy Clin Immunol 1982; 70:88–93.
31. Cluzel M, Damon M, Chanez P, Bousquet J, Crastes de Paulet A, Michel FB, Godard Ph. Enhanced alveolar cell luminol-dependent chemiluminescence in asthma. J Allergy Clin Immunol 1987;80:195–201.
32. Arnoux B, Joeph M, Simoes AH, Tonvel AB, Duraux P, Capron A, Benveniste J. Antigenic release of PAF-acether and beta-glucuronidase from alveolar macrophages of asthmatics. Bull Eur Physiopathol Respir 1987; 23:119–124.
33. Chanez P, Dent G, Yukawa T, Chung KF, Barnes PJ. Increased eosinophil

responsiveness to platelet-activating factor in asthma. Am Rev Respir Dis 1988; 137:281.
34. Peters SP, Kagey-Sobtka A, MacGlashan DW, Lichtenstein LM. Effect of prostaglandin D2 in modulating histamine from human basophils. J Pharmacol Exp Ther 1984; 228:400–406.
35. Dessein AJ, Lee TH, Elsas P, et al. Enhancement of monokines of leukotriene generation by human eosinophils and neutrophils stimulated with calcium ionphere A23187. J Immunol 1986; 136:3829–3838.
36. Silberstein DS, David JR. The regulation of human eosinophil function by cytokines. Immunol Today 1987; 8:380–385.
37. Copas JL, Borgeat P, Gardiner PJ. The actions of 5-, 12-, and 15-HETE on tracheobronchial smooth muscle. Prost Leuk Med 1982; 8:105–114.
38. Lee TH, Austen KF, Corey EJ, Drazen JM. LTE4-induced airway hyperresponsiveness of guinea pig tracheal smooth muscel to histamine and evidence for 3 separate sulfidopeptide leukotriene receptors. Proc Natl Acad Sci (USA) 1984; 81:4922–4925.
39. Chung KF, Evans TW, Graf PD, Nadel JA. Modulation of cholinergic neurotransmission in canine airways by thromboxane-mimetic U 46619. Eur J Pharmacol 1985; 117:373–375.
40. Tanaka DT, Grunstein MM. Effect of substance P on neurally mediated contraction of rabbit airway smooth muscle. J Appl Physiol 1986; 60: 458–463.
41. Walters EH, Parrish RW, Bevan C, Smoth AP. Induction of bronchial hypersensitivity: evidence for a role of prostaglandins. Thorax 1981; 36:571–574.
42. Fuller RW, Dixon CMS, Dollery CT, Barnes PJ. Prostaglandin D2 potentiates airway responses to histamine and methacholine. Am Rev Respir Dis 1986; 133:252–254.
43. Cuss FM, Dixon CMS, Barnes PJ. Effects of inhaled platelet activating factor on pulmonary function and bronchial responsiveness in man. Lancet 1986; 2:189–192.
44. Williams TJ, Morley J. Prostaglandins as potentiators of increased vascular permeability in inflammation. Nature 1973; 246:215–217.
45. O'Byrne PM, Dolovich J, Hargreave FE. Late asthmatic responses. Am Rev Respir Dis 1987; 136:740–751.
46. Chung KF, Osborne ML, Corrales R, Evans TW, McCabe L, Frick OL, Gold WM. Histamine release and circulating cells after antigen inhalation in allergic dogs. J Appl Physiol 1987; 62:253–258.
47. Murray JJ, Tonnel AB, Brash AR, Roberts LJ, Gosset P, Workman R, Cafron A, Oates JA. Release of Prostaglandin D2 into human airways during acute antigen challenge. N Engl J Med 1986; 315:800–804.
48. Creticos PS, Peters SP, Adkinson NF, et al. Peptide leukotriene release after antigen challenge in patients sensitive to ragweed. N Engl J Med 1984; 310:1626–1630.
49. Proud D, Togias A, Naclerio RM, Crush SA, Norman PS, Lichtenstein LM. Kinins are generated in vivo following nasal airway challenge of allergic individuals with allergen. J Clin Invest 1983; 72:1678–1685.

50. Gravelyn TR, Pan PM, Eschenbacher WL. Mediator release in an isolated airway segment in subjects with asthma. Am Rev Respir Dis 1988; 137: 641–646.
51. Henderson WR, Jorg A, Klebanoff SJ. Eosinophil peroxidase-mediated inactivation of leucotrienes B4, C4 and D4. J Immunol 1982; 128:2609–2613.
52. Paredes J-M, Weiss SJ. Human neutrophils transform prostaglandins by a myeloperoxidase-dependent mechanism. J Biol Chem 1982; 257:2738–2740.
53. Lam S, Chan H, Leriche JC, Chan-Yeung M, Salari H. Release of leukotrienes in patients with bronchial asthma. J Allergy Clin Immunol 1988; 81:711–717.
54. Morris HR, Taylor GW, Clinton PM, et al. Measurement of leukotrienes in asthma. Adv Prost Throm Leuk Res 1983; 11:221–228.
55. Latrigue-Mattei C, Godeneche D, Chabard JL, Petie J, Berger JA. Pharmakokinetic study of ^{3}H-labelled Paf-acether. II. Comparison with ^{3}H-labelled lyso-Paf-acether after intravenous administration in the rabbit and protein binding. Ag Act 1984; 15:643–648.
56. Haroldsen PE, Voelkel NF, Henson JE, Henson PM, Murphy RC. Metabolism of platelet-activating factor in isolated perfused rat lung. J Clin Invest 1987; 79:1860–1867.
57. Barnes NC, Piper PJ, Costello J. The effect of an oral leukotriene antagonist L-649, 923 on histamine and leukotriene D4-induced bronchoconstriction in normal man. J Allergy Clin Immunol 1987; 79:816–821.
58. Fujimura M, Sasaki F, Nakatsumi Y, Takahashi Y, Hifumi S, Taga K, Mifune JI, Tanaka T, Matsuda T. Effects of thromboxane synthetase inhibitor (OKY-046) and a lipoxygenase inhibitor (AA-861) on bronchial responsiveness to acetylcholine in asthmatic subjects. Thorax 1986; 41:955–959.
59. Casterline CL, Evans R, Ward GW. The effect of atropine and albuterol aerosols on the human bronchial response to histamine. J Allergy Clin Immunol 1976; 58:607–613.
60. Simonsson BG, Jacobs FM, Nadel JA. Role of autonomic nervous system and the cough reflex in the increased responsiveness of airways in patients with obstructive airway disease. J Clin Invest 1967; 46:1812–1818.
61. Evans TW, Chung KF, Rogers DF, Barnes PJ. Effect of platelet-activating factor on airway vascular permeability: possible mechanisms. J Appl Physiol 1987; 63:479–484.
62. Baumgarten CR, Nichold RC, Naclerio RM, Lichtenstein LM, Norman PS, Proud D. Plasma kallikrein during experimentally-induced allergic rhinitis: Role in kinin formation and contribution to TAME-esterase activity in nasal secretions. J Immunol 1986; 137:977–982.
63. Shelhamer J, Marom Z, Kaliner M. Immunologic and neuropharmacologic stimulation of mucous glycoprotein release from human airways in vitro. J Clin Invest 1980; 66:1400–1408.
64. Clark RAF, Sandler JA, Gallin JI, Kaplan AP. Histamine modulation of eosinophil migration. J Immunol 1977; 118:137–145.

65. Barnes PJ, Ind PW, Brown MJ. Plasma histamine and catecholamines in stable asthmatic subjects. Clin Sci 1982; 62:661-665.
66. Barnes PJ, Brown MJ. Venous plasma histamine in exercise and hyperventilation induced asthma in man. Clin Sci 1981; 61:159-162.
67. Howarth PH, Durham SR, Lee TH, Kay AB, Church MK, Holgate ST. Influence of albuterol, cromolyn sodium and ipratropium bromide on the airway and circulating mediator responses to allergen bronchial provocation in asthma. Am Rev Respir Dis 1985; 132:986-992.
68. Nagy L, Lee TH, Kay AB. Neutrophil chemotactic activity in antigen-induced late asthmatic reactions. N Engl J Med 1982; 306:497-501.
69. Keyser JJ, Kauffman HF, Demonchy JGR, Keyzer-Udding JJ, De Vries K. Urinary N+-methylhistamine during early and late allergen-induced bronchial obstructive reaction. J Allergy Clin Immunol 1984; 74:240-245.
70. Morgan DJR, Moodley I, Phillips MJ, Davies RJ. Plasma histamine in asthmatic and control subjects following exercise: influence of circulating basophils and different assay techniques. Thorax 1983; 38:771-777.
71. Eiser NM, Mills J, Snashall PD, Guz A. The role of histamine receptors in asthma. Clin Sci 1981; 60:363-370.
72. Nogrady SG, Hartley JPR, Handslip PDJ, Hurst NP. Bronchodilatation after inhalation of an antihistamine, Clemastine. Thorax 1978; 33:396-404.
73. Dowdrd AJ, Patel KR. A comparison of Ketotifen with clemastine, ipratropium bromide and sodium cromoglycate in exercise-induced asthma. Clin Allergy 1982; 12:355-361.
74. Phillips MJ, Ollier S, Gould C, Davies RJ. Effect of antihistamines and antiallergic drugs on responses to allergen and histamine provocation tests in asthma. Thorax 1984; 39:345-351.
75. Curzen N, Rafferty P, Holgate ST. Effects of cyclo-oxygenase inhibitor, flurbiprofen and on Hl histamine recepter antagonist, terfenadine alone and in combination an allergen induced immediate bronchoconstriction in man. Thorax 1987; 42:946-952.
76. Chan TB, Shelton DM, Eiser NM. Effect of an oral H1-receptor antagonist, terfenadine, on antigen-induced asthma. Br J Dis Chest 1986; 80:375-384.
77. Holgate ST, Emmanuel MB, Howarth PH. Astemizole and other H1-antihistaminic drug treatments of asthma. J Allergy Clin Immunol 1985; 76: 375-380.
78. Karlin JM. The use of antihistamines in asthma. Ann Allergy 1972; 30: 342-347.
79. Lewiston NJ, Johnson S, Sloan E. Effect of antihistamine on pulmonary function of children with asthma. J Pediatr 1982; 101:458-460.
80. Smith AP, Cuthbert MF, Dunlop LS. Effects of inhaled prostaglandins E1, E2, and F2α on the airway resistance of healthy and asthmatic man. Clin Sci Mol Med 1975; 48:421-430.
81. Harding CC, Robinson C, Tattersfield AE, Holgate ST. The bronchoconstrictor effect of inhaled prostaglandin D2 in normal and asthmatic men. N Engl J Med 1984; 311:209-213.
82. Beasley R, Varley J, Robinson C, Holgate ST. Cholinergic-mediated bronchoconstriction induced by prostaglandin D2, its initial metabolite

9α, 11B-PGF2 and PGF2α in asthma. Am Rev Respir Dis 1987; 136:1140–1144.
83. Svensson J, Stranberg GK, Tuvemo T, Hamberg M. Thromboxane A2: Effects on airway and vascular smooth muscle. Prostaglandins 1977; 14: 425–437.
84. Kawakami Y, Uchiyama K, Irie T, Murao M. Evaluation of aerosols of prostaglandins E1 and E2 on bronchodilators. Eur J Clin Pharmacol 1973; 6:127–32.
85. Herxheimer H, Roetscher I. Effects of prostaglandin E1 on lung function in bronchial asthma. Eur J Clin Pharm 1971; 3:123–125.
86. Costello JF, Dunlop LS, Gardiner PJ. Characteristics of prostaglandin-induced cough in man. Br J Clin Pharmacol 1985; 20:355–359.
87. Lopez-Vidriero MI, Das I, Smith AP, Picot R, Reid L. Bronchial secretion from normal human airways after inhalation of prostaglandin F2alpha, acetylcholine, histamine and citric acid. Thorax 1977; 32:734–739.
88. Flower RJ, Harvey EA, Kingston WP. Inflammatory effects of prostaglandin D2 in rat and human skin. Br J Pharmacol 1976; 56:229–233.
89. Green K, Hedqvist P, Svanborg N. Increased plasma levels of 15-keto 13,14-dihydro-prostaglandin F2a after allergen-provoked asthma in man. Lancet 1974; 1419–1421.
90. Shephard EG, Malon L, Macfarlane CM, Mouton W, Joubert JR. Lung function and plasma levels of thromboxane B2, 6-keto-prostaglandin F1alpha, beta-thromboglobulin in antigen-induced asthma before and after indomethacin pretreatment. Br J Clin Pharmacol 1985; 19:459–470.
91. Fish JE, Ankin MG, Adkinson Jr NF, Peterman VI. Indomethacin modification of immediate-type immunologic airway responses in allergic asthmatic and nonasthmatic subjects. Am Rev Respir Dis 1981; 123:609–614.
92. Ogilvy CS, Dubois AB, Douglas JS. Effects of ascorbic acid and indemethacin on the airways of healthy male subjects with and without induced bronchoconstriction. J Allergy Clin Immunol 1981; 67:363–369.
93. Szczeklik A, Gryglewski RJ, Czerniawska-Mysik G. Relationship of inhibition of prostaglandin biosynthesis by analgesics to asthma attacks in aspirin-sensitive patients. Br Med J 1975; 1:67–69.
94. O'Byrne PM, Jones GL. The effect of indomethacin on exercise-induced bronchoconstriction and refractiveness after exercise. Am Rev Respir Dis 1986; 134:69–72.
95. Fairfax AJ, Hanson JM, Morley J. The late reaction following bronchial provocation with house dust mite allergen: Dependence on arachidonic acid metabolism. Clin Exp Immunol 1983; 52:393–398.
96. Kirby JG, Hargreave FE, Cockcroft DW, O'Byrne PM. Effect of indomethacin on allergen-induced asthmatic responses. J Appl Physiol 1989; 66:578–583.
97. Chung KF, Aizawa H, Becker AB, Frick O, Gold WM, Nadel JA. Inhibition of antigen-induced airway hyperresponsiveness by a thromboxane synthetase inhibitor (OKY-046) in allergic dogs. Am Rev Respir Dis 1986; 134: 258–261.
98. Weiss JW, Drazen JM, McFadden ER, et al. Airway constriction in normal

humans produced by inhalation of leukotriene D: potency, time, course, and effect of aspirin therapy. JAMA 1983; 249:2814-2817.

99. Barnes NC, Piper PJ, Costello JF. Comparative effects of inhaled leukotrine C4, leukotriene D4, and histamine in normal human subjects. Thorax 1984; 39:500-504.

100. Davidson AB, Lee TH, Scanlon PD, Solway J, McFadden ER, Ingram RH, Corey EJ, Austen KF, Drazen JM. Bronchoconstrictor effects of leukotriene E4 in normal and asthmatic subjects. Am Rev Respir Dis 1987; 135:333-337.

101. Smith LJ, Greenberger PA, Patterson R, Krell RD, Bernstein PR. The effect of inhaled leukotriene D4 in humans. Am Rev Respir Dis 1985; 131: 368-372.

102. Adelroth E, Morris MM, Hargreave FE, O'Byrne PM. Airway responsiveness to leukotrienes C4 and D4 and to methacholine in patients with asthma and normal controls. N Engl J Med 1986; 315:480-484.

103. Marom Z, Schelhamer JH, Bach MK, Morton DR, Kaliner M. Slow reacting substances LTC4 and D4 increases the release of mucus from human airways in vitro. Am Rev Respir Dis 1982; 126:449-451.

104. Hua X-Y, Dahlen S-E, Lundberg JM, Hammerstrom S, Hedqvist P. Leukotrienes C4 and E4 cause widespread and extensive plasma extravasation in the guinea-pig. Naunyn-Schmiedeberg's Arch Pharmacol 1985; 330: 136-141.

105. Bjork J, Hedqvist P, Afors K-E. Increase of vascular permeability induced by leukotriene B4 and the role of polymorphonuclear leukocytes. Inflammation 1982; 6:189-200.

106. Ford-Hutchinson AW, Bray MA, Doig MV, Shipley ME, Smith MJH. Leukotriene B4, a potent chemokinetic and aggregating substance released from polymorphonuclear leukocytes. Nature 1981; 286:264-265.

107. Wardlaw AJ, Moqbel R, Cromwell O, Kay AB. Platelet-activating factor. A potent chemotactic and chemokinetic factor for human eosinophils. J Clin Invest 1986; 78:1701-1706.

108. Martin TR, Pistorese BP, Matthay MA. Leukotriene B4 recruits active neutrophils into normal human lungs (abstr). Am Rev Respir Dis 1988; 137:372.

109. Feinemark SJ, Lindgren JA, Claesson H-E, Malmsten C, Samuelsson B. Stimulation of human leukocyte degranulation by leukotriene B4 and its omega-oxidized metabolites. FEBS Letters 1981; 136:141-144.

110. Serhan CN, Radin A, Smolen JE, Korchak H, Samuelsson B, Weissmann G. Leukotriene B4 is a complete secretagogue in human neutrophils: a kinetic analysis. Biochem Biophys Res Commun 1982; 107:1006-1012.

111. Nagy L, Lee TH, Goetzl EJ, Pickett W, Kay AB. Complement receptor enhancement and chemotaxis of human neutrophils and eosinophils by leukotrienes and other lipoxygenase products. Clin Exp Immunol 1982; 47:541-547.

112. O'Byrne PM, Leikauf GD, Aizawa H, Bethel RA, Ueki IF, Holtzman MJ, Nadel JA. Leukotriene B4 induces airway hyperresponsiveness in dogs. J Appl Physiol 1985; 59:1941-1946.

113. Black PN, Fuller RW, Taylor GW, Barnes PJ, Dollery CT. Inhalation of LTB4 together with PGD2 does not lead to an increase in bronchial reactivity (abstr). Am Rev Respir Dis 1988; 137:508.
114. Arm JP, Spur BW, Lee TH. The effects of inhaled leukotriene E_4 on the airway responsiveness to histamine in subjects with asthma and normal subjects. J Allergy Clin Immunol 1988; 82:654–660.
115. Arm JP, Horton CE, Mencia-Huerta J-M, House F, Eiser NM, Clark TJH, Spur BW, Lee TH. Effect of dietary supplementation with fish oil in asthma. Thorax 1988; 43:84–92.
116. Van Inwegen RG, Khandwala A, Gordon R, Sonnind P, Coutts S, Jolly S. Rev 5901: An orraly effective peptidoleukotriene antagonist, detailed biochemical/pharmacological profile. J Pharmacol Exp Ther 1987; 241: 117–124.
117. Adams GK, Lichtenstein LM. Antagonism of antigen-induced contraction of guinea pig and human airways. Nature 1977; 270:255–257.
118. Dahlen SE, Hansson G, Heqvist P, Bjorck T, Granstrom E, Dahlen B. Allergen challenge of lung tissue from asthmatics elicits bronchial contraction that correlates with the release of leukotrienes C4, D4 and E4. Proc Natl Acad Sci (USA) 1983; 80:1712–1718.
119. Mann JS, Robinson C, Sheridan AQ, Clement P, Bach MK, Holgate ST. Effect of inhaled Piriprost (U-60257), a novel leukotriene inhibitor, on allergen and exercise induced bronchoconstriction in asthma. Thorax 1986; 41:746–752.
120. Britton JR, Hanley SP, Tattersfield AE. The effect of an oral leukotriene D4 antagonist L-649,923 on the response to inhaled antigen in asthma. J Allergy Clin Immunol 1987; 79:811–816.
121. Rubin A-H, Smith LJ, Patterson R. The bronchoconstrictor properties of platelet-activating factor in humans. Am Rev Respir Dis 1987; 136:1145–1151.
122. Chung KF, Barnes PJ. Effects of platelet-activating factor on airway calibre, airway responsiveness and circulating cells in asthmatic subjects. Thorax 1989; 44:108–115.
123. Lellouch-Tubiana A, Lefort J, Simon M-T, Pfister A, Vargaftig BB. Eosinophil recruitment into guinea pig lungs after PAF-acether and allergen administration: modulation by prostacyclin, platelet depletion and selective antagonists. Am Rev Respir Dis 1988; 137:948–954.
124. Wardlaw AJ, Chung KF, Moqbel R, Hartnell A, McCusker M, Barnes PJ, Kay AB. Effect of inhaled platelet-activating factor on lung cells and circulating neutrophils in-vivo: Relationship to changes in lung function. Am Rev Respir Dis 1989; in press.
125. Chung KF, Aizawa H, Leikauf GD, Ueki IF, Evans TW, Nadel JA. Airway hyperresponsiveness induced by platelet-activating factor: role of thromboxane generation. J Phrmacol Exp Ther 1986; 236:580–584.
126. Henocq E, Vargaftig BB. Skin eosinophilia in atopic patients. J Allergy Clin Immunol 1988; 81:691–695.
127. Bruijnzeel PLB, Koenderman L, Kok PTM, Hamelink ML, Verhagen JL. Platelet activating factor (PAF-acether) induced leukotriene C4 formation

and luminol dependent chemi-luminescence of human eosinophils. Pharm Res Comm 1986; 18:61–69.
128. Kroegel C, Yukawa T, Chanez P, Dent G, Chung KF, Barnes PJ. Release of eosinophil peroxidase by platelet-activating factor from human eosinophils. Immunology 1988; 64:559–562.
129. Court EN, Goadby P, Hendrick DJ, Kelly CA, Kingston W, Stenton SC, Walters EH. Platelet-activating factor in bronchoalveolar lavage fluid from asthmatic patients (abstr). Br J Clin Pharmacol 1987; 24:258.
130. Nakamura T, Morita Y, Kuriyama M, Ishihara K, Ito K, Miyamoto T. Platelet-activating facter in late asthmatic response. Int Arch Allergy Appl Immunol 1987; 82:57–61.
131. Chung KF, Barnes PJ. PAF antagonists: their therapeutic role in asthma. Drugs 1988; 35:93–103.
132. Chung KF, Dent G, McCusker M, Guinot PM, Page CP, Barnes PJ. Effect of a ginkgolide mixture (BN 52063) in antagonising skin and platelet responses to platelet activating factor in man. Lancet 1987; 1:248–251.
133. Roberts NM, Page CP, Chung KF, Barnes PJ. The effect of a specific PAF antagonists, BN 52063, on antigen-induced cutaneous responses in man. J Allergy Clin Immunol 1988; 82:236–241.
134. Roberts NM, McCusker MT, Barnes PJ. Effect of a PAF antagonist BN 52063 on PAF-induced bronchoconstriction and neutropenia in man. Br J Clin Pharmacol 1988; 26:65–72.
135. Touvay C, Etienne A, Braquet P. Inhibition of antigen-induced lung anaphylaxis in the guinea-pig by BN 52021 a new specific PAF-acether receptor antagonist isolated from Ginkgo biloba. Ag Act 1985; 17:371–372.
136. Casals-Stenzel J. Effects of WEB 2086, a novel antagonist of platelet-activating factor in active and passive anaphylaxis. Immunopharmacology 1987; 3:7–24.
137. Metzger WJ, Sjoersma K, Borwn L, Coyle T, Page C, Touvay C. The late phase asthmatic response in the allergic rabbit: A role for PAFG and modification by PAF antagonist, Ginkgolide BN5201. The role of platelet-activating facter in immune disorders. New Trends Lipid Med 1988; 2:40–58.
138. Simonsson BG, Skoogh BE, Bergh NP, Anderson R, Svedmyr N. In vivo and in vitro effect of bradykinin on bronchial motor tone in normal subjects and in patients with airway obstruction. Respiration 1973; 30:378–388.
139. Fuller RW, Dixon CMS, Cuss FMC, Barnes PJ. Bradykinin-induced bronchoconstriction in man: mode of action. Am Rev Respir Dis 1987; 135:176–180.
140. Kaufman MP, Coleridge HM, Coleridge JCG, Baker DG. Bradykinin stimulates afferent vagal C-fibers in intrapulmonary airways of dogs. J Appl Physiol 1980; 48:511–517.
141. Ueda N, Maramatsu I, Fujiwara M. Capsaicin and bradykin-induced substance P-ergic responses in the iris sphincter muscle of the rabbit. J Pharmacol Exp Ther 1984; 230:469–473.

142. Saria A, Lundberg JM, Skofitsch G, Lembeck F. Vascular protein leakage in various tissues induced by substance P, capsaicin, bradykinin, serotonin, histamine and by antigen challenge. Naunyn-Schmiedeberg's Arch Pharmacol 1983; 324:212-218.
143. Proud D, Reynolds CJ, Lacapra S, Kagey-Sobotka A, Lichtenstein LM, Naclerio RM. Nasal provocation with bradykinin induces symptoms of rhinitis and a sore throat. Am Rev Respir Dis 1988; 137:613-616.
144. Abe K, Watanab N, Kumagai L, Moumi T, Steki T, Yosunga K. Circulating plasma kinin in patients with bronchial asthma. Experientia 1967; 22:626-627.
145. Christiansen SC, Proud D, Cochrane CG. Detection of tissue kallikrein in the bronchoalveolar lavage fluid of asthmatic patients. J Clin Invest 1987; 79:188-197.
146. Fuller RW, Maxwell DL, Dixon CMS, McGregor GP, Barnes VF, Bloom SR, Barnes PJ. The effects of substance P on cardiovascular and respiratory function in human subjects. J Appl Physiol 1987; 62:1473-1479.
147. Joos G, Pauwels R, Van Der Straeten M. Effect of inhaled substance P and neurokinin A on the airways of normal and asthmatic subjects. Thorax 1987; 42:779-783.
148. Coles SJ, Neill KH, Reid LM. Potent stimulation of glycoprotein secretion in canine trachea by substance P. J Appl Physiol 1984; 57:1323-1327.
149. Barnes PJ, Brown MJ, Dollery CT, Fuller RW, Heavey DJ, Ind PW. Histamine is released from skin by substance p but does not act as the final vasodilator in the axon reflex. Br J Pharmacol 1986; 88:741-745.
150. Payan GP, Levine JD, Goetzl EJ. Modulation of immunity and hypersensitivity by sensory neuropeptides. J Immunol 1984; 132:1601-1604.
151. Barnes PJ. Asthma as an axon reflex. Lancet 1986; 1:242-245.
152. Lundberg JM, Saria A. Capsaicin-induced desensitization of the airway mucosa to cigarette smoke, mechanical and chemical irritants. Nature 1983; 302:251-253.
153. Thompson JE, Scypinski L, Gordon T, Sheppard D. Tackykinins mediate toluene diisocyanate induced airway hyperresponsiveness in guinea pigs. Am Rev Respir Dis 1987; 136:43-49.
154. Chung KF, Barnes PJ. Bronchial hyperresponsiveness and inflammation in asthma. In: *Asthma Reviews*, Morley J, ed. Academic Press, New York, 1987, pp 25-41.

9

Cough as a Manifestation of Asthma

E. H. RAMSDALE

St. Joseph's Hospital and McMaster University
Hamilton, Ontario, Canada

Classically, attacks of asthma are characterized by breathlessness and wheezing, but clinically it is obvious that cough is a frequent accompaniment (1) and the paroxysmal cough may be as distressing as the dyspnea. The exact mechanism producing cough, however, is not always apparent although relief by beta-agonists is suggestive that the cough is secondary to bronchospasm. Cough can be secondary to sputum production or related to the irritation from impacted mucus plugs. In addition to the classical wheezy presentation of asthma, over the last 15 years it has become apparent that cough may be the sole symptom of asthma, in both adults and children (2-11).

This chapter discusses the physiology of cough and possible pathological changes leading to cough in asthma.

CLINICAL STUDIES

There is increasing evidence in the literature that isolated chronic cough may be the sole manifestation of asthma in both adults (3-5) and children (6-11). In these studies, the diagnosis has been made on the basis of airflow obstruction reversible after administration of a beta-agonist, or by the demonstration of airway hyperresponsiveness using methacholine inhalation or exercise testing. It has been shown that the cough in these patients has often been present for some time, with repeated unsuccessful treatment with antihistamines, cough suppressants, or antibiotics. Uniformly the patients have been shown to respond to treatment with antiasthmatic medications. Thus an increased suspicion of the possible diagnosis of asthma in patients presenting with cough would lead to decreased morbidity.

The prevalence of cough either as the sole manifestation of asthma, or in association with other symptoms of asthma is not certain, partly due to the difficulty of defining asthma in population surveys (12). In adults presenting to tertiary referral centers with a chronic cough of unknown cause, about 40% were found to have asthma (4,5). In a university pediatric clinic, chronic cough due to asthma was found in 5% of all new patients (8). Chronic cough with or without sputum is surprisingly common in nonsmoking children and young adults (13,14). In a survey of over 15,000 children aged 8-19 in the north of England (13), 35% of boys under 11 reported frequent coughs, and the prevalence decreased with age (18% age 11-13, 10% over age 14 years). The frequency for girls was only slightly less (32%, 17% and 7%). The frequency of cough increased to 50% if there was parental smoking. This could be related to the proportion with asthma, as parental smoking is a known risk for increased symptoms of asthma in childhood (15). There was a similar frequency of chronic cough and phlegm in a cohort of over 10,000 young adults age 23 years born during one week in Britain in 1958 (14). In those who had a history of asthma at age 16, 30% of the nonsmokers and 57% of smokers had chronic cough, whereas in the nonasthmatic group, only 28% of smokers and 8% nonsmokers had cough. The interesting feature of these figures is the similarity to the prevalence of wheeze of over 30% in a population survey in the United States (16).

In those with cough, it is often difficult to separate by history those with an increase in airway responsiveness to histamine or methacholine (i.e., asthma) from those whose responsiveness is normal (6,17-19). In both instances the cough is precipitated by cold air, exercise, and smoke or other irritant fumes. In addition, it is often worse first thing in the morning. In more classical asthmatics these are the factors associated with increased wheeze. In a population study concerning airway responsiveness to an inhaled pharmacological bronchoconstrictor, histamine, there was considerable overlap between normal and increased airway responsiveness in patients presenting with isolated cough (20). This could be explained either because "chronic cough" is a disease separate from asthma, with a range of airway hyperresponsiveness overlapping asthma and nonasthma, or alternatively that all patients with chronic cough have the pathological features of asthma, with an increase in smooth muscle responsiveness in some, and hyperresponsiveness of the cough receptors in others. There is currently not enough information available to distinguish between these two possibilities.

GENERAL MECHANISM OF COUGH

Cough Reflex

Normal cough is a protective mechanism (21) designed to expel foreign bodies from the tracheobronchial tree and warn that irritant gases or smoke are being inhaled. Irritant receptors are located in the oropharynx, larynx, and tracheobronchial tree with an increased density at the carina. Afferent nerves run in the glossopharyngeal, superior laryngeal, and vagus nerves. The cough center is located in the dorsolateral region of the medulla close to the respiratory center. Central connections are made with the respiratory center, and cough is also under voluntary control. Efferent impulses pass from the cough center to coordinate movements of the glottis, diaphragm, and abdominal intercostal muscles (22).

The Irritant Receptor

The physiology of the receptors of the lung can be confusing. Depending on the method used to define them, the myelinated fibers can be referred to as irritant, rapidly adapting stretch receptors, deflation receptors, or cough receptors. In addition, nonmyelinated 'C' fibers have been described in the airway epithelium as well as deeper in the lung (23). The receptors have been identified from single vagal nerve fibers. The activity of the receptors in response to drugs, inhaled irritants, or mechanical probing of the epithelium can be recorded. They have been localized to the trachea and larger bronchi, but also occur in the larynx and pharynx (24). The receptors lie in the paracellular spaces between epithelial cells, separated only by tight junctions from the airway lumen. They are responsive to stimulation by inhaled irritants such as sulfur dioxide, cigarette smoke, dust, ammonia, and in addition pulmonary edema, anaphylaxis, and microembolism. The mechanism of the latter is not clear, but may be related to changes in the interstitial fluid composition (25), and the release of histamine or prostaglandins could have a direct effect on the receptor endings (26). The actual mode of excitation, however, is not known (24).

Role of the Epithelium and Extracellular Fluid

The lining of the airway is permeable to low-molecular weight solutes. There is free interchange between the airway surface liquid and the paracellular spaces so that the irritant receptors sample changes occurring in the surface liquid (24). There appears to be some species difference in the composition of the airway surface liquid [hypotonic in humans (27), hypertonic in dog (28)], so some caution has to be exercised in extrapolating across species. In humans, however, stimuli which change the osmolarity of the surface liquid lead to cough. Hyperventilation of dry air will reproducibly cause cough (29,30), probably due to increasing osmolarity of the surface liquid (28). Inhalation of a mist of distilled water is a potent cause of cough, and appears to be due to the loss of a permeant anion (chloride) (31). Dilution of permeant anions depolarizes afferent nerve receptors by causing an outward anion flux. In addition, osmotic gradients across the epithelium can cause mechanical disruption of the epithelial tight junction by either a fall in electrical resistance or solute diffusion and swelling (32).

The composition of the fluid in the paracellular space between epithelial cells appears to be controlled by the level of cyclic adenosine monophosphate (AMP) in the epithelial cell (33). Elevation of cell cyclic AMP levels causes a reversible increase in transepithelial resistance, suggesting a drop in permeability, and is associated with an increase in the area of cell membrane involved in the tight junction. Epithelial cell levels of cyclic AMP can be increased by direct beta-adrenergic stimulation (34) and, in addition, epinephrine causes the paracellular spaces to decrease in volume (35). This is one possible mechanism for the effectiveness of inhaled fenoterol in the protection of normal subjects against cough induced by distilled water (25), and inhaled terbutaline in the treatment of chronic cough in those with normal airway responsiveness (36). Cough is also attenuated by pretreatment with ipratropium bromide (25) and since anti-muscarinic agents are not believed to act directly on vagal sensory receptors (37), suggests that antimuscarinics, as well as beta-agonists, may have a direct effect on airway epithelium.

Role of Mediators

Prostaglandins are a potent cause of cough in both humans and animals. Prostaglandin $F_2\alpha$ has been shown to stimulate both rapidly adapting stretch "irritant" receptors, and afferent C fiber endings (38,39). Even the bronchodilator prostaglandins PGE_1 and PGE_2 stimulate cough in both humans (40,41) and animals (38). In animals, PGE_2 appears to stimulate C fiber endings rather than irritant receptors (38), which is in keeping with the inability of isoprenaline to prevent cough produced by PGE_2 in humans (40).

In the rat, irritation of the respiratory tract mucosa by cigarette smoke, light mechanical stimuli, or local chemicals (ether, formalin, histamine, bradykinin, or capsaicin) induces subepithelial edema (42). This increase in vascular edema appears to be due to capsaicin-sensitive neurons, which by local axon reflexes release substance P. Substance P has a potent direct stimulating effect on vascular permeability in the airway. Capsaicin produces cough in both animals (43) and humans (44), presumably because capsaicin releases substance P from sensory nerve endings.

Bronchoconstriction

Bronchoconstriction is a potent cause of cough (17). In dogs, histamine aerosol causes both stimulation of irritant receptors and coincident bronchoconstriction (26). Pretreatment with isoprenaline blocks the bronchoconstriction, but the receptors are still activated, indicating a direct action of histamine on the irritant receptor. In contrast, locally applied acetylcholine was able to produce localized bronchoconstriction, but did not stimulate the irritant receptors (26). Hence histamine, but not acetylcholine directly stimulates irritant receptors. In addition, cough and bronchoconstriction can be separated in humans when cough is stimulated by inhaled solutions of different ionic content (31). The absence of a permeant anion led to cough, but not bronchoconstriction, whereas changes from isosmolar led to bronchoconstriction in those with mild asthma. In addition, lidocaine will block the cough but not the bronchoconstriction produced by inhaled distilled water in those with asthma (45). Thus, although bronchoconstrictor agents cause cough, the mechanism has not been established.

Experimental Cough

During the evaluation of new cough suppressants, antitussive potencies of new drugs were compared with codeine using experimentally induced cough in both animals and humans (22). Recently, citric acid (46-48), distilled water (25), and hyperventilation with dry air (29,30) have been used not only to evaluate drugs, but also examine the mechanism of cough production in ***normal*** subjects. Citric acid is thought specifically to stimulate irritant receptors, and inhaled lidocaine will inhibit cough produced by both citric acid (49) and distilled water (45). In contrast, oropharyngeal anesthesia will not inhibit citric acid-induced cough, confirming that the receptors causing cough with citric acid are in the tracheobronchial tree or larynx (50).

MECHANISM OF COUGH IN ASTHMA

In theory, increased sensitivity of any part of the cough reflex could produce an increase in the symptom of cough (51). Thus, cough could be explained by increased receptor sensitivity, lowered threshold of response of the cough center, or increased response of the effector muscles. It is questionable whether any one disease could increase the response of such a diverse variety of muscles as are involved in the production of cough. Cough suppressant medications, such as codeine and analogues, rely on depression of the cough center in the medulla. It has been well documented that these are of no benefit in cough subsequently found to be due to asthma (8). Thus, in asthma, it is likely that the pathological changes in the respiratory tract are responsible for cough. There is also the possibility that cough produced reflexly by stimulation of the vagal afferents, in areas other than the respiratory tract, could be triggered more easily in asthmatics.

Increased Sensitivity of the Irritant Receptors

Apparent increases in sensitivity of the irritant receptors could be brought about either because of a change in the receptor itself, or because of a change in the local environment. Disruption of the epithelium, or increases in leakiness of the tight junction would bring the receptor closer to the events in the airway, leading to a response with a smaller stimulus. The receptors could be stimulated either by changes in the fluid environment or presence of mediators, or there may be intrinsic changes in the receptors themselves resulting in a lower firing threshold. Locally produced inflammatory mediators could potentially lower the firing threshold of the irritant receptor in response to exogenous stimuli.

Damage to the Epithelium

Disruption of the epithelial lining of the airway has been known for many years to be present in patients who died from exacerbations of asthma (52). It has not been easy to obtain pathological specimens from mild asthmatics who do not die from their disease. Recently however, bronchial biopsies have been obtained from a small group of asthmatics, whose asthma varied from mild to severe (53). It was difficult to find normal areas of epithelium in these biopsies. Epithelial desquamation was common. Even when present, the ciliated cells appeared abnormal with swelling apparent on light microscopy, and vacuolization of the endoplasmic reticulum and mitochondria with loss of cilia on electron microscopy. The intercellular spaces were widened. Thus the epithelial damage was prominent enough in even mild asthmatics to expose epithelial nerve endings. In this situation cough could occur more easily in response to exogenous stimuli such as smoke or cold air.

The desquamation of the epithelium can be explained by the presence of eosinophils in the airway lumen, which in addition to being present in sputum in asthmatic exacerbations (54), have been found in bronchoalveolar lavage specimens (55), even in mild asthmatics (56). The major basic protein in eosinophilic granules has been shown to be toxic to respiratory epithelium in the guinea pig with concentrations as low as 10 μg/ml producing ciliostasis at 48 hours and disruption of the epithelium, with damaged cells lying free in the lumen (57). It has also been confirmed that human major basic protein can damage human airway epithelium in the same manner (54). The pathological findings in vitro were similar to the pathological changes observed in bronchial asthma. Major basic protein is present in the sputum of asthmatics and increases during the acute attack (54,58), and in some patients hospitalized with asthma the concentration of the major basic protein was above the minimum known to cause epithelial damage in vitro (57,58).

Viral infections produce cough in nonasthmatic subjects, and the cough threshold measured with citric acid is lower during a viral infection than that after recovery, suggesting that there might be a decreased firing threshold for the irritant receptors in the airway (59). The likely explanation for this change is the airway epithelial damage known to be produced by viral infections such as influenza (60). Viral infections are often precursors for severe exacerbations of asthma in both adults (61) and children (62,63), where cough is particularly troublesome, and the exposure of the cough receptors by both the viral infection and the asthmatic pathology would both lead to epithelial disruption and exposure of the irritant receptors.

Beta-Adrenergic Receptor Function

In the past it has been postulated that there is a defect in beta-receptor function in asthma (64). It currently seems unlikely that this is the fundamental defect in asthma since normal subjects do not develop asthma or airway hyperresponsiveness when treated with beta-blockers. However it is still possible that there is a defect in beta-receptor function secondary to the disease, since leukocyte beta-receptor density and responses are reduced after antigen challenge in asthmatics (65). Since it appears that cyclic AMP levels regulate the permeability of the airway epithelium (33), and that beta-adrenergic stimulation will decrease the volume of paracellular space (35), thus protecting the cough receptor, it is possible that a defect in beta-receptor function could increase the permeability of the epithelium and hence increase cough.

Axon Reflex

A more recent theory concerning the origin of airway hyperresponsiveness in asthma relates to the axon reflex (66). C-fiber afferent nerve endings (nonmyelinated) would be exposed by damage to airway epithelium. These endings could then be stimulated by inflammatory mediators such as bradykinin to produce a local axon reflex, such as occurs with the wheal and flare reaction in the skin. Substance P is responsible for the flare due to local vasodilatation, and is released from the afferent nerves following the local reflex. In addition to its other activities such as producing bronchoconstriction, it is also thought to be a potent cause of cough. Capsaicin (the active ingredient in hot peppers) releases substance P from nerve endings, and is a potent cause of cough in both animals (43) and humans (44). Thus cough in asthma could be secondary to the effect of substance P on the afferent nerve endings.

Sputum Production

A common stimulus to cough in those with respiratory disease is the formation of sputum in the respiratory tract, and the cough process is an essential element in keeping the tract clear (1). When mucus is produced in excess of the capacity of the cilia to move, there is an accumulation of mucus which can only be removed by cough, and sputum is produced. In asthma exacerbations sputum production is common, with eosinophils being the predominant cell type (54,58, 67,68). Chemical mediators released during allergic reactions can also increase the rate of either mucus secretion or water influx into the lumen (69).

Bronchoconstriction

As described in the previous section, although cough can be separated from bronchoconstriction (26,31,45), airway narrowing is a potent cause of cough (17). It has been suggested that those in whom cough is the predominant symptom have disease in the central airways, whereas more peripheral airflow obstruction will cause breathlessness (2). If bronchoconstrictor or inflammatory responses occur in the central airways, mechanical stimulation of the receptors can cause cough.

Gastroesophageal Reflux

Cough of unknown etiology is associated with gastroesophageal reflux (5,70), and treatment of the reflux leads to resolution of the symptom of cough (5). There is an increased incidence of gastroesophageal reflux in asthmatics (71,72). Reflux could cause cough either directly through stimulation of the cough receptors if aspiration occurs, or indirectly through a reflex following stimulation of the vagal afferents in the esophagus. Cough has been reported to be caused by stimulation of vagal afferents in other areas (51,73,74). In addition, acute acid stimulation of the esophagus has been shown to increase airway responsiveness (75,76), so that any exogenous stimulus would be expected to produce a more significant response. However, a controlled study of treatment of the symptoms of reflux in asthmatic subjects had no significant effect on airway responsiveness (77).

TREATMENT

One of the common experiences in medicine is that a symptom is usually not well treated unless a definitive diagnosis can be made (5). With wheeze, the symptom is not appropriately treated by physicians unless a label of asthma has been given (78). It is important therefore to recognize that cough may be the sole symptom of asthma and use appropriate drugs for treatment. Antiasthmatic medications should be used rather than antibiotics and/or antitussives, which are ineffective (8). Both bronchodilators and inhaled steroids have been shown to be effective (5,6,19,36,79,80) in the treatment of cough, whether or not airway responsiveness is increased.

REFERENCES

1. Crofton JC, Douglas A. *Respiratory Diseases* 2nd edition. Blackwell Scientific Publications Ltd., Oxford, 1975; p. 439.
2. McFadden ER Jr. Exertional dyspnea and cough as preludes to acute attacks of bronchial asthma. N Engl J Med 1975; 292:555-559.
3. Corrao WM, Braman SS, Irwin RS. Chronic cough as the sole presenting manifestation of bronchial asthma. N Engl J Med 1979; 300:633-637.
4. Poe RH, Israel RH, Utell MJ, Hall WJ. Chronic cough: Bronchoscopy or pulmonary function testing? Am Rev Respir Dis 1982; 126:160-162.
5. Irwin RS, Corrao WM, Pratter MR. Chronic persistent cough in the adult: the spectrum and frequency of causes and successful outcome of therapy. Am Rev Respir Dis 1981; 123:413-417.
6. Galvez RA, McLaughlin FJ, Levison H. The role of the methacholine challenge in children with chronic cough. J Allergy Clin Immunol 1987; 79:331-335.
7. Hannaway PJ, Hopper DK. Cough variant asthma in children JAMA 1982; 247:206-208.
8. Konig P. Hidden asthma in childhood. Am J Dis Child 1981; 135:1053-1055.
9. Glauser FL. Variant asthma. Ann Allergy 1972; 30:457-459.
10. Cloutier MM, Loughlin GM. Chronic cough in children: a manifestation of airway hyperreactivity. Paediatrics 1981; 67:6-12.
11. Yahav Y, Katznelson D, Benzaray S. Persistent cough–a forme-fruste of asthma. Eur J Respir Dis 1982; 63:43-46.
12. Sears MR. Epidemiology of asthma. In: *Recent Advances in Respiratory Medicine*. Flenley DC, Petty TL, eds. Churchill Livingstone, Edinburgh, 1986; pp. 1-11.
13. Charlton A. Children's coughs related to parental smoking. Br Med J 1984; 1647-1649.
14. Strachan DP, Anderson HR, Bland JM, Peckham C. Asthma as a link between chest illness in childhood and chronic cough and phlegm in young adults. Br Med J 1988; 296:890-893.
15. Murray AB, Morrison BJ. The effect of cigarette smoke from the mother on bronchial responsiveness and severity of symptoms in children with asthma. J Allergy Clin Immunol 1986; 77:575-581.
16. Dodge RR, Burrows B. The prevalence and incidence of asthma and asthma-like symptoms in a general population sample. Am Rev Respir Dis 1980; 122:567-575.
17. Chausow AM, Banner AS. Comparison of the tussive effects of histamine

and methacholine in humans. J Appl Physiol: Respir Environ Exercise Physiol 1983;55:541-546.
18. Peress L, Mintz S, Silverman F. Methacholine challenge and chronic cough. Ann R Coll Phys Surg Can 1978; 11:90.
19. Ramsdale EH, Morris MM, Roberts RS, Hargreave FE. Inhaled glucocorticoids in chronic cough. In: *Glucocorticoids, Inflammation and Bronchial Hyperreactivity*. Hogg JC, Ellul-Micallef R, Brattsand R, eds. Exerpta Medica, Amsterdam, 1985; pp. 91-6.
20. Cockcroft DW, Killian DN, Mellon JA, Hargreave FE. Bronchial reactivity to inhaled histamine: a method and clinical survey. Clin Allergy 1977; 7:235-243.
21. Crofton JC, Douglas A. *Respiratory Diseases*, 2nd ed. Blackwell Scientific, Oxford, 1975; p. 80.
22. Eddy NB, Friebel H, Hahn K-J, Halbach H. *Codeine and Its Alternates for Pain and Cough Relief*. Geneva, World Health Organization, 1970; pp. 127-156.
23. Coleridge HM, Coleridge JCG. Impulse activity in afferent vagal cell fibres with endings in the intrapulmonary airways of dogs. Respir Physiol 1977; 29:143-150.
24. Widdicombe JG. Nervous receptors in the respiratory tract and lungs. In: *Regulation of Breathing Part 1*. Hornbein T, ed. Marcel Dekker, New York, 1981; pp. 429-72.
25. Higenbottam T. Cough induced by changes of airway composition of airway surface liquid. Bull Eur Physiopathol Respir 1984; 20:553-562.
26. Sampson SR. Sensory neurophysiology of airways. Am Rev Respir Dis 1977; 115:107-115.
27. Mentz WM, Knowles JB, Brown JB, Gatzy JT, Boucher RC. Measurement of airway surface liquid (ASL) composition of normal human subjects. Am Rev Respir Dis 1984; 129(suppl):A315.
28. Man SFF, Adams GK, Proctor DF. Effect of temperature, relative humidity and mode of breathing on canine airway secretion. J Appl Physiol: Respir Environ Exercise Physiol 1979; 46:205-210.
29. Banner AS, Chausow A, Green J. The tussive effect of hyperpnea with cold air. Am Rev Respir Dis 1985; 131:362-367.
30. Banner AS, Green J, O'Connor M. Relation of respiratory water loss to coughing after exercise. N Engl J Med 1984; 311:883-886.
31. Eschenbacher WL, Boushey HA, Sheppard D. Alteration in osmolarity of inhaled aerosols cause bronchoconstriction and cough, but absence of a permeant anion causes cough alone. Am Rev Respir Dis 1984; 129:211-215.
32. Hogg JB, Eggleston PE. Is asthma an epithelial disease? Am Rev Respir Dis 1984; 129:207-208.
33. Duffey ME, Hainau B, Ho S, Bentzel CJ. Regulation of epithelial tight junctions permeability by cyclic AMP. Nature 1981; 294:451-453.

34. Al-Bazzaz FJ. Role of cyclic AMP in regulation of chloride secretion by canine tracheal mucosa. Am Rev Respir Dis 1981; 123:295–298.
35. Al-Bazzaz FJ, Veech J. Narrowing of intercellular spaces by epinephrine in canine tracheal mucosa. Am Rev Respir Dis 1984; 129(suppl):A314.
36. Ramsdale EH, Fester D. Terbutaline is effective in the treatment of chronic cough. Clin Invest Med 1987; 10(suppl):B117.
37. Nadel JA. Autonomic control of airway smooth muscle and airway secretions. Am Rev Respir Dis 1977; 115:117–26.
38. Coleridge HM, Coleridge JCG, Ginzel KH, Baker DG, Banzett RB, Morrison MA. Stimulation of irritant receptors and C-fibres in the lungs by prostaglandins. Nature 1976; 264:451–453.
39. Bergren DR, Gustafson JM, Myers DL. Effect of prostaglandin F2alpha on pulmonary rapidly-adapting-receptors in the guinea pig. Prostaglandins 1984; 27:391–405.
40. Herxheimer H, Roetscher I. The effect of prostaglandin E on lung function in bronchial asthma. Eur J Clin Pharmacol 1971; 3:123–125.
41. Kawakami Y, Uchiyama K, Irie T, Murao M. Evaluation of aerosols of prostaglandins E1 and E2 as bronchodilators. Eur J Clin Pharmacol 1973; 6:127–32.
42. Lundberg JM, Saria A. A capsaicin-induced desensitization of airway mucosa to cigarette smoke, mechanical and chemical irritants. Nature 1983; 302:251–3.
43. Coleridge HM, Coleridge JCG, Luck JC. Pulmonary afferent fibres of small diameter stimulated by capsaicin and by hyperinflation of the lungs. J Physiol 1965; 179:248–262.
44. Collier JG, Fuller RW. Capsaicin inhalation in man and the effects of sodium cromoglycate. Br J Clin Pharmacol 1984; 81:113–7.
45. Sheppard D, Rizk NW, Boushey HA, Bethel RA. Mechanism of cough and bronchoconstriction induced by distilled water aerosol. Am Rev Respir Dis 1983; 127:691–694.
46. Bickerman HA, Barach AL, Itkin S, Drimmer F. The experimental production of cough in humans by citric acid. The evaluation of anti-tussive agents. Am J Med Sci 1954; 228:156–163.
47. Bickerman HA, Cohen BM, German E, Itkin S. The cough response of healthy human subjects induced by citric acid aerosol. Alterations produced by anti-tussive agents. Am J Med Sci 1956; 232:57–66.
48. Pounsford JC, Birch MJ, Saunders KB. Effect of bronchodilators on the cough response to inhaled citric acid in normal and asthmatic subjects. Thorax 1985; 40:662–667.
49. Thomson NC. The effect of different pharmacological agents on respiratory reflexes in normal and asthmatic subjects. Clin Sci 1979; 56:235–241.
50. McNally JF Jr, Enright P, Hirsch JE, Souhrada JF. The attenuation of exercise-induced broncoconstriction by oropharyngeal anesthesia. Am Rev Respir Dis 1979; 119:247–52.

51. Irwin RS, Rosen MJ, Braman SS. Cough: a comprehensive review. Arch Intern Med 1977; 137:1186.
52. Dunnill MS. The pathology of asthma with special reference to changes in the bronchial mucosa. J Clin Pathol 1960; 13:27-33.
53. Laitinen LA, Heino M, Laitinen A, Kava T, Haahtela T. Damage of the airway epithelium and bronchial reactivity in patients with asthma. Am Rev Respir Dis 1985; 131:599-606.
54. Frigas E, Loegering DA, Solley GO, Farrow GM, Gleich GJ. Elevated levels of the eosinophil granule major basic protein in the sputum of patients with bronchial asthma. Mayo Clin Proc 1981; 56:345-353.
55. Flint KC, Leung KBP, Hudspith BN, Brostoff J, Pearce FL, Johnson NM. Bronchoalveolar mast cells in extrinsic asthma: a mechanism for the initiation of antigen specific bronchoconstriction. Br Med J 1985; 291:923-6.
56. Kirby JG, Hargreave FE, Gleich GJ, O'Byrne PM. Bronchoalveolar cell profiles of asthmatic and nonasthmatic subjects. Am Rev Respir Dis 1987; 136:379-383.
57. Frigas E, Loegering DA, Gleich GJ. Cytotoxic effects of the guinea pig eosinophil major basic protein on tracheal epithelium. Lab Invest 1980; 42:35-43.
58. Dor PJ, Ackerman SJ, Gleich GJ. Charcot-Leyden crystal protein and eosinophilic granule major basic protein in sputum of patients with respiratory disease. Am Rev Respir Dis 1984; 130:1072-1077.
59. Empey DW, Laitinen LA, Jacobs L, Gold WM, Nadel JA. Mechanisms of bronchial hyperreactivity in normal subjects after upper respiratory tract infections. Am Rev Respir Dis 1976; 113:131-139.
60. Hers JFPH. Disturbances of the ciliated epithelium due to influenza virus. Am Rev Respir Dis 1966;93:162-171.
61. Beasley R, Coleman ED, Hermon Y, Holst PE, O'Donnell TV, Tobias M. Viral respiratory tract infection and exacerbations of asthma in adult patients. Thorax 1989;43:679-683.
62. Horn MEC, Brain EA, Gregg I, Inglis JM, Yealland SJ, Taylor P. Respiratory viral infection and wheezy bronchitis in childhood. Thorax 1979; 34:23-28.
63. Minor TE, Dick EC, Baker JW, Ouellette JJ, Cohen M, Reed CE. Rhinovirus and influenza type A infections as precipitants of asthma. Am Rev Respir Dis 1976; 113:149-153.
64. Barnes PJ. Cell receptors and airway function in asthma. In: *Recent Advances in Respiratory Medicine*. Flenley DC, Petty TL, eds. Churchill Livingstone, Edinburgh, 1986; pp. 25-43.
65. Meurs H, Koeter GH, De Vries K, Kauffman HF. The beta adrenergic system and allergic bronchial asthma: changes in lymphocytes beta adrenergic receptor number and adenylate cyclase activity after an allergen-induced attack. J Allergy Clin Immunol 1982; 70:272-280.
66. Barnes PJ. Asthma as an axon reflex. Lancet 1986; i:242-245.
67. Thurlbeck WM, Hogg JC. Pathology of asthma. In: *Allergy Principles and*

Practice, 3rd ed. Middleton E Jr, Reed CE, Ellis EF, Adkinson NF, Yunginer JW, eds. C. V. Mosby, St. Louis, 1988; pp. 1008–1017.
68. Gibson PG, Girgis-Gabardo A, Hargreave FE, Morris MM, Mattoli S, Kay JM, Dolovich J, Denburg J. Cellular characteristics of sputum from patients with asthma and chronic bronchitis. Am Rev Respir Dis 1989; 139:A326.
69. Pavia D, Lopez-Vidriero MT, Clarke SW. Mediators and muco-ciliary clearance in asthma. Bull Eur Physiopathol Respir 1987; 23(suppl 10):89S.
70. Fitzgerald JM, Allen CJ, Craven MA, Newhouse MT. Chronic cough and gastrooesophageal reflux. CMAJ 1989; 140:520–524.
71. Sontag SJ, Skorodin M, O'Connell S, Schnell T, Chintam R, Nemchausky B, Greenlee H. Ambulatory 24 hour oesophageal pH monitoring in patients with asthma. Gastroenterology 1984; 86:1261.
72. Goodall RJ, Earis JE, Cooper DN, Bernstein A, Temple JG. Relationship between asthma and gastro-oesophageal reflux. Thorax 1981; 36:116–121.
73. Wolff AP, May M, Nuelle D. The tympanic membrane. JAMA 1973; 223: 1269.
74. Bowton DL, Katz PO. Esophageal cyst as a cause of chronic cough. Chest 1984; 86:150–152.
75. Wilson NM, Charette L, Thomson A, Silverman M. Gastro-oesophageal reflux and childhood asthma: the acid test. Thorax 1985; 40:592–597.
76. Herve P, Denjean A, Jian R, Simonneau G, Duroux P. Intraesophageal perfusion of acid increases the bronchomotor response to methacholine and to isocapnic hyperventilation in asthmatic subjects. Am Rev Respir Dis 1986; 134:986–989.
77. Ekstrom T, Lindgren BR, Tibbling L. Effects of ranitidine treatment on patients with asthma and history of gastro-oesophageal reflux: a double blind crossover study. Thorax 1989; 44:19–23.
78. Speight ANP, Lee DA, Hey EN. Underdiagnosis and undertreatment of asthma in childhood. Br Med J 1983; 286:1253–1258.
79. Gibson PG, Dolovich J, Denburg J, Ramsdale EH, Hargreave FE. Chronic cough: eosinophilic bronchitis without asthma. Lancet 1989; i:1346–1348.
80. Ellul-Micallef R. Effect of terbutaline sulphate in chronic "allergic" cough. Br Med J 1983; 287:940–943.

10

The Pharmacology of Antiasthma Medications

FRANCIS M. C. CUSS

Schering-Plough Research
Kenilworth, New Jersey

INTRODUCTION

This chapter details the history, pharmacology, and safety of the major classes of drugs available for the treatment of asthma today. In addition, there is discussion of the value and relevance of various human models of asthma and of how they contribute to our understanding of drug action and therapeutic drug use in this chapter.

As the number of antiasthmatic drugs have increased and the theories on the underlying causes of asthma changed, so have there been attempts to classify medication either by their clinical or pharmacological effects. Clearly, classification of mechanisms of drug action and establishment of a treatment hierarchy should be the basis of rational therapy. However, with the ever-increasing information from research and improvements in experimental techniques, both in animals and humans, rigid classification could prove more limiting than useful. It is now widely agreed that asthma is associated with airway wall inflammation and it has been suggested that antiasthma drugs could be broadly divided into those that are symptomatic or prophylactic. Bronchodilators such as beta-adrenoceptor agonists, xanthines, and anticholinergics would be termed "symptomatic" while "antiallergic drugs" and corticosteroids would be "prophylactic." Recently the term anti-inflammatory has been used interchangeably with prophylactic. Since it is difficult to directly measure the effect of drugs on airway inflammation in asthma, the classification has evolved from indirect indices such as observations of the effects of various agents on inflammatory cells in vitro, antigen-induced asthma, and clinical trials. However, as more information becomes available, the distinctions become blurred. For instance, ketotifen is considered to have some of the features of a prophylactic drug in vitro and in models of asthma, but has proved relatively ineffective in clinical trials. Conversely, xanthines and beta-agonists, which are usually considered symptomatic medication have recently been shown to have inhibitory effects on some inflammatory cells in vitro and to attenuate the late response to antigen. Clearly, blockade of the late response alone may not indicate antiinflammatory activity as convincingly as reduction of inflammatory cells in the airway after antigen challenge. However, because of the technical difficulties of this sort of study, a direct anti-inflammatory effect has yet to be demonstrated even for medications such as corticosteroids or cromolyn sodium, which consistently block late responses. The use and value of models of asthma in predicting therapeutic efficacy will be discussed in greater detail later in this chapter.

There is always a temptation to extrapolate from the results of small clinical studies in selected patients to the management of an asthmatic population. However, while it may be preferable to determine optimal treatment from long-term, large-scale clinical trials, the cost in terms of finance and time, and the difficulties of administration and of interpretation of these trials should not be underestimated. Thus, since long-term, well-controlled, comparative trials of antiasthmatic drugs are relatively rare, it may be prudent to consider claims of either long-term benefits or detrimental effects with some degree of caution if they are only based on small or short-term trials. However, it remains the belief of some and the hope of many respiratory physicians that the prolonged use of anti-inflammatory medication for asthma, in particular inhaled corticosteroids, will lead to modifications in the natural history of the disease.

BETA-ADRENOCEPTOR AGONISTS

History

Herbal remedies with beta-adrenoceptor agonist activity have been used in China (Ma Huang) and Greece (Ephedra vulgaris) for millenia. A greater appreciation of their value in asthma began in the 1900s with the successful use of adrenal tablets (1) and adrenaline injections (2). The active principal of Ma Huang, ephedrine, when isolated and characterized (3), offered both oral activity and longer action. Later, the discovery of isoproterenol (4), not only brought the major therapeutic advance of effective bronchodilatation without the vascular effects of epinephrine, but also stimulated the characterization of adrenoceptors into alpha and beta subtypes (5). Receptor classification into $beta_1$, and $beta_2$ subtypes (6) and the discovery of the first $beta_2$-selective adrenoceptor, albuterol (7) improved the therapeutic index of these drugs still further. Other drugs with a similar selectivity soon followed (e.g., terbutaline) and these now form the most widely used group of beta-adrenoceptor agonists. However, the search for compounds with an improved affinity for $beta_2$-receptors, a greater selectivity for lung tissue, and an extended duration of action continues.

Structure and Activity

The catechole moiety is a constant feature of beta-adrenoceptor agonists although small substitutions either on the benzene ring or the amine group lead to dramatically different properties (Fig. 1). The catecholamines, both natural (epinephrine) and synthetic (isoproterenol), have a relatively short duration of action because they are rapidly taken up by nerve terminals or metabolized. Noncatecholamines (metaproterenol, albuterol) are resistant to these processes, so are both orally active and longer lasting. Beta selectivity is modified by substi-

Name	Alternative	Structure	Inactivated by MAO/COMT	Duration
Epinephrine	Adrenaline	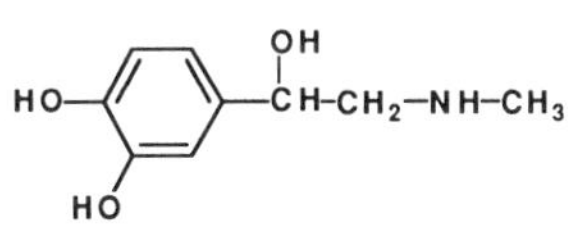	Yes	1/2-1
Isoproterenol	Isoprenaline	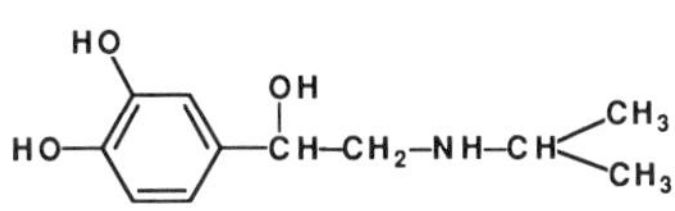	Yes	1-2
Metaproterenol	Orciprenaline	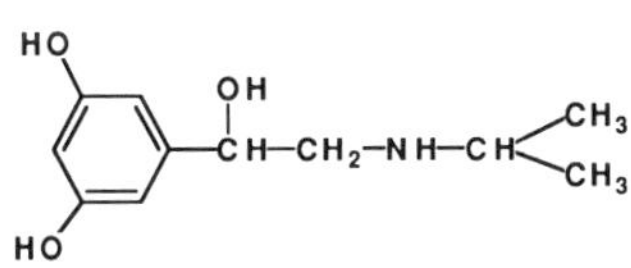	No	3-4
Albuterol	Salbutamol	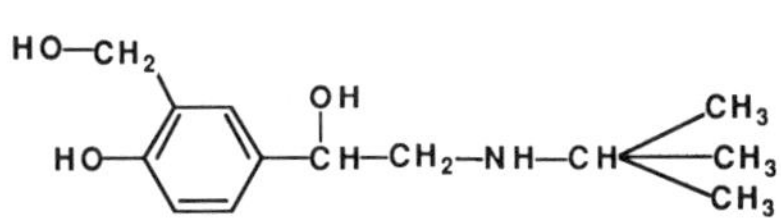	No	4-6
Salmeterol	–	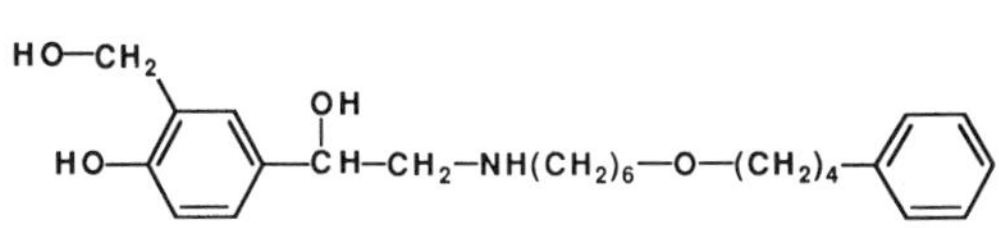	No	12+

FIGURE 1 Structure and activity of beta-adrenoceptor agonists.

tutions on the amine group. The addition of a carbon spacer to the molecule (salmeterol) considerably increases the duration of effect both in vitro (8) and in vivo (9). The prolonged effect may be the result of interaction of the molecule with an exoreceptor (10).

Pharmacokinetics

Catecholamines whether endogenous or synthetic are rapidly removed from the systemic circulation by being taken up both into sympathetic nerve terminals (Uptake 1) and other cells (Uptake 2). Catechol 3-O-methyl transferase (COMT) and monoamine oxidase (MAO), which are found throughout the body, also quickly metabolize these compounds. Noncatecholamines (e.g., albuterol, terbutaline) are well absorbed orally and conjugated to varying degrees in the liver. Because they are not subject to the uptake mechanisms or to metabolism by COMT and MAO, they have a longer duration of action and are usually excreted unchanged or as conjugates in the urine.

Administration of beta-adrenoceptor agonists by inhalation rather than by the oral route produces a considerable margin between beneficial pulmonary effects and unwanted systemic effects. However, attempts have been made to improve yet further the therapeutic index of beta-adrenoceptor agonists. Unfortunately, few of these have translated into significant advantages in clinical practice. For instance, procaterol, which has a markedly greater affinity for $beta_2$ than $beta_1$ receptors and exhibits considerable selectivity for lung tissue in vitro (11), has proved to have a similar side effect profile to albuterol when given to humans (12). Attempts to reduce tremor while maintaining pulmonary efficacy by separating $beta_2$ effects in the lung from those in skeletal muscle, have had little success to date. Another attempt at producing tissue selectivity has been the synthesis of prodrugs such as biltoterol and bambuterol. These compounds are inactive when administered and utilize enzymatic degradation in the target tissue (i.e., the lung) to liberate the active drug. Thus, inactive biltoterol is transformed, when inhaled, to colterol, by lung esterases. Unfortunately, colterol, being a catecholamine, has a short duration of action. However, a recent review of the clinical data (13) suggests that biltoterol has a longer duration of action than isoproterenol and similar degree and incidence of adverse effects. Bambuterol may be somewhat more resistant to first-pass activation in the liver than biltoterol and is transformed in the lung to terbutaline, a noncatecholamine (14).

Mechanism of Action

Cellular

The beta-adrenoceptor agonist binds directly to the beta-receptor on the cell surface. The receptor then links onto the adenylate cyclase catalytic unit

(ACCU) via the guanine nucleotide-binding complex (N). The N complex occurs in either an inhibitory (N_i) or in the case of beta-receptors in stimulatory form (N_s). Thus, a beta-agonist/receptor interaction leads to activation of N_s, stimulation of adenylate cyclase and conversion of adenosine triphosphate (ATP) to cyclic 3′,5′-adenosine monophosphate (cAMP). Cyclic AMP then binds to specific protein kinases. In smooth muscle cells, where the biochemistry is best characterized, these activated protein kinases then phosphorylate myosin light chain kinase (MLCK) leading to reduced phosphorylation of the myosin light chain. This causes smooth muscle relaxation (Fig. 2). Other protein kinases may, in addition, directly reduce the intracellular Ca^{2+} concentration. Obviously, in other cells, increased concentrations of cAMP and protein kinase activation will have other effects.

Pharmacological Action

The ubiquity of $beta_2$-receptors and their presence on many different cells explains the many therapeutic actions for adrenoceptor agonists. Postulated mechanisms are:

a. Bronchial smooth muscle relaxation
b. Inhibition of inflammatory mediator release
c. Modulation of cholinergic neurotransmission (15)
d. Increase in mucociliary clearance (16)
e. Reduction inmicrovascular permeability (17)
f. Increased contractility of fatigued diaphragmatic muscle (18)
g. Reduction in pulmonary artery pressure (19)

It is probable, however, that a major proportion of the therapeutic effect of these drugs is achieved through mechanisms (a) and (b). However, because of their potent effect on these mechanisms, it is technically difficult to gather evidence to show that the minor mechanisms make a significant contribution to the overall therapeutic effect.

BRONCHIAL SMOOTH MUSCLE RELAXATION Beta$_2$-receptors are present on airway smooth muscle throughout the respiratory tract with a greater density distally (20). Thus, beta-adrenoceptor agonists are extremely potent relaxants of both spontaneously and pharmacologically contracted human bronchi and bronchioles in vitro (21,22). They are functional antagonists of smooth muscle contraction for all contractile stimuli, although they are less effective when there is a high degree of contraction, particularly from cholinoceptor agonists (23).

INHIBITION OF INFLAMMATORY MEDIATOR RELEASE Beta-adrenoceptor agonists are very potent inhibitors of the release of histamine, prostaglandin D_2, and leukotrienes from human lung (24). Beta$_2$-receptors have been identified on human mast cells and albuterol blocks IgE-dependent histamine release in vitro (25) and in vivo (26). New longer-acting beta-adrenoceptor agonists may offer

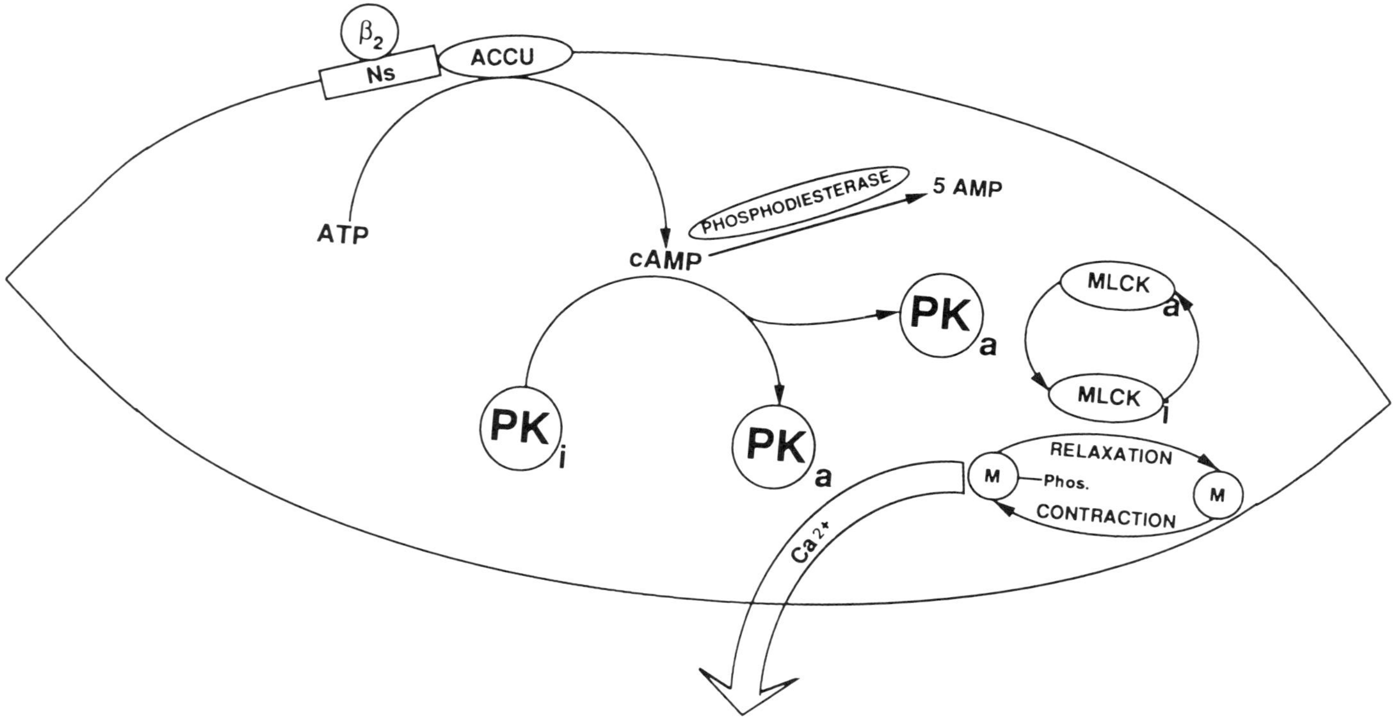

FIGURE 2 Schematic representation of the intracellular events in airway smooth muscle after beta$_2$-receptor stimulation or phosphodiesterase inhibition. Beta$_2$-receptor (B_2); guanine nucleotide-binding stimulatory complex (N_S); adenylate cyclase catalytic unit (ACCU); adenosine triphosphate (ATP; cyclic 3,5-adenosine monophosphate (cAMP); 5-adenosine monophosphate (5-AMP); protein kinase (PK_i) inactivated and (PK_a) activated; myosin light chain kinase ($MLCK_a$) activated and ($MLCK_i$) inactivated; phosphorylated myosin (M-phos).

further therapeutic possibilities (27). Other inflammatory cells such as lymphocytes and leukocytes have beta-adrenoceptors on their cell surface, but the therapeutic significance of beta-agonist action on these cells is unknown.

Clinical Effects

Beta-adrenoceptor agonists cause dose-dependent bronchodilatation in both normal and asthmatic subjects. They are also the most effective inhibitors of exercise and allergen-induced early asthmatic responses. In contrast, the late asthmatic response and the increase in airway responsiveness which occurs with it are not blocked by a dose of a conventional beta agonist given before antigen challenge (28). However, a recent study suggests that fomoterol, which is long acting and a large dose of albuterol may attenuate the late response (29). Airway challenge with pharmacological agonists, and irritant gases and dusts are blocked by beta-adrenoceptor agonists. However, long-term treatment with beta-adrenoceptor agonists do not improve airway responsiveness (see section on airway challenge).

Adverse Effects

Adverse effects occur as a result of extrapulmonary beta-adrenoceptor stimulation. These become more frequent and severe with increasing systemic concentrations of beta-adrenoceptor agonists. Usually, however, adequate efficacy can be achieved with a minimum .of adverse effects by the inhaled route. If the dose required is large, then significant systemic absorption may occur and dose-related pharmacological effects will be noted (30). Oral and parenteral administration produces greater systemic effects while achieving comparable pulmonary efficacy.

TREMOR There are beta$_2$-receptors on skeletal muscle fibers, although the exact type of tremor depends on whether fast or slow muscle fibers are the predominant type being stimulated. Most evidence suggests that the beta$_2$-receptors on skeletal muscle are the same as those on bronchial smooth muscle (31), and therefore the degree of tremor and bronchodilatation are closely related after systemic administration of beta-adrenoceptor agonists. However, individuals vary considerably in the amount of tremor they experience, and over time, some degree of tolerance to the tremor, but not the bronchodilatation may occur (32).

CARDIOVASCULAR EFFECTS Drugs such as isoproterenol, with high affinity for beta$_1$ receptors, cause increases in heart rate and cardiac output. However, similar cardiovascular effects can be induced when beta$_2$-selective agonists are administered systemically. It is likely that this is mainly due to reflex changes following beta$_2$-mediated vasodilatation (33). However, those beta$_2$-receptors which have been identified in the human myocardium by autoradiographic and binding studies (34), may have some inotropic and chronotropic effects after large parenteral doses (35).

METABOLIC EFFECTS Systemic beta-adrenoceptor agonists have many biochemical effects including increases in glycogenolysis, insulin release, plasma glucose, lactate, pyruvate, and high-density lipoprotein cholesterol and reductions in plasma potassium, calcium, and magnesium (36). However, after administration of a therapeutically equivalent dose of an aerosol preparation, only small changes in glucose are observed (37). Administration of large inhaled doses (30), or less $beta_2$-selective drugs (38) may be associated with reductions in plasma potassium concentrations.

TACHYPHYLAXIS Over time, constant stimulation of a receptor leads to down regulation and reduction of the elicited response. Thus, a number of studies have been performed to investigate whether clinically significant tachyphylaxis occurs in asthmatics, and if so, which of the actions of beta-adrenoceptor agonists are affected. These studies differ in trial design, duration, choice of control groups, and prestudy washout period, and these differences make interpretation of the results difficult (39,40). It appears that the effects of beta-adrenoceptor agonists on tremor, metabolic parameters, lymphocytes, and leukocytes become reduced after continued usage while bronchodilator responses are maintained (41). Even if bronchodilator tolerance does occur, there remains the question of whether this is of clinical significance. Overall, it appears that the majority of patients taking standard doses of beta-adrenoceptor agonists do not exhibit bronchodilator tachyphylaxis. Whether administration of large doses after prolonged periods may be associated with problems in a small number of patients remains to be seen.

DRUG COMBINATIONS Combination of beta-adrenoceptor agonists with other drugs is common in the treatment of asthma. The addition of ipratropium bromide (42), theophylline, and corticosteroids (43) to beta-adrenergic agonists can give additive improvements in lung function, but may also increase adverse effects. The improvement in efficacy is less and the increase in adverse effects greatest after systemic administration of theophylline and beta-adrenoceptor agonists together. A review of the cardiovascular toxicity of drug combinations in animals noted that the effect of large concentrations of isoproterenol was accentuated by concomitant administration of theophylline, although the effects of $beta_2$-selective agents were less severe in these models (44). Although the relevance of these observations for human subjects is unclear, the conclusion that oral theophylline should not be added to oral beta-adrenoceptor agonist therapy is a prudent one. The combination of inhaled beta-adrenoceptor drugs and oral theophylline has not been associated with an excess of adverse events or cardiovascular side effects (45,46).

METHYL XANTHINES

History

A recent historical review (47) suggests that Dr. Hyde Salter should receive the distinction of recording the first use of xanthines in asthma. Salter wrote in 1859, "To the question 'Have you tried strong coffee?' the asthmatic is pretty sure to answer 'yes' and he is also pretty sure to add that it gives him relief" (48).

Caffeine was noted to relax airways in vitro in 1912 (49), but it was not until the early 1920s that the effects of xanthines in vitro were correlated with their antiasthmatic properties (50). Despite its effectiveness as a bronchodilator, the subsequent use of theophylline was generally limited to the treatment of acute asthma probably because its relatively short duration of action and narrow margin of safety made its use difficult. With the advent of plasma theophylline assays and extended release formulations, dosing has become both easier and more rational (51,52). Despite their extrapulmonary effects, xanthines, and particularly theophylline, are now widely used for the treatment of chronic asthma.

Structure and Activity

During the 1950s, small changes were made to the xanthine structure (N_7 substitutions, see Fig. 3) in an attempt to improve the safety and efficacy of these drugs. Dyphylline is renally excreted (53) with a short half-life, but is less potent than theophylline (54) and there is no reliable plasma assay. Similarly prophylline, although possessing a longer half-life (55), is much less potent. None of these analogues offer any significant advantage over theophylline and are not widely used. A fuller study of the structure/activity relationships of xanthines (56) resulted in the development of enprophylline. This drug is more potent than theophylline, is excreted renally, and does not antagonize the effects of adenosine which may give it some advantages in terms of safety (57). At present, theophylline is the "gold standard" among xanthines; partly because of the large amount of data on its use, but also on account of the wide selection of controlled-release formulations and the ready availability of plasma assays. It remains to be seen whether the different pharmacological profile of enprophylline will offer therapeutic advantage in clinical practice.

Pharmacokinetics

Since theophylline and its salts (which are absorbed as theophylline) represent the vast majority of xanthine usage, only their pharmacokinetics will be considered here. Theophylline is rapidly and completely absorbed after oral admin-

		Half-life (hours)	Potency
Caffeine	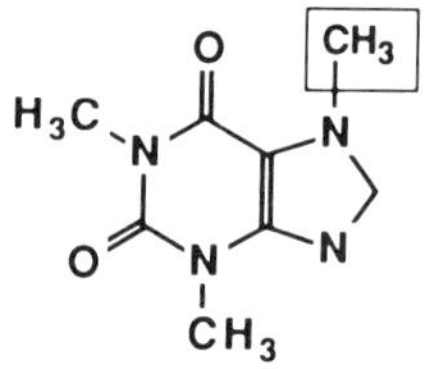	4	<Theo
Theophylline	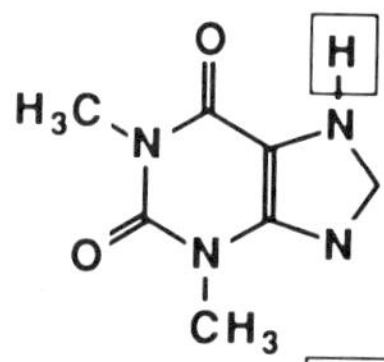	8	-
Dyphylline (Diprophylline)	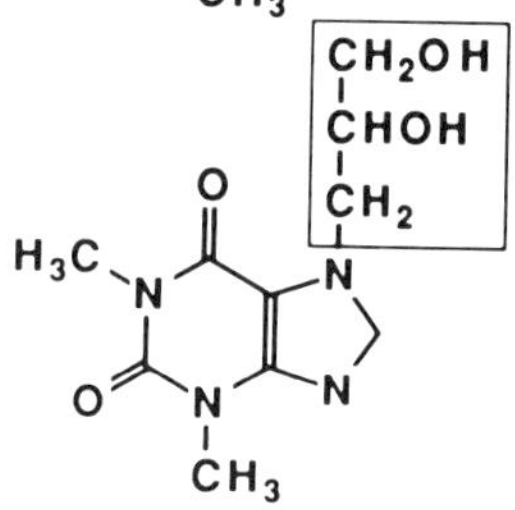	2 (Renal excretion)	<Theo
Proxphylline	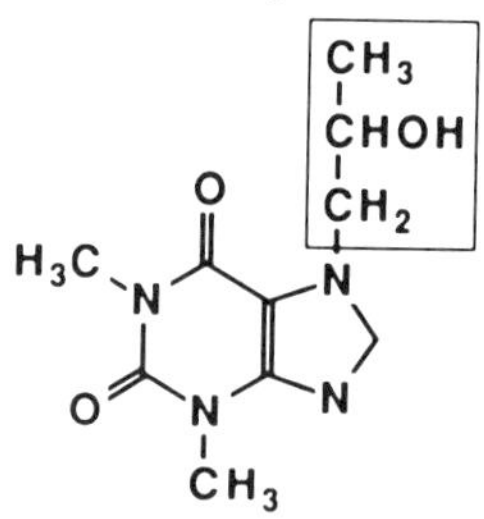	8-12	<<Theo
Enprophylline	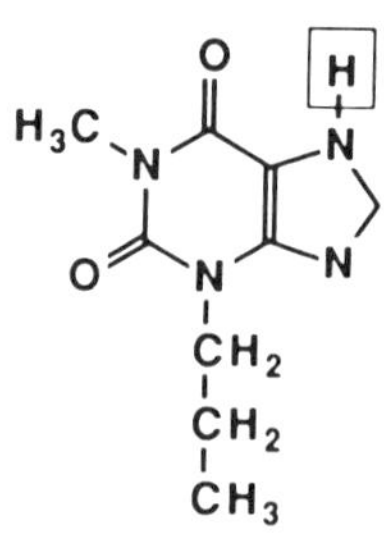	1.5 (Renal excretion)	>Theo

FIGURE 3 Structure and activity of xanthines. N_7 substitutions shown in box.

istration. Some preparations particularly taken with food can be associated with erratic absorption and "dose dumping" (52). Theophylline has a volume of distribution of approximately 0.45 L/kg and quickly reaches equilibrium with body tissues including the brain. Theophylline is metabolized in the liver, predominately by oxidation, and little is excreted unchanged in the urine. Metabolism varies considerably between individuals and can be effected by many factors including smoking, concomitant diseases such as heart failure and hepatitis, and medication including macrolide antibiotics, cimetidine, and anticonvulsants. Biotransformation is very rapid in young children and becomes slower in the elderly. In view of the narrow therapeutic index for theophylline it is prudent to monitor plasma levels on a regular basis (58).

Mechanism of Action

Intracellular Effects

At present the exact intracellular mechanism of xanthines is unclear. Xanthines are phosphodiesterase inhibitors and it has been proposed that the concentration of intracellular cAMP would be increased by this action, thereby causing smooth muscle relaxation (59) (Fig. 1). However, careful comparison of the concentrations which are effective in vitro with those achieved in vivo suggested that very little phosphodiesterase inhibition occurs in the therapeutic range (60). It was then suggested that theophylline's potent adenosine antagonism might explain its antiasthmatic action. However, enprophylline, a xanthine devoid of adenosine antagonistic activity, was shown to be both more potent than theophylline as a bronchodilator (57) and to share other antiasthmatic properties (61). However, some of the unwanted effects, particularly in the central nervous system, may be caused by adenosine antagonism. Other mechanisms have been considered. Theophylline does not have any effect on phosphatidylinositol turnover induced by cholinergic agonists (62), but has been shown to cause intracellular calcium sequestration without changes in cyclic nucleotide concentrations (63).

Interestingly, it has recently been shown that phosphodiesterase inhibitors in vitro produce smooth muscle relaxation without measurable changes in tissue content of cyclic nucleotides (64). These data when considered with earlier, apparently conflicting observations of the lack of correlation between contraction and cyclic nucleotide concentrations, may after all indicate that phosphodiestrase inhibition plays some part in the action of xanthines.

Pharmacological Effects

Several clinical effects have been identified which may contribute to the effectiveness of xanthines in the treatment of asthma. These include:

a. Bronchial smooth muscle relaxation
b. Inhibition of mediator release and inflammatory cells

c. Improved munociliary clearance
d. Reduction in microvascular permeability
e. Improved contractability of fatigued diaphragm
f. Reduction in pulmonary artery pressure and increase in right heart function
g. Increase in endogenous catecholamines
h. Stimulation of respiratory drive

Xanthines are considerably less potent than beta-agonists as relaxants of precontracted bronchial smooth muscle but may be more effective at higher tensions (23). They do share with beta-agonists the capability to functionally antagonize the effects of many different constrictive agents. Xanthines have been shown to reduce the activity of several types of inflammatory cell including mast cells, macrophages and leukocytes (65-67). However, these studies need to be interpreted with care since in some cases the beta-adrenoceptor agonists administered concomitantly may have produced a major proportion of the inhibitory effect. Xanthines do not provide the same degree of protection in vivo as beta-adrenoceptor against allergen-induced asthmatic responses. Xanthines also reduce the plasma leakage induced by inflammatory mediators in the airways (17). Mucociliary clearance is increased by xanthines (68) although overall this is of little clinical significance. Improvements in right ventricular function and reductions in pulmonary artery pressure observed after acute administration probably have little relevance in asthma but may have therapeutic effects in patients with chronic obstructive airways disease. Similarly, the clinical significance of improvements in diaphragmatic function observed after theophylline administration is debatable (69). Infusion of theophylline in humans causes an increase in cAMP which is blocked by propranolol, which suggests that theophylline stimulates the release of endogenous catecholamines (70). While epinephine concentrations increase after acute administration (71), they do not appear to change with chronic dosing (72). Theophylline also stimulates ventilation probably by inhibiting the suppressive effects of adenosine on the breathing center in the brain stem.

Clinical Effects

Theophylline is a bronchodilator and as would be expected of any pharmacological effect, the degree of bronchodilatation is proportional to the logarithm of the plasma concentration. Theophylline, particularly at higher doses, appears to offer some protection against exercise-induced bronchospasm (73) and although the majority of studies have shown significant protection against bronchial challenge (74-76) the effect is small compared to other drugs. The effect of theophylline on the immediate response to allergen is variable, but a constant infusion significantly reduces the late response (77). Theophylline is mainly used for the oral therapy of chronic asthma where it reduces symptoms and the need for concomitant medication (78).

Adverse Effects

Xanthines have a number of extrapulmonary effects which may be troublesome at therapeutic concentrations, but become dangerous at higher levels (58,79). Many factors reduce the elimination of theophylline and, therefore, because of the narrow therapeutic index, the potential for toxicity is high, particularly in the absence of plasma monitoring. In rare cases, overdosage has been fatal (80). Enprophylline because it lacks adenosine antagonism does not have all the adverse effects of other xanthines (62).

GASTROINTESTINAL EFFECTS The most common theophylline-related adverse effects are probably anorexia, nausea, and vomiting. These occur with increasing frequency above 15 mg/L, but also occur at lower concentrations at the start of treatment. Theophylline causes increased gastric secretion and relaxation of the esophageal sphincter. Enprophylline has no effect on gastric secretion, but otherwise has similar gastrointestinal (GI) effects as theophylline.

NEUROLOGICAL EFFECTS High plasma concentrations of theophylline may precipitate epileptic fits which can lead to death (80). Generally, but not always, these are preceded by other adverse effects such as GI disturbance. These may be related to central adenosine inhibition because enprophylline does not cause seizures in animals (62). Both cause headaches which are pulsatile in nature. Recently it has been suggested that some children receiving chronic theophylline treatment have learning and behavioral problems (81), although this remains controversial.

CARDIOVASCULAR EFFECTS Theophylline and enprophylline have similar inotropic effects, but enprophylline may have a slightly smaller chronotropic effect. When toxicity occurs, tachycardia is a common sign and various arrhythmias have been noted (73).

MISCELLANEOUS EFFECTS Theophylline particularly at high concentrations is associated with naturesis, diuresis, hyperglycemia, and increases in free fatty acids, plasma, and urinary calciums and uric acid (46,82). When combined with systemic beta-agonists, many of the extra pulmonary effects of these drugs are increased.

CHOLINOCEPTOR ANTAGONISTS

History

In a fashion similar to other antiasthma drugs, cholinoreceptor antagonists often called anticholinergic agents, have been used for centuries in the form of herbal remedies. Their use in respiratory diseases was recorded during the eleventh century in India (83) and species of the Datura plant were brought back to England for medicinal use in the early 1800s. The smoking of cigarettes made from stramonium leaves (i.e., inhaled anticholinergics) was fairly widespread during the nineteenth century although the efficacy of the treatment was controversial (48). However, with the advent of adrenergic agents in the early twentieth century, anticholinergic remedies lost favor. However, their use has increased again with a better understanding of the cholinergic innervation of the lungs and the availability of more selective compounds.

Structure and Activity

Anticholinergic agents are competitive inhibitors of acetylcholine at muscarinic receptors in the lung. Atropine, the active principal of herbal remedies such as stramonium leaves and the deadly nightshade fungus, has a similar structure (ammonium group and ester linkage) to muscarinic agonists (Fig. 4). Thus, all antagonists have the same basic structure. There are at least two types of muscarinic recepters (M_1 and M_2) of which M_2 appears to be the subtype which mediates contraction in airway smooth muscle (84). There may also be M_1 recepters on presynaptic terminals of postganglionic neurones (85). Atropine and ipratropium bromide are effective antagonists for both recepter subtypes, and therefore these compounds do not have any tissue selectivity. The valency of the nitrogen atom determines the capacity of the molecule to be absorbed. Tertiary amines such as atropine cross membranes easily and are therefore well absorbed across the gut wall, the lungs and can enter the brain. In contrast, quaternary amines are ionized and therefore reach the systemic circulation much less readily. Since they cannot cross the blood-brain barrier, they do not have CNS effects. Thus, functionally tissue selectivity is achieved by administration of quaternary amines by the inhaled route.

Pharmacokinetics

Atropine, a tertiary amine, is well absorbed and rapidly distributed throughout the body. It has a half-life of approximately 3 hours and is excreted unchanged in the urine. In contrast, only 0.2% of an oral dose and 0.3% of an inhaled dose of ipratropium bromide is absorbed after 3 hours (86).

The plasma half-life of parenteral ipratropium is approximately 4 hours and the majority of the drug is excreted in the urine.

Mechanism of Action

Pharmacological Effects

Since these drugs are specific receptor antagonists their action is restricted to inhibiting those cell types that are activated by muscarinic agents. Muscarinic receptors have been identified on bronchial smooth muscle, submucosal glands, mast cells, and prejunctional, postganglionic nerves (87,88). Receptors are plentiful in the larger airways and become less dense distally. However, in

		Duration of action (hr)	Systemic effects
Atropine	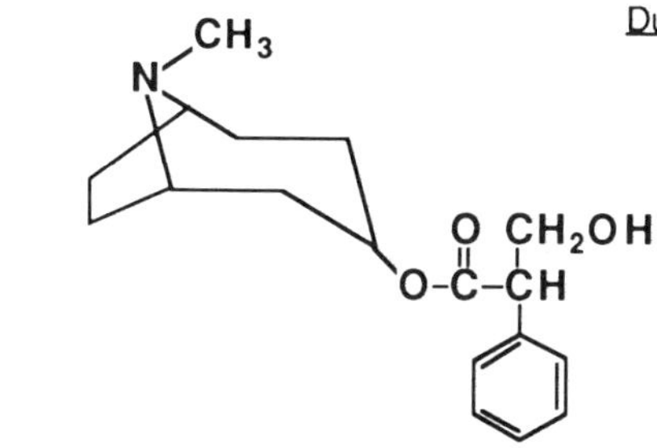	3-4	Dry mouth Problems with: Micturation Glaucoma CNS Effects
Ipratropium Bromide	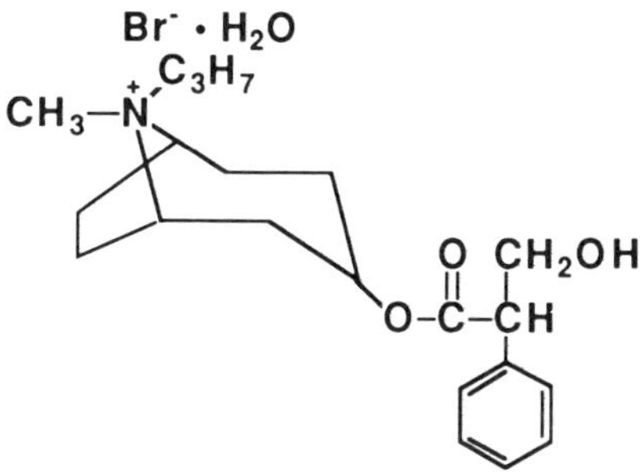	5-6	Negligible
Oxitropium Bromide	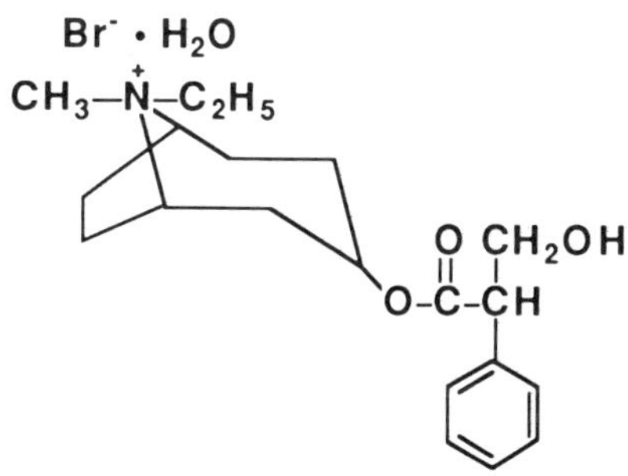	8	Negligible
Acetylcholine	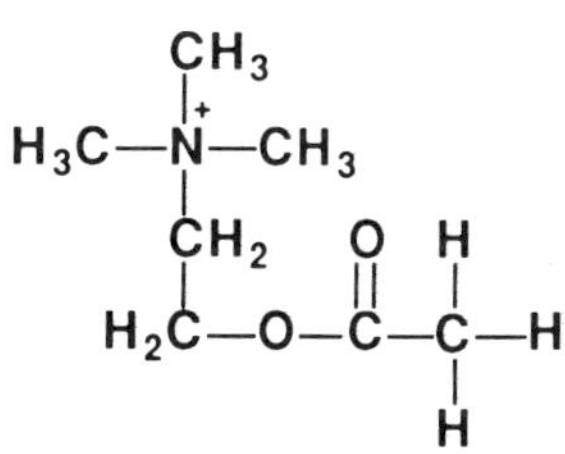	1/4-1	—

FIGURE 4 Structure and activity of cholinoceptor antagonists.

practice, anticholinergic drugs cause bronchodilation of both large and small airways (89). Quaternary amines have a longer effect than tertiary amines although duration is also dose dependent (90,91).

Clinical Effects

There have been many studies of anticholinergic agents in induced asthma, but these give conflicting results (92). Generally they do not appear to provide significant protection against exercise, allergen, or cold air challenges, and apart from antagonizing cholinergic challenge, offer relatively little protection against histamine and other pharmacological constrictor agents. The effects of gases and dusts are attenuated to a moderate degree by anticholinergic drugs. They cause bronchodilatation which is slower in onset, but longer lasting than conventional beta-agonists. Anticholinergic agents are useful both in preventing (93) and reversing (94) bronchoconstriction induced by beta-adrenoceptor antagonists.

Adverse Effects

Administration of atropine is associated with systemic effects such as glaucoma and bladder neck dysfunction. Ipratropium bromide even at high doses does not appear to cause these effects (95,96).

GLANDULAR SECRETION AND MUCOCILIARY CLEARANCE Atropine administration is associated with reductions in glandular secretion (97) and ciliary beat frequency (98), but ipratropium bromide has little effect (99). Similarly, mucociliary clearance is reduced by atropine and hyoscine (100,101), but not by ipratropium bromide (95,102). Sputum volume a crude measure of mucociliary function does not appear to be affected (103).

CARDIOVASCULAR Atropine is associated with bradycardia and a small change in right right ventricular and pulmonary artery pressure, but even large doses of ipratropium bromide do not change cardiac output (104) or have any effect on gas exchange (105).

PARADOXICAL BRONCHOCONSTRICTION Bronchoconstriction has been reported on rare occasions after inhalation of ipratropium bromide both from metered dose inhaler (106) and from a nebulizer (107). Several mechanisms for this effect have been suggested, including hypotonicity of the solution, the presence of preservatives (107), or blockade of postganglionic presynaptic M_1 receptors (88). Although there are several published reports of paradoxical bronchoconstriction after ipratropium bromide, it can also occur after other inhaled medications.

ANTIALLERGIC DRUGS

Any drug which blocks antigen-induced responses or has an effect on IgE/antigen interactions, mast cell activation, mediator release, or their effect can be considered "antiallergic." This section will be limited to consideration of cromolyn sodium, nedocromil sodium, ketotifen, and H_1-receptor antagonists. The success of cromolyn sodium (disodium cromoglycate; DSCG) stimulated the development of many similar drugs with greater potency in animal models of "allergy" such as the rat passive cutaneous anaphylaxis test or the sensitized rat peritoneal mast cell test. Unfortunately, many lacked clinical efficacy or were unsafe. At present, there is another generation of "antiallergic" drugs in development which could better be termed "antimediator" drugs. However, since they are all, at present, in clinical development they will not be discussed here.

Cromolyn Sodium

History

In the 1950s the screening of a number of plant derivatives with smooth muscle relaxant properties led to the synthesis of a biscromone, DSCG. DSCG was found to be devoid of bronchodilator activity, but did appear to inhibit mast cell mediator release following IgE/antigen interactions (108). At the same time, Altounyan, discovered that DSCG blocked both the immediate and late antigen responses (109). A small clinical trial confirmed the efficacy and safety of DSCG (110) and further reports of its effectiveness in asthma in children (111), in adults (112), in preventing allergen-induced responses (113), and in preventing exercise-induced bronchospasm (114) followed soon after.

Structure-Activity Relationships

DSCG is a *bis*-cromone (Fig. 5). Chemical modification of this structure has led to compounds with higher in vitro mast cell-stabilizing activity, but with little or no antiasthma activity in asthma. Thus to date, structure/activity analysis has not led to further compounds with superior clinical properties.

Pharmacokinetics

DSCG is highly ionized at physiological pH, so it is poorly absorbed both orally (1%) or by the inhaled route. Given parenterally, DSCG is not metabolized but excreted partly in the urine and partly in the bile (115).

Mechanism of Action

PHARMACOLOGICAL EFFECTS DSCG is unique in that the antiasthmatic effect of the drug was proved in humans very early in its development (109) and the putative mode of action was established later (116). Thus, mast cell stabilization, its most prominent pharmacological effect in animal models, was considered to be the underlying mechanism of its therapeutic effect in humans. Subsequently, it was realized that more potent analogues lacked clinical efficacy, that beta-agonists were more potent mast-cell stabilizers (24,117), but had a different clinical profile to DSCG, and that DSCG had effects in induced asthma

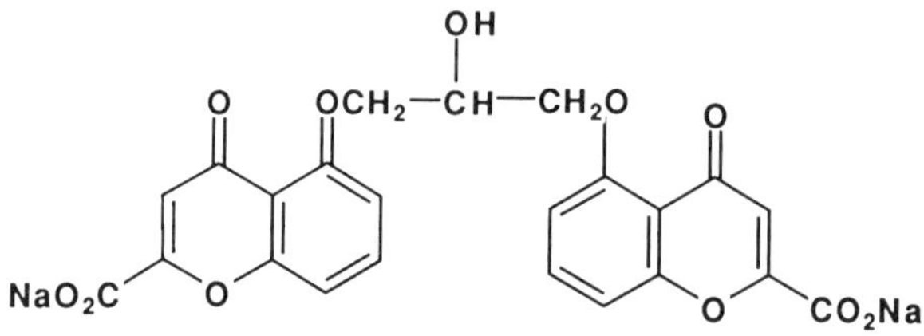

DISODIUM CROMOGLYCATE

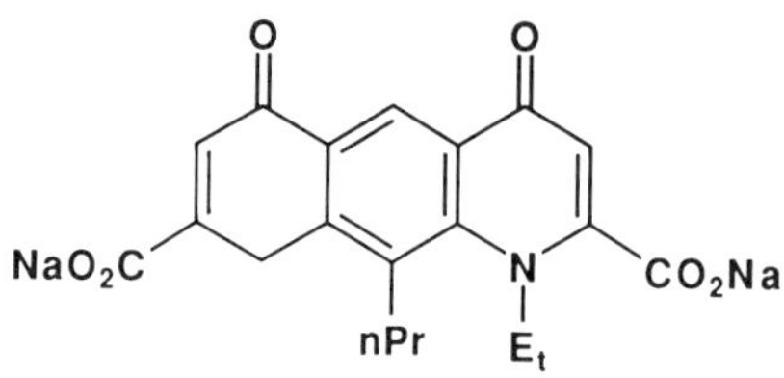

NEDOCROMIL SODIUM

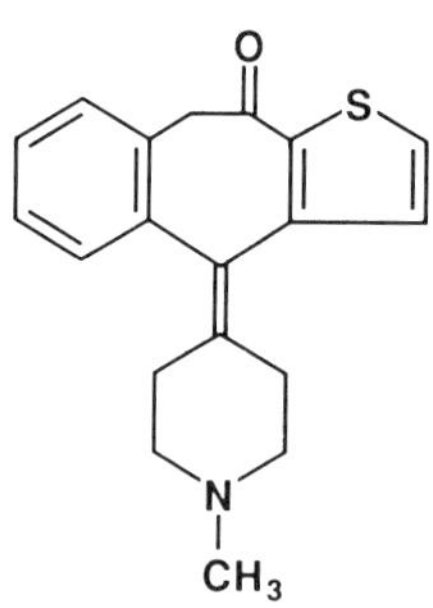

KETOTIFEN

FIGURE 5 Structure of antiallergic drugs.

where mast cells were not involved. This led to other mechanisms of action being considered.

As well as high affinity IgE receptors on mast cells, there appears to be low affinity IgE binding sites on other inflammatory cells such as neutrophils, macrophages, and platelets (118) which are blocked by DSCG (119,120). DSCG has inhibitory effects on neutrophils, monocytes, and eosinophils activated by F-Met-Leu-Phe or Zymosan, but not by LTB_4 (121,122). The clinical relevance of these observations remains to be established.

DSCG has been shown to block irritant nerves (C fibers) stimulated with serotonin or capsaicin in dogs (123). However, in humans neither bronchoconstriction (124) nor cough (125) induced by capsaicin was blocked by DSCG. However, DSCG does block the effects of some stimuli where bronchoconstriction is probably mediated through neurogenic mechanisms. Sulfur dioxide (126), fog (125), cold air (127), and bradykinin (128) induced asthma are all blocked by DSCG. Interestingly, the effect of SO_2 can be blocked by parenteral DSCG in concentrations that do not block mast cell degranulation (129).

CLINICAL EFFECTS DSCG has mast-cell-stabilizing effects in vitro and clearly reduces circulating mast cell mediators following antigen challenge in humans (26). It also abolishes late responses (130) and the airway hyperresponsiveness that is associated with it (28). DSCG blocks exercise-induced bronchoconstriction. In long-term controlled clinical studies in noncorticosteroid-dependent adults (131) and children (132) the DSCG-treated groups did significantly better than the placebo groups. Overall, DSCG is more effective in this type of patient rather than more severe nonatopic asthmatics.

ADVERSE EFFECTS Adverse effects related to its pharmacological actions are rare with DSCG. Mild throat discomfort has been reported after use of the dry powder formulation, and in very rare cases, severe bronchospasm has been associated with administration of DSCG.

Nedocromil Sodium

Since the discovery of DSCG, the search for more potent and orally active analogues has continued. From these programs a novel, more potent but topically active pyranoquinoline dicarboxylic acid derivative (Fig. 5), nedocromil sodium, has emerged (133). The drug has a profile similar to DSCG in some of the animal models but is more potent or active where DSCG is not in others. For instance in the *Ascaris*-sensitive macaque monkey following administration of antigen, it blocks bronchoconstriction and histamine, LTC_4 and PGD_2 release, whereas DSCG does not (134). Nedocromil, like DSCG, blocks the bronchoconstricter effects of exercise (135), cold air (136), and SO_2 (137), but not capsaicin (138). Nedocromil may be effective in chronic nonsteroid-dependent asthma (139), and in protecting against airway hyperresponsiveness in the pollen season (140). It appears to have no steroid-sparing effect (141). Although more potent, it is not yet clear whether it is any more effective than DSCG in clinical practice.

H_1 Receptor Antagonists

Histamine was probably the first mediator of "allergic" responses to be identified, have its action characterized, and specific antagonists of its action synthesized (142). While H_1 receptor antagonists (antihistamines) have proved useful in allergic rhinitis and have been shown to block the immediate antigen response

(143) they have been surprisingly ineffective in asthma. The older antihistamines such as chlorpheniramine maleate are relatively weak H_1 antagonists and are less effective at blocking histamine challenge than functional antagonists such as beta-adrenoceptor agonists (144). However, compounds have now been synthesized with greater potency and less effects on the central nervous system. Thus, terfenadine (145) and citirizine (146) not only provide greater protection against histamine-induced bronchoconstriction, but also cause bronchodilatation. At high concentrations, these drugs can have mast cell stabilizing effects (147), however, it is not clear whether these actions have any clinical relevance. Other potent nonsedating and long-acting antihistamines such as astemazole are now becoming available and their therapeutic use in asthma is being reassessed.

Ketotifen

Ketotifen is a benzocycloheptathiophene (Fig. 5) with good bioavailability, which has been shown to have activity against anaphylaxis, histamine and platelet-activating factor (PAF)-induced effects in animal models (119). However, the results of bronchial challenge testing and clinical studies have been variable. In some studies, ketotifen has proven effective against antigen-induced responses (148,149), but in others it has no effect (150), or is inferior to other antihistamines (143). Although some subjects have reduced exercise-induced bronchospasm following administration of ketotifen (149,141), the majority of studies have demonstrated no significant effect (152–154). Also although ketotifen will block the effects of PAF injected in the skin, it is without effect on PAF-induced pulmonary responses (155).

The results of clinical studies are equally varied, with significant improvement in symptoms, lung function (156), and steroid usage (157) in some and no difference from placebo in others (154,158,159). The variability of therapeutic effect in clinical trials could be due to choice of patient, trial design, or length of treatment, although more recent studies have been randomized placebo-controlled trials of three months duration or more. It has also been suggested the therapeutic clinical effects are the result of ketotifen's antihistaminic properties and that the actions observed in vitro occur at much higher concentrations than can be achieved in humans (160). The most common adverse effect is drowsiness, which is a feature of other older antihistamines. Weight gain has also been noted in some studies (158,159). Whether ketotifen at therapeutic doses in humans possesses any therapeutic effects beyond those of an H_1 receptor antagonist remains unclear. However, with the recent availability of more potent H_1 receptor blockers also with in vitro "antiallergic" properties, the role of these drugs in the treatment of asthma may be clarified.

CORTICOSTEROIDS

History

After many years of effort cortisone was characterized (161) and synthesized. Cortisone and adrenocorticotrophic hormone (ACTH) were initially used in the 1940s in the treatment of arthritis, but as soon as their therapeutic efficacy was appreciated they were studied in many other diseases including asthma (162–164). A rapid appreciation of the effects of large systemic doses of corticosteroids led investigators to administer hydrocortisone by inhalation in an attempt to maximize pulmonary effects while reducing systemic absorption (165–167). Unfortunately, while therapeutically effective, the low topical potency and high oral bioavailability of inhaled hydrocortisone offered few advantages over oral therapy. Later, with the discovery of highly potent topical corticosteroids with low systemic absorption and high plasma clearance, and with their formulation into aerosols and dry powders for inhalation, the use of corticosteroids in asthma was revolutionized. Beclomet/hasone dipropionate (BDP) was the first such compound (168,169), subsequently followed by betamethasone valerate and budesonide in Europe and flunisolide and triamcinolone acetonide in the United States. Similar improvements were made in the 1950s with oral corticosteroids. Compounds with higher potency such as prednisone and prednisolone were developed (170). Other more potent drugs such as dexamethasone, triamcinolone, and methyl prednisolone followed, but prednisone and prednisolone remain the most widely used for oral treatment.

Structure and Activity

There has been considerable interest in the modification of the main steroid structure to improve topical potency, reduce mineralocorticoid effects, and increase systemic clearance. Much of this work was performed to improve the safety and efficacy of dermatological corticosteroids and therefore dermatological methods became the standard for assessing the relative potencies of different compounds. The McKenzie vasoconstriction test is the most common (171), although measured potencies depend considerably on the ease with which the compounds get through the epidermis. Thus, the most potent corticosteroids tend to be those that are most lipophilic. Whether this attribute has any importance for inhalational corticosteroids in asthma is not known, although the results of the vasoconstrictor skin test do correlate fairly well with the relative efficacy of these compounds in asthma. However, because of the many different variables involved in inhalation therapy relative potencies of inhalational corticosteroids are better compared by clinical trials in asthma. Many modifications of the steroid nucleus have been made in order to improve the characteristics of the compound (Fig. 6). Substitutions or additions to the steroid ring also modify the metabolism of the compound.

Pharmacokinetics

The pharmacokinetics of these drugs have recently been reviewed (172), but, in general, inhalational corticosteroids have a low oral bioavailability and high plasma clearance in contrast to those used orally. The biological effects of potent oral corticosteroids such as dexamethasone can endure beyond the disappearance of the drug from the plasma, but inhaled corticosteroids achieve measurable systemic concentrations only at high doses. The amount that reaches the systemic circulation depends partly on the completeness of first-pass hepatic metabolism of the swallowed portion, and partly on the amount absorbed across the lung. Concomitant medication such as rifampicin and troleandomycin can affect the metabolism of oral corticosteroids, but physical factors such as the method of administration and severity of the disease are more likely to affect the pharmacokinetics of inhaled corticosteroids.

Mode of Action

Intracellular Effects

The intracellular actions of corticosteroids are complex (173). The corticosteroid molecule diffuses into the target cell and binds to a cytoplasmic receptor. This complex then translocates to the cell nucleus where it interacts with specific areas of the genome to produce messenger RNA. The mRNA is translated into proteins which then produce the anti-inflammatory effects. The many other effects of this class of drugs are produced by the same mechanisms, but in different tissues. The time taken to produce these regulatory proteins explains the slow onset of action of corticosteroids which persists after their removal from the systemic circulation. The effects of one group of proteins, the lipocortins, on inflammatory responses is particularly important and will be discussed below.

Pharmacological Effects

As would be expected from the ubiquity of steroid hormone receptors, corticosteroids have many effects which could potentially be beneficial in asthma. Some of these effects are "antiallergic" (174) and others are anti-inflammatory.

Dexamethasone has been shown to prevent sensitization in the skin by IgE and thereby prevent subsequent type 1 allergic reactions (175). In addition, corticosteroids have numerous effects on cells involved in allergic and inflammatory reactions. Although they do not appear to have a direct action on human mast cells (176), they do reduce the production of mediators from sensitized lung fragments (174). Corticosteroids reduce eosinophilic chemotaxis and ad-

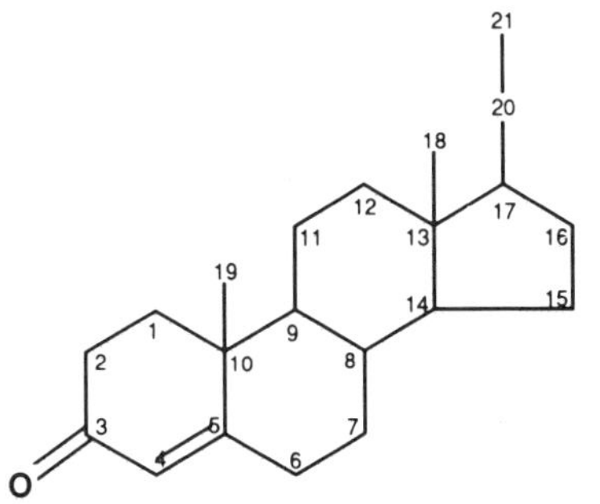

CORTICOSTEROID MOIETY

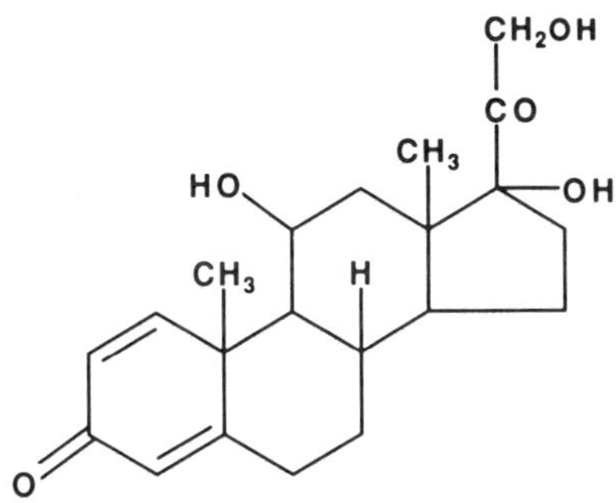

PREDNISOLONE

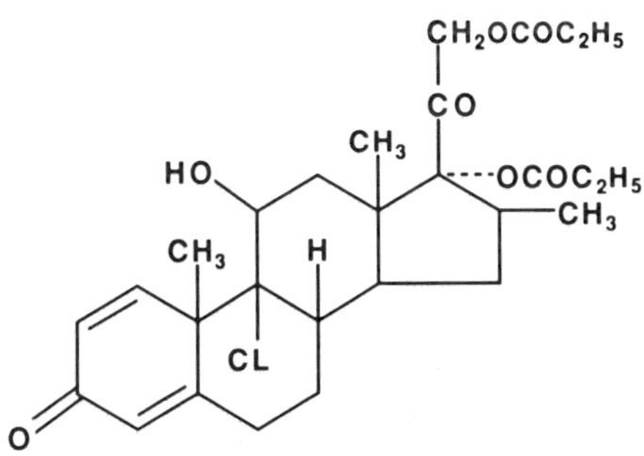

BECLOMETHASONE DIPROPIONATE

FIGURE 6 Structure of corticosteroid moiety. Increases in potency follow addition of a double bond between positions 1 and 2, 9 alpha esterification, or 16 alpha and/or 17 alpha substitutions. Addition of a methyl group at position 16 alpha reduces otherwise increased mineralocorticoid activity.

herence (177), which causes a circulating eosinopenia. In contrast, although neutrophil adherence is also reduced, leukocytosis occurs because of an additional release of leukocytes from the bone marrow (178). Transient lymphopenia occurs after corticosteroid administration, T-cell responses are reduced (179), as is the $T_4:T_8$ ratio (180). At high doses, IgE and IgG production can be attenuated (181). Macrophage functions, namely migration, expression of Ia antigens and production of IL-1 and mediators are all modified by corticosteroids (182). The exact clinical significance of these many effects in the treatment of asthma remains to be elucidated. A major breakthrough in understanding the anti-inflammatory effects of corticosteroids came about with the establishment of a link between corticosteroid-induced intracellular synthesis of lipocortins and the inhibition of phospholipase A_2 (PLA_2) (183). PLA_2 is responsible for the production of inflammatory mediators such as prostaglandins, leukotrienes, and PAF. With increased knowledge of the mechanism of action of corticosteroids and the cloning of lipocortin (184), the synthesis of nonsteroidal drugs with specific anti-inflammatory actions becomes a possibility.

Corticosteroids do not appear to have a direct effect on bronchial smooth muscle, but may reverse beta-receptor subsensitivity. They reduce mucous glycoprotein secretion from cells in culture (185), reduce sputum, and increase cough and mucociliary clearance in asthmatic patients (186).

Clinical Effects

Corticosteroids have been shown to have relatively acute effects in severe asthma. Bronchodilatation and improvement in gas exchange occur after oral and inhaled corticosteroids (172). Late antigen responses and the airway hyperresponsiveness that accompany them are blocked by inhaled corticosteroids (28) although it requires longer treatment to prevent the immediate response (187), or exercise-induced asthma (188). Long-term administration particularly of inhaled corticosteroids improves airway hyperresponsiveness (189), as well as the signs and symptoms of asthma (190).

Adverse Effects

The adverse effects of high concentrations of systemic corticosteroids for prolonged periods are well recognized (e.g., Cushing's syndrome). The dramatic effects of prolonged treatment with oral corticosteroids were appreciated soon after their introduction and led to a reappraisal of their use in chronic diseases (191). The introduction of inhaled corticosteroids established that good asthma control could be maintained without significant side effects. The effects of inhaled BDP, the most studied inhaled drug, on hypothalmic pituitary adrenal function have recently been reviewed (192). It appears that up to a "threshold dose" (BDP 1200–1500 μg/day), the majority of patients do not exhibit any changes in HPA function but above this dose there is dose-dependent suppression. As would be expected, this threshold dose is lower in children. Growth retardation in children, which occurs with oral corticosteroids, has not been seen in the majority of trials of inhaled corticosteroids. However, the interpretation of these trials is complicated by the effect of asthma on growth (193) and the choice of control groups. There are no well-controlled studies on other potential systemic effects of inhaled corticosteroids such as osteoporosis, deranged carbohydrate metabolism, and hypertension. Unlike topical corticosteroids on the skin, long-term inhalational use for as long as 10 years is not associated with connective tissue changes, and improvements in the degree of inflammation may be seen (194). Oral colonization with candida is a regular occurrence with inhaled corticosteroids although symptomatic oral candidiasis is much less common. Dysphonia can occur particularly with higher doses of inhaled corticosteroids and in some cases may be associated with a characteristic abnormality of the vocal cords (195).

MEASUREMENT OF EFFICACY

Study Design

There are a number of principles of clinical trial design that should be observed in the measurement of efficacy of antiasthma drugs if the results are to be easily interpreted. Blinding a study is accepted as crucial to prevent bias, however, random administration of treatments and comparison with a matched-placebo treatment arm (not just a prestudy control run) are equally important. Absolute efficacy can be shown by demonstration of significant positive superiority to placebo, demonstration of superiority to an active comparator, which need be no better than placebo, or by demonstration of a significant relationship between dose (or concentration) and effect. Showing clinical bioequivalence with a drug of proven efficacy is acceptable if the design and power of the study is sufficient to show a difference between the treatments (i.e., the chances of a type II error are small). Perhaps the most difficult and contentious area is deciding what constitutes clinical significance. As the models of asthma become more complex or further removed from clinical experience, it is difficult to determine the therapeutic implications of "significant" results. Finally, there are many inherent characteristics which make asthma trials particularly difficult to perform. For example, the pattern of exacerbations and remissions in asthmatic patients, the effects of repeated drug administration, either tachyphylaxis or "carry over," and the variability of individual responses all contribute to difficulty in completing a satisfactory study.

Bronchodilator Response

The acute effects of drugs on pulmonary function have been the traditional and most easily determined measurement of efficacy of antiasthmatic medication.

Choice of optimal dose and dose frequency have been determined by balancing bronchodilatation against side-effect liability. This is perhaps understandable since the major advances in asthma therapy during the first half of this century have concerned drugs where the most obvious action is smooth muscle relaxation. With the discovery of effective, nonbronchodilator drugs such as cromolyn and corticosteroids and the appreciation that the underlying problem of asthma is not just bronchial muscle constriction, other measurements of antiasthmatic efficacy have been required. The measurement of bronchodilator responses may offer important diagnostic or prognostic information in clinical practice. However, in the assessment of new drugs they provide limited, albeit quick and conveniently measured, information concerning their effectiveness. Many factors have to be taken into account when interpreting the data from bronchodilator trials. The type of patient selected, the severity of their asthma, the route of administration of the drug and the "washout" period from other drugs need to be carefully considered. Similarly, the drug's pharmacokinetics, particularly if inhaled, its pharmacodynamics, and the type of physiological measurement used may all influence the results particularly in comparative trials. Cholinocepters are distributed mainly in the central airways and beta-receptors are mainly distal (196) so deposition of aerosols to one part of the bronchial tree or measurement of predominantly large or small airway responses might show different though clinically irrelevant results. Also specific antagonists such as anticholinergics and antihistamines may only cause bronchodilation if the respective agonists are involved in maintaining bronchial tone, whereas functional antagonists such as beta-agonists and methyl xanthines will reverse constriction due to all causes. Although acute changes in pulmonary function usually represent smooth muscle relaxation (symptomatic arc), after prolonged drug usage improvement in lung function, its maintenance at the same level or a reduction in its loss may represent amelioration of more fundamental processes (prophylactic arc) (Fig. 7). While improvement in other indices of inflammation may also be useful, interpretation of pulmonary function data from long-term studies remains extremely difficult.

Airway Challenge Testing

Airway hyperresponsiveness to a variety of stimuli is one of the hallmarks of asthma (174) and the degree of airway responsiveness is correlated with the severity of asthma as measured by lung function, asthma attacks and concomitant medication (197). With the growing dissatisfaction with the predictive value of animal models and bronchodilator testing in the development of antiasthma drugs, airway challenge testing has been widely used to identify potentially useful compounds, to investigate their mechanism of action and latterly to study their pharmacokinetics. Perhaps the most notable example of this approach was

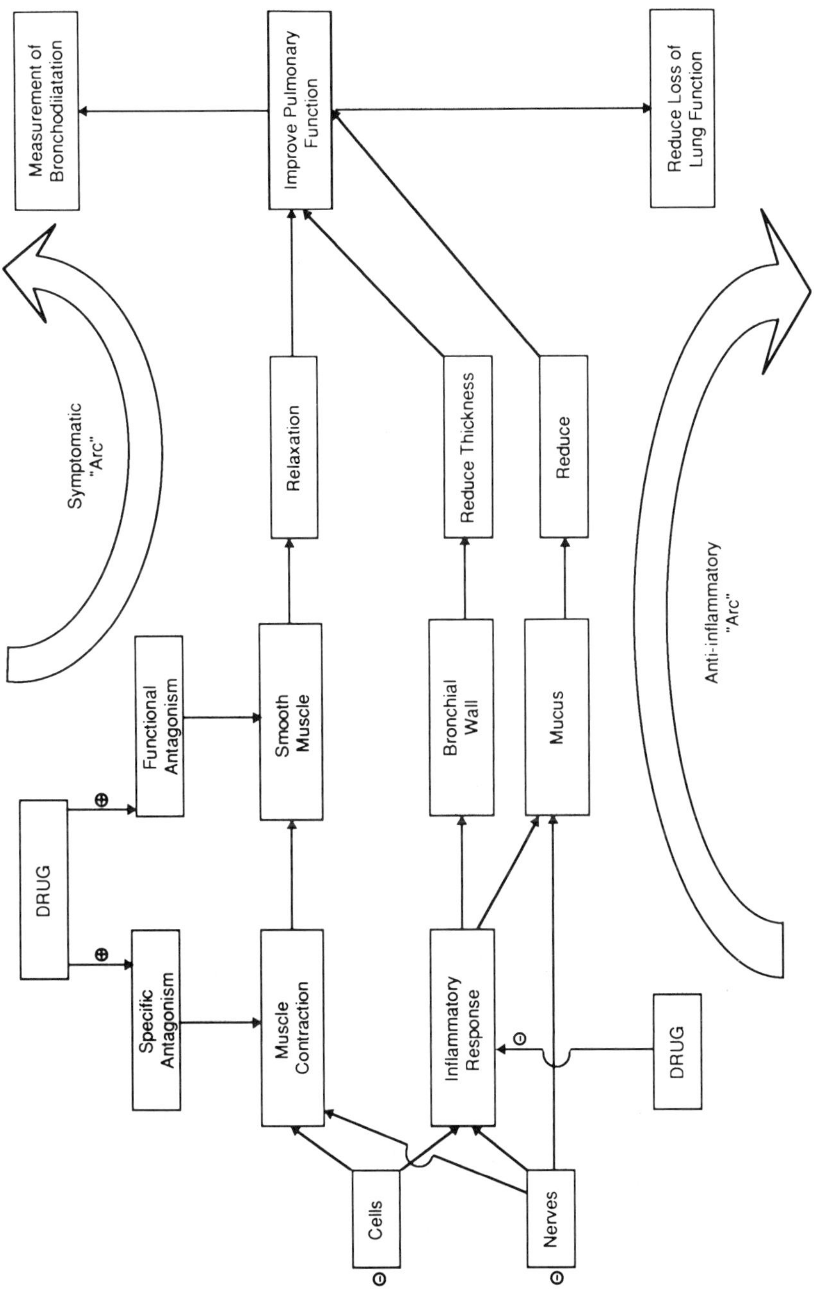

FIGURE 7 Schematic representation of the effects of symptomatic and anti-inflammatory drugs on pulmonary function.

the characterization of clinical pharmacology of cromolyn by Altounyan using his own antigen-induced responses (109). In addition, the effects of various compounds on the human models of asthma have offered an insight into its causes. Using these observations, attempts have been made to classify drugs as symptomatic, prophylactic, antiallergic, or anti-inflammatory. However, as the number of different pharmacological actions identified for any one drug increases, these divisions become blurred and more difficult to sustain. It is perhaps more useful to regard these challenges as simple stimulus-response "arcs" with the afferent limb representing the stimulus and the efferent limb the measurement of changes in pulmonary function. The sensitivity to the stimulus and the strength of the response can be considered as being modulated by the degree of asthmatic inflammation. Therefore, pharmacological modification of the challenge test may occur through a direct effect somewhere in the stimulus-response "arc" or else through a more fundamental but indirect effect on the degree of inflammation. In the succeeding sections schematic "arcs" for various challenges have been constructed and the effects of antiasthma drugs on these will be briefly summarized. The value of the effects in predicting therapeutic usefulness will be considered.

Exercise Challenge

Study of the pharmacological modulation of exercise-induced bronchospasm (EIB) has served to determine not only a therapeutic approach but has also provided some insights into the mechanism of EIB. Exercise or hyperventilation leads to heat and/or water loss from the airways which in turn through a mechanism as yet undetermined causes smooth muscle contraction (Fig. 8) (198,199). Although late asthmatic responses are observed (200), there appears to be no increase in airway responsiveness (201) after exercise. Several methods have been suggested for evaluating the effect of drugs on exercise-induced bronchospasm but those suggested by Anderson's group probably give the best description of the data while retaining some clinical relevance (153). EIB is considered totally blocked by a drug if a subject's lung function remains within the normal range after exercise (reduction in $FEV_1 \leqslant 10\%$ and PEFR $\leqslant 12.5\%$). A drug produces clinically effective protection if the postexercise drop in lung function is $<50\%$ of that after placebo. In addition, the group mean reduction in lung function on active and placebo medication is tested for statistically significant differences. These three indices have been compared for several drugs from published studies (Fig. 9). This analysis allows not only comparison of the protective effects of various drugs but also consideration of what is therapeutically useful. Inhaled beta-adrenergic agonists appear to offer the best protection against EIB with cromolyn having a beneficial effect in the majority of subjects. Inhaled anticholinergic agents and chronic oral theophylline offer a degree of clinical protection although this is less predictable. The effects of oral beta-agonists are small compared to those of inhaled. Calcium channel blockers offer some significant

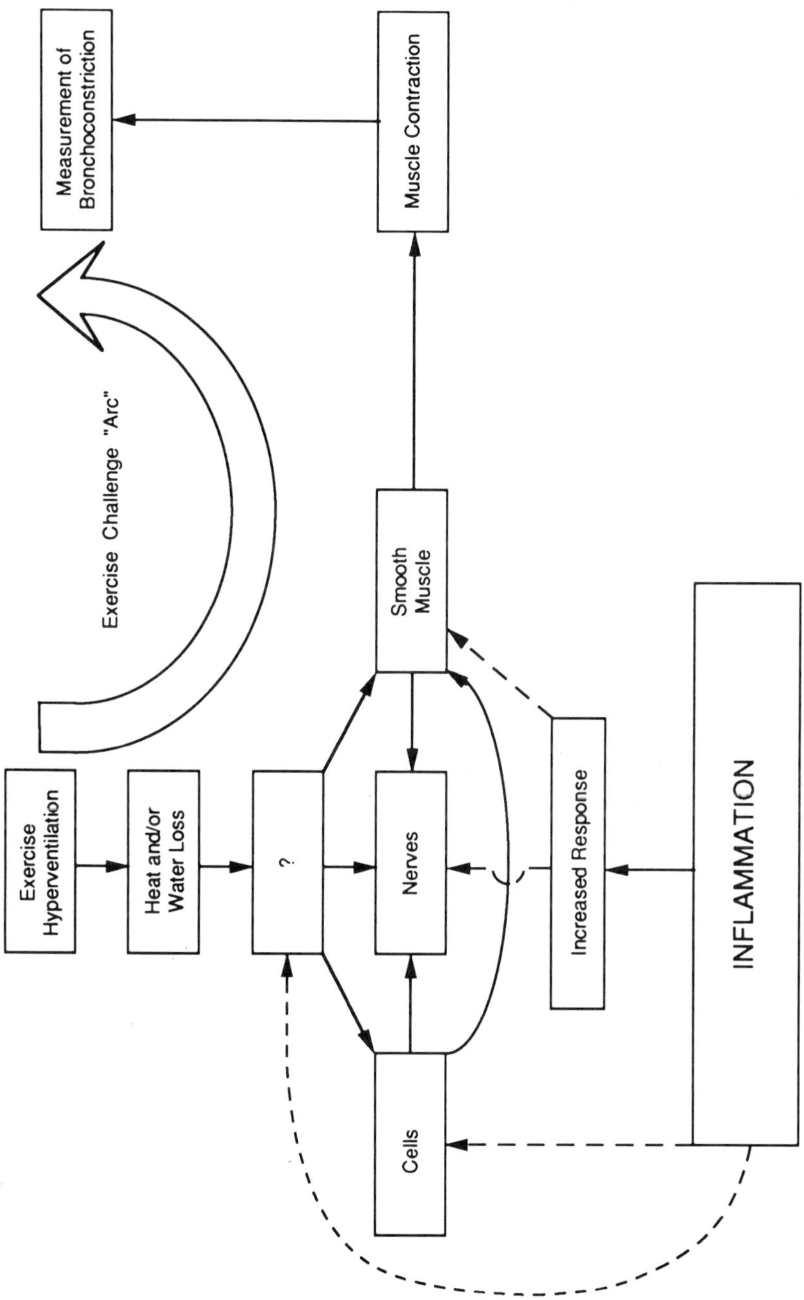

FIGURE 8 Schematic representation of the exercise challenge arc. It is as yet unclear exactly how heat and/or water loss leads to smooth muscle contraction. Pharmacological modulation of the stimulus–response arc is most effective in presenting EIB, but reduction of inflammation may also be beneficial.

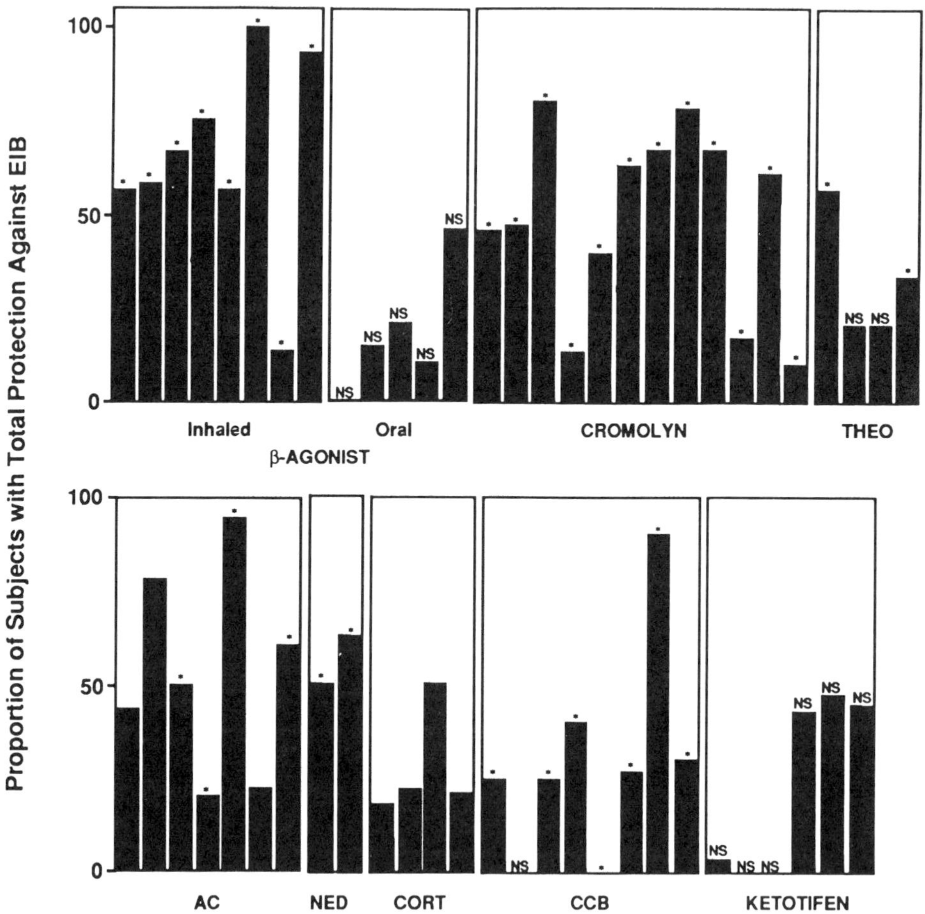

FIGURE 9 The proportions of subjects with total protection against exercise-induced bronchospasm (EIB) (drop in FEV_1, <10%; PEFR <12.5%) after administration of antiasthma medication in published studies. * = Significant difference between mean reductions after active and placebo; NS = not significant; blank = not tested; THEO = theophylline; AC = anticholinergic agent; NED = nedocromil; CORT = corticosteroid; CCB = calcium channel blocker.

reduction in postexercise falls in lung function but little in the way of clinically useful protection, while ketotifen appears to offer little at all. These results suggest that the drugs that attenuate the stimulus-response arc are most effective at blocking EIB. Interestingly, prolonged use of inhaled corticosteroids gives a degree of protection against EIB (189), although not as much as inhaled beta-agonists and cromolyn.

Airway Challenge with Constrictor Mediators

The up-regulation of the "stimulus-response arc" (Fig. 10) in asthmatic subjects, presumably as a result of bronchial inflammation, results in the airway hyperresponsiveness that is one of the diagnostic features of asthma. Therefore, as well as its use in diagnosis and epidemiology, it has been suggested that measuring airway responsiveness would be a more valuable means of comparing the effectiveness and duration of action of different drugs (202), than bronchodilator responses. Bronchodilator responses may poorly discriminate between two effective drugs if both are able to achieve maximal bronchodilatation. In contrast, airway challenge testing which relies on the shifts in stimulus-effect curves, at least in theory, has no upper limit and thus may better discriminate between drugs. It is also argued that the duration of protection against pharmacologically induced bronchoconstriction, which is shorter than the duration of bronchodilatation, might offer a more rational basis for the choice of dose frequency of an investigational drug (203). It is as yet unclear what clinical relevance continuous protection against induced bronchoconstriction might offer or whether indeed it is a worthwhile goal.

A large number of studies have investigated the effects of various drugs on bronchial challenge testing. Many stimuli have been used, but the most common and best documented are histamine and methacholine. Despite the many different methods of performing the challenge (204), it is possible to compare the results from different studies. The shift in the dose-effect curves after drug administration is represented by a change in the dose of histamine or methacholine which provokes an arbitrary but significant fall in lung function (PD_{sig}). The dose ratio (predrug PD_{sig}/post PD_{sig}) gives an indication of the inhibitory effect of a drug and can be calculated from most published studies. This is more conveniently represented as the change in doubling doses (LN [dose ratio]/LN2). This has the advantage of not only being a linear measurement but also of having some relevance to the method of its generation. The change in doubling doses of histamine and methacholine after antiasthma drugs varies considerably (Fig. 11a,b). The specific antagonists (anticholinergic agents and antihistamines) are very effective at blocking their respective agonists. Inhaled beta-adrenoceptor agonists, however, are the most effective agents at protecting against both these stimuli. It is interesting to note that calcium channel blockers provide protection to much the same degree as in EIB, although their clinical efficacy is

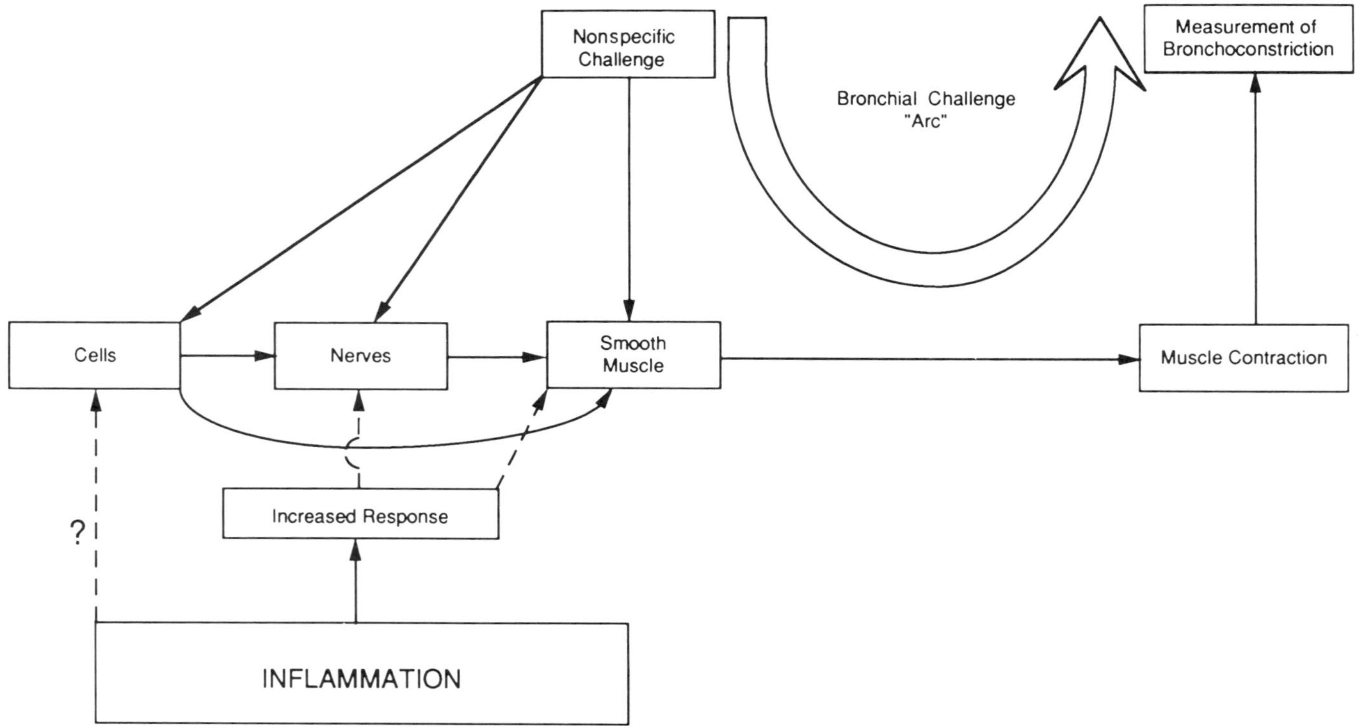

FIGURE 10 Schematic representation of the bronchial challenge arc. Pharmacological modulation of the stimulus-response arc acutely is most effective at reducing bronchial response to nonspecific stimuli. Long-term anti-inflammatory treatment may also reduce the response usually by smaller amounts presumably by reducing inflammation.

probably negligible. Drugs such as cromolyn and corticosteroids appear to have little acute effect on this stimulus-response arc compared to beta-adrenoceptor agonists despite their proven efficacy in the treatment of asthma. The longer term use particularly of inhaled corticosteroids is associated with small but significant changes in bronchial responsiveness (205,206). Some studies have shown significant changes after cromolyn (207) while others have not (208). Prolonged use of inhaled corticosteroids produces significantly greater improvements in responsiveness than theophylline (209), cromolyn (210), and oral corticosteroids (190). It is proposed that over longer periods inhaled corticosteroids ameliorate bronchial wall inflammation and reduce the sensitivity of the stimulus-response arc (Fig. 10). This hypothesis suggests that although the changes in responsiveness are small, they may represent a significant reduction in inflammation. This further implies that inhaled corticosteroids may be able to modify the natural history of the asthma. Airway challenge testing during longer term administration of beta-agonists, after their acute effects have worn off (more than 8 hr) shows no improvement. Indeed, two studies showed small but significant increases in airway responsiveness from prestudy baseline values (<1 doubling doses) during regular treatment with a beta-adrenoceptor agonist (211,212). A placebo-controlled study showed a significantly greater airway responsiveness after stopping the beta-adrenoceptor agonist compared to placebo, but the absolute amount was no greater than prestudy values (213). There has only been one other trial studying the effects on airway responsiveness after stopping antiasthma medication. In this case, there was a transient increase in methacholine sensitivity after cessation of ipratropium bromide (214). What happens to airway responsiveness after stopping other antiasthma medication is not known, however, clinical experience and published studies would suggest that when inhaled corticosteroids are stopped, some patients deteriorate (215). It may be that suddenly stopping any effective antiasthma medication can be associated with clinical deterioration (and perhaps increase in airway responsiveness). While it is true that there is a good correlation between asthma severity and the degree of airway hyperresponsiveness, it is impossible to be sure that small changes in airway responsiveness in either direction represent a significant improvement or deterioration of bronchial inflammation without other confirmatory evidence, particularly when the stimulus-response arc can be affected by many other variables including the pharmacological agents themselves.

Finally, airway challenge testing may be useful in assessing the pharmacokinetics of an investigational drug. For instance if an oral antihistamine does not block inhaled histamine, it either lacks efficacy or sufficient oral bioavailability.

Allergen-Induced Responses

The inhalation of allergen in susceptible individuals leads to mast cell degranulation, mediator release and bronchoconstriction (Fig. 12) which is called the

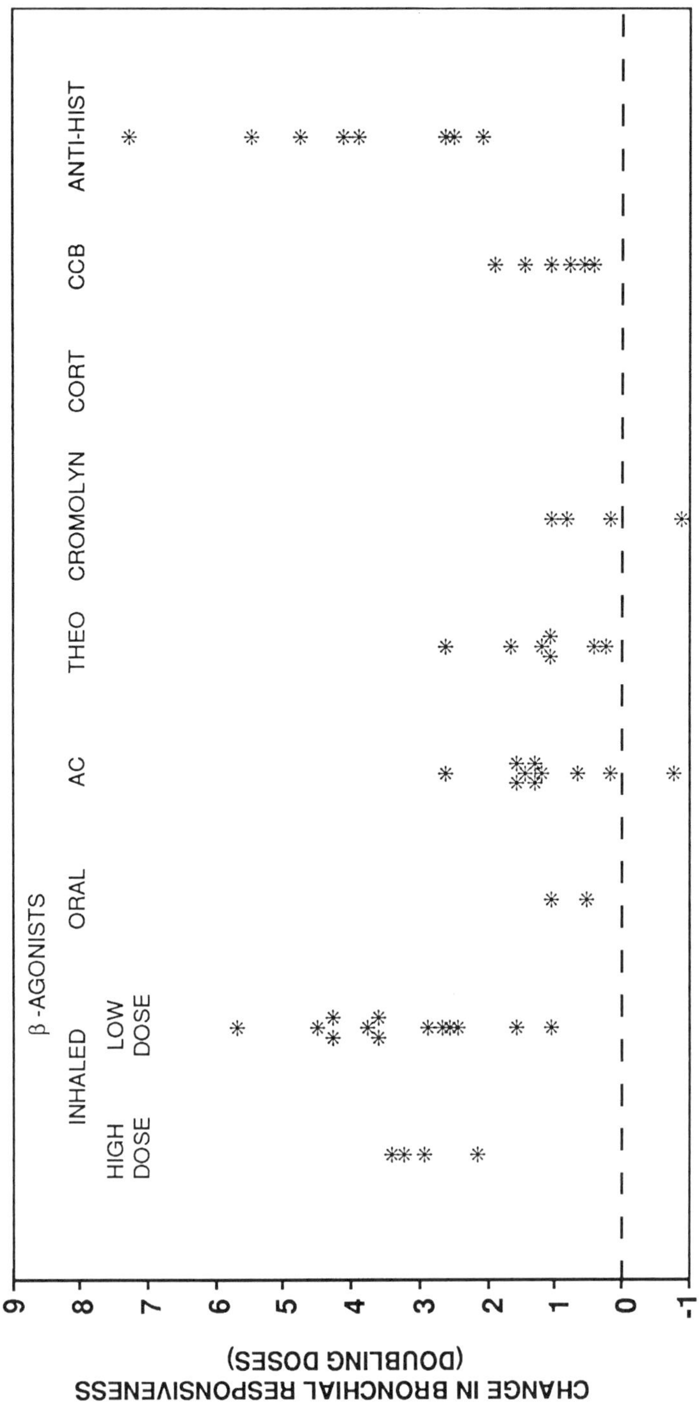
β-AGONISTS
INHALED
HIGH DOSE
LOW DOSE
ORAL
AC
THEO
CROMOLYN
CORT
CCB
ANTI-HIST
9
8
7
6
5
4
3
2
1
0
-1
CHANGE IN BRONCHIAL RESPONSIVENESS
(DOUBLING DOSES)

(a)

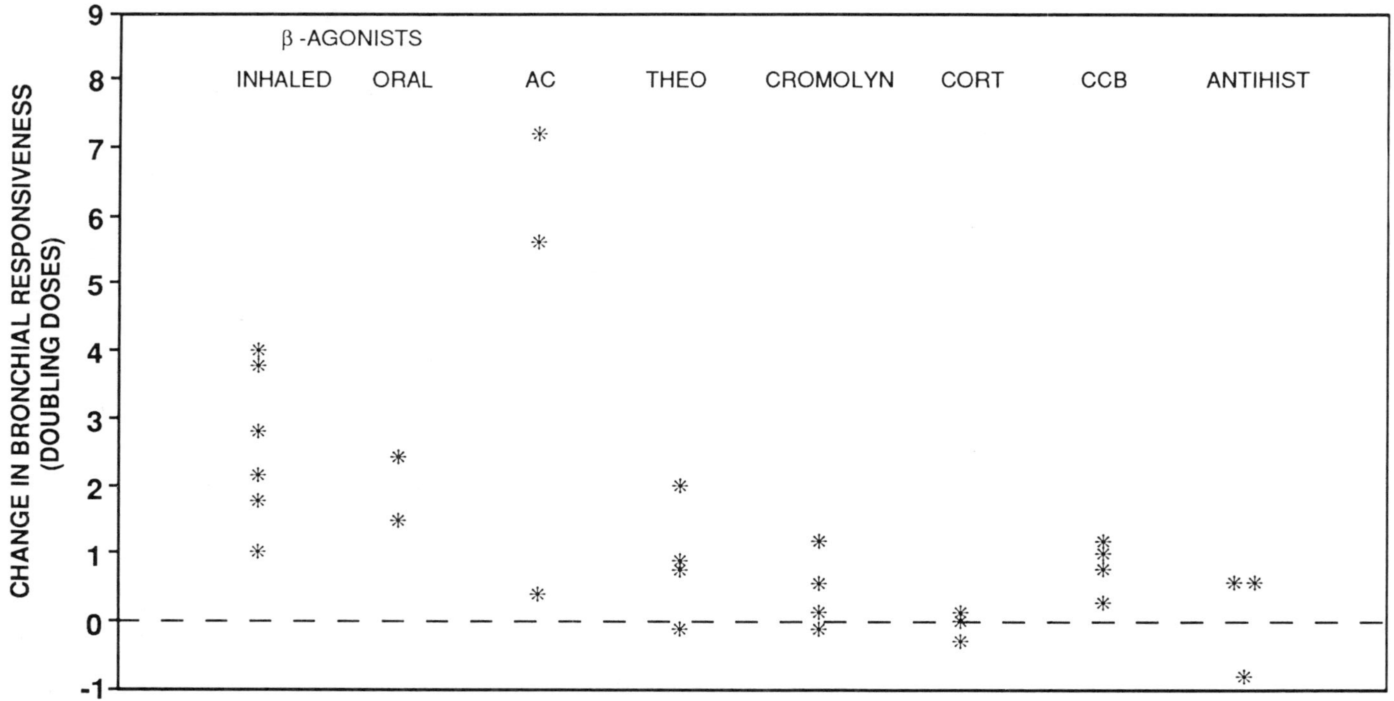

(b)

FIGURE 11 The change in provocative dose of histamine (a) and methacholine (b) represented in doubling dose after administration of antiasthma drugs from published studies. * = Significant difference from control or placebo; NS = not significant; blank = not tested; THEO = theophylline; AC = anticholinergic agent; NED = Nedocomil; CORT = corticosteroid; CCB = calcium channel blocker; Doubling dose = LN (predrug PD/postdrug PD)/LN2.

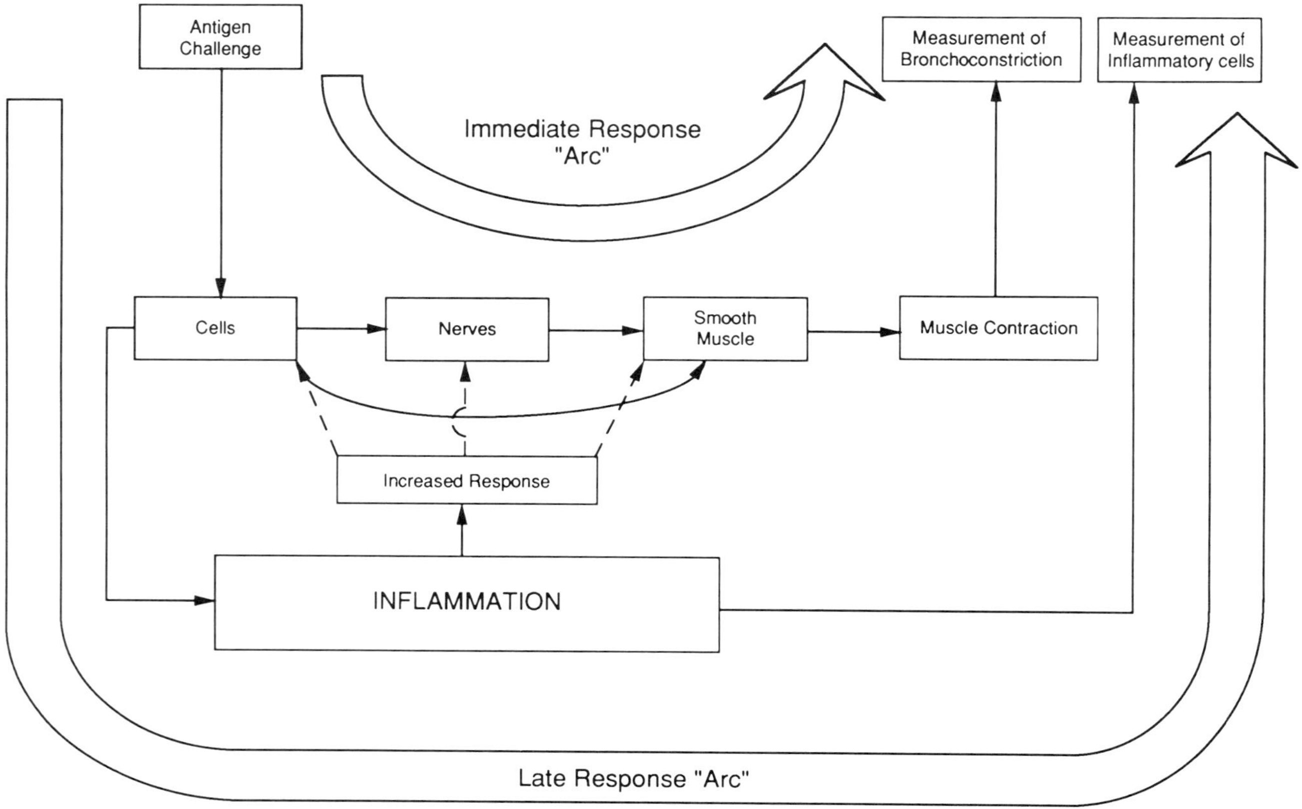

FIGURE 12 Schematic representation of the antigen challenge arc. Pharmacological modulation of the immediate response arc predominantly involves antagonism of smooth muscle contraction. The late response arc involves bronchial wall inflammation as well as changes in pulmonary function.

immediate response. In some individuals after recovery from the immediate response there is further reduction in lung function termed the late response (216). This late response is associated with an increase in airway responsiveness (217), and bronchoalveolar eosinophilia (218), presumably as a result of bronchial inflammation. Since this experimental model has many of the features of clinical asthma, its pharmacological modulation has excited considerable attention. Since administration of antigen is the most technically demanding and potentially the most dangerous challenge, properly designed studies are particularly difficult to perform. In addition, differences in techniques and presentation of results makes interpretation and comparison of results from different studies difficult. The most effective inhibitors of the immediate response are beta-adrenoceptor agonists followed in effectiveness by cromolyn (Fig. 13). Anticholinergics, antihistamines, theophylline, and corticosteroids have a variable effect. Although ineffective when given immediately before antigen challenge, inhaled corticosteroids do provide some degree of protection when given for several days (219). Inhibition of the immediate response does not prevent the late response and its sequelae. In this case, cromolyn and corticosteroids are more effective in blocking both the changes in lung function (Fig. 13) and airway responsiveness (28). Anticholinergic agents, antihistamines, and conventional beta-agonists given before antigen challenge have no significant effect on the late response (Fig. 13). This distinction has led to compounds which block late responses being termed prophylactic or anti-inflammatory, and those that do symptomatic. However, in one study, xanthines when given as an infusion before antigen challenge and continued for several hours afterward, attenuated the late response (77). Also, formoterol a long-acting beta-adrenoceptor agonist, and a large dose of albuterol also significantly reduced the late response (29). Other drugs such as cyclo-oxygenase inhibitors have been shown to block the late response in some studies (220), but not others (221). The most direct measurement of a late "inflammatory" response, albeit the most difficult to study, is bronchoalveolar eosinophilia. Thus, the acid test for any drug will remain not just the inhibition of epiphenomena, but the suppression of the inflammatory response. Other models of airway inflammation have been used to explore the actions of antiasthmatic medication. Nature's own antigen challenge, namely airborne pollen, has been used to test the protective effects of drugs over a prolonged period. For instance, oral corticosteroids prevented increases in symptoms and airway responsiveness in pollen sensitive asthmatic patients during the season (222) as did cromolyn (208), but not ketotifen (223). Sensitization with toluene diisocyanate, an industrial chemical, with subsequent rechallenge causes immediate and late responses, increased airway responsiveness and airway inflammation. Unlike antigen challenge only high-dose inhaled corticosteroids inhibited the late response and concomitant increase in airway responsiveness (224). Similarly, administration of either PAF (225) or

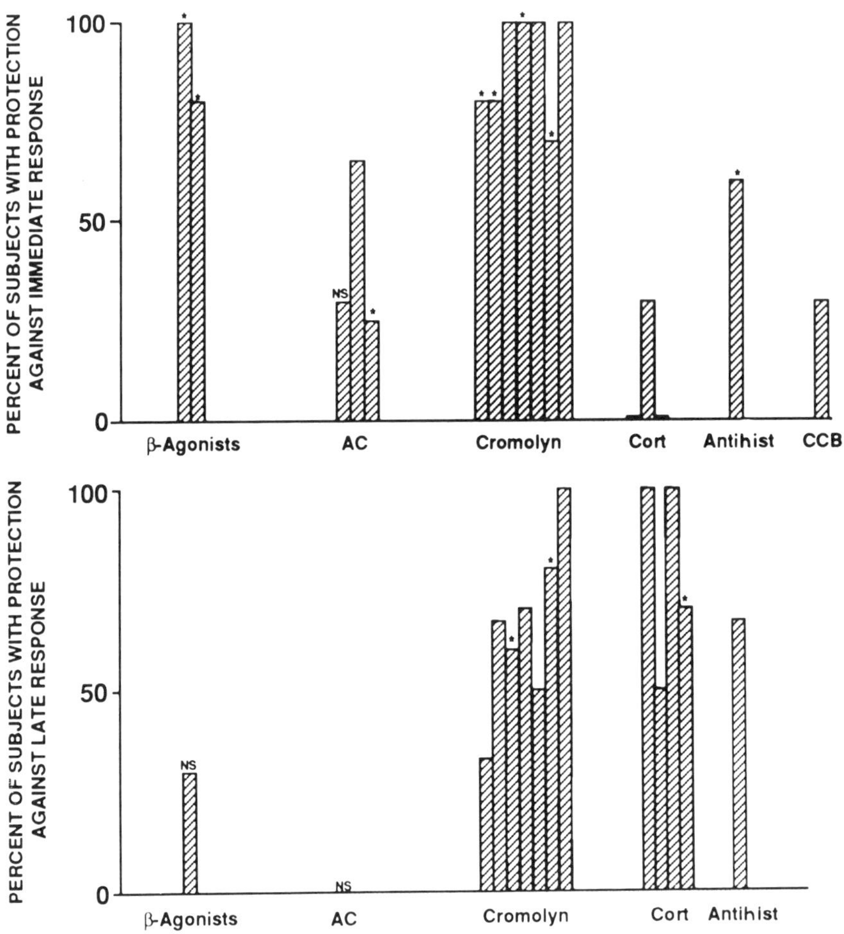

FIGURE 13 The proportion of subjects with clinically effective protection after antiasthma medication (<50% of reduction in pulmonary function after placebo) in published studies. Upper panel is for the immediate response and the lower for the late response. * = Significant difference from control or placebo; NS = not significant; blank = not tested; AC = anticholinergic agents; CORT = corticosteroids; Antihist = antihistamines; CCB = calcium channel blockers.

leukotriene E_4 (226) cause airway hyperresponsiveness and perhaps also airway inflammation. It is possible that these additional models of induced airway responsiveness and inflammation may offer further opportunities for the assessment of investigational drugs.

ACKNOWLEDGMENTS

I am most grateful to Brenda Jordan for typing the manuscript, Russ Maxwell for producing the artwork, to Jeno Marton, Duncan Richards, and Eva Beaule for bibliographic services.

REFERENCES

1. Solis-Cohen S. The use of adrenal substance in the treatment of asthma. J Am Med Assoc 1900; 34:1164–1166.
2. Bullowa JGM, Kaplan DM. The hypodermatic use of adrenalin chloride in the treatment of asthmatic attacks. Med News 1903; 83:787–790.
3. Chen KK, Schmidt CF. The action of ephedrine: the active principle of the Chinese drug Ma Huang. J Pharmacol Exp Ther 1924; 24:339-357.
4. Konzett H, Neve broncholytisch hochwirksame Körper der Adrenalinreihe. Arch Exp Path Pharm 1940; 197:27–40.
5. Ahlquist RP. A study of adrenotropic receptors. Am J Physiol 1948; 153: 586–600.
6. Lands AM, Arnold A, McAuliff JP, Luduena P, Brown TG Jr. Differentiation of receptor systems activated by sympathomimetic amines. Nature 1967; 214:597–598.
7. Brittain RT, Farmer JB, Jack D. a-[(t-butylamino)methyl] -4-hydroxy-m-xylene-al, a3-diol, (AH3365): a selective B-adrenergic stimulant. Nature 1968; 219:862–863.
8. Ball DI, Coleman RA, Denyer LH, Nials AT, Sheldrick KE. In vitro characterization of the B2 adrenoceptor-agonist salmeterol (abstr). Br J Pharmacol 1987; 92:591P.
9. Ullman A, Svedmyr N. Salmeterol, a new long-acting inhaled B2 adrenoceptor agonist: comparison with salbutamol in adult asthmatic patients. Thorax 1988; 43:674–678.
10. Bradshaw J, Brittain RT, Coleman RA, Jack D, Kennedy I, Lunts LH, Skidmore IF. The design of salmeterol, a long acting selective Beta2 adrenoceptor agonist. (Abstract). Br J Pharmacol 1987; 92:590P.
11. Yabuuchi Y. The B-adrenoceptor stimulant properties of OPC-2009 on guinea-pig isolated tracheal, right atrial, and left atrial preparations. Br J Pharmacol 1977; 61:513–521.
12. Petty TL, Brandon ML, Busse WW, Chervinsky P, Schoenweter W, Beaupre A, Boulet LP, Mazza J. A comparison of oral procaterol and albuterol in reversible airflow obstruction. Am Rev Resp Dis 1988; 138:1504–1509.
13. Friedel HA, Brogden RN. Bitolterol: a preliminary review of its pharmacological properties and therapeutic efficacy in reversible obstructive airways disease. Drugs 1988; 35:22–41.
14. Svensson LA. Bambuterol, a bronchodilator prodrug with sustained action, enhances delivery of active drug to the lung. Agents Actions 1988; 23(Suppl):271–276.

15. Skoogh BE. Transmission through airway ganglia. Eur J Respir Dis 1983; 64(Suppl 131):159–170.
16. Pavia D, Bateman JRM, Clarke SW. Deposition and clearance of inhaled particles. Clin Respir Physiol 1980; 16:335–366.
17. Erjefalt I, Persson CGA. Anti-asthma drugs attenuate inflammatory leakage of plasma into airway lumen. Acta Physiol Scand 1986; 128:653–654.
18. Howell S, Roussos C. Isoproterenol and aminophylline improve contractility of fatigued canine diaphragm. Am Rev Respir Dis 1984; 129:118–124.
19. Winter RJ, Langford JA, Rudd RM. Effects of oral and inhaled salbutamol and oral pirbuterol on right and left ventricular function in chronic bronchitis. Br Med J [Clin Res] 1984; 288:824–825.
20. Carstairs JR, Nimmo AJ, Barnes PJ. Autoradiographic visualization of beta-adrenoceptor subtypes in human lung. Am Rev Resp Dis 1985; 132:541–547.
21. Goldie RG, Spina D, Henry PJ, Lulich KM, Paterson JW. In vitro responsiveness of human asthmatic bronchus to carbachol, histamine, beta-adrenoceptor agonists and theophylline. Br J Clin Pharmacol 1986; 22: 669–676.
22. Palmer JB, Cuss FM, Barnes PJ. VIP and PHM and their role in non-adrenergic inhibitory responses in isolated human airways. J Appl Physiol 1986; 61:1322–1328.
23. Karlsson JA, Persson CGA. Influence of tracheal contraction on relaxant effects in vitro of theophylline and isoprenaline. Br J Pharmacol 1981; 74:73–79.
24. Butchers PR, Fullerton JR, Skidmore IF, Thompson LE, Vardey CJ, Wheeldon A. A comparison of the anti-anaphylactic activities of salbutamol and disodium cromoglycate in the rat, the rat mast cell and in human tissue. Br J Pharmacol 1979; 67:23–32.
25. Church MK, Hiroi J. Inhibition of IgE-dependent histamine release from human dispersed lung mast cells by anti-allergic drugs and salbutamol. Br J Pharmacol 1987; 90:421–429.
26. Howarth PH, Durham SR, Lee TH, Kay AB, Church MK, Holgate ST. Influence of albuterol, cromolyn sodium and ipratropium bromide on the airway and circulating mediator responses to allergen bronchial provocation in asthma. Am Rev Respir Dis 1985; 132:986–992.
27. Butchers PR, Cousins SA, Vardey CJ. Salmeterol: a potent and long-acting inhibitor of the release of inflammatory and spasmogenic mediators from human lung (Abstr). Br J Pharmacol 1987; 92:745P.
28. Cockcroft DW, Murdock KY. Comparative effects of inhaled salbutamol, sodium cromoglycate, and beclomethasone dipropionate on allergen-induced early asthmatic responses, late asthmatic responses, and increased bronchial responsiveness to histamine. J Allergy Clin Immunol 1987; 79: 734–740.
29. Palmqvist M, Balder B, Lowhagen O, Melander B, Svedmyr N, Wahlander L.

Late asthmatic reaction prevented by inhaled salbutamol and formoterol (Abstr). J Allergy Clin Immunol 1989; 83:224.

30. Lipworth BJ, Clark RA, Dhillon OP, Brown RA, McDevitt DG. B-adrenoceptor responses to high doses of inhaled salbutamol in patients with bronchial asthma. Br J Clin Pharmacol 26:527–533.
31. Waldeck B, Jeppsson AB, Widmark E. Partial agonism and functional selectivity: a study on beta-adrenoceptor mediated effects in tracheal, cardiac and skeletal muscle. Acta Pharmacol Toxicol Copenh 1986; 58:209–218.
32. Larsson S, Svedmyr N, Thiringer G. Lack of bronchial B-adrenoceptor resistance in asthmatics during long-term treatment with terbutaline. J Allergy Clin Immunol 1977; 59:93–100.
33. Arnold JMO, McDevitt DG. Heart rate and blood pressure responses to intravenous boluses of isoprenaline in the presence of propranolol, practolol and atropine. Br J Clin Pharmacol 1983; 16:175–184.
34. Heitz A, Schwartz J, Velly J. B-adrenoceptors of the human myocardium: determination of B1 and B2 subtypes by radioligand binding. Br J Pharmacol 1983; 80:711-717.
35. Levine MAH, Leenan FHH. Role of B1-receptors and vagal tone in cardial inotropic and chronotropic responses to B2-agonist in humans. Circulation 1989; 79:107–115.
36. Phillips PJ, Vedig AE, Jones PL, Chapman MG, Collins M, Edwards JB, Seaton TC, Duncan BMcL. Metabolic and cardiovascular side effects of beta-adrenoceptor agonists, salbutamol and rimiterol. Br J Clin Pharmacol 1980; 9:483–491.
37. Neville A, Palmer JBD, Gaddie J, May CS, Palmer KNV, Murchison LE. Metabolic effects of salbutamol: comparison of aerosol and intravenous administration. Br Med J 1977; 1:413–414.
38. Scheinin M, Koulu M, Laurikainen E, Allonen H. Hypokalaemia and other non-bronchial effects of inhaled fenoterol and salbutamol: a placebo-controlled dose-response study in healthy volunteers. Br J Clin Pharmacol 1987; 24:645–653.
39. Jenne JW. Wither beta-adrenergic tachyphylaxis. J Allergy Clin Immunol 1982; 70:413–416.
40. Tattersfield AE. Tolerance to beta-agonists. Bull Eur Physiopathol Respir 1985; 21:1s–5s.
41. Harvey JE, Tattersfield AE. Airway response to salbutamol: effect of regular salbutamol inhalations in normal, atopic and asthmatic subjects. Thorax 1982; 37:280–287.
42. Ruffin RE, Fitzgerald JD, Rebuk AS. A comparison of the bronchodilator activity of SCH-1000 and salbutamol. J Allergy Clin Immunol 1977; 59: 136–141.
43. Harrison AR, Richards R, Howarth P, Tattersfield AE. Interaction of inhaled corticosteroids and beta2-agonists in asthmatic subjects. Thorax 1984; 39:710–711.
44. Nicklas RA, Whitehurst VE, Donohoe RF, Balazs T. Concomitant use of beta-adrenergic agonists and methylxanthines. J Allergy Clin Immunol 1984; 73:20–24.

45. Joad JP, Ahrens RC, Lindgren SD, Weinberger MM. Extrapulmonary effects of maintenance therapy with theophylline and inhaled albuterol in patients with chronic asthma. J Allergy Clin Immunol 1986; 78:1147–1153.
46. Kemp JP, Chervinsky P, Orgel HA, Meltzer EO, Noyes JH, Mingo TS. Concomitant bitolterol mesylate aerosol and theophylline for asthma therapy, with 24-hour electrocardiographic monitoring. J Allergy Clin Immunol 1984; 73:32–43.
47. Persson CGA. On the medical history of xanthines and other remedies for asthma. A tribute to H. H. Salter. Thorax 1985; 40:881-886.
48. Salter H. On some points in the treatment and clinical history of asthma. Edinb Med J 1859; 4:1109–1115.
49. Trendelenburg P. Physiologische und pharmakologische Untersuchungen an der isolierten Bronchialmuskulatur. Naunyn-Schmiedebergs Arch Pharmakol Exp Pathol 1912; 69:79–107.
50. Hirsch S. Klinischer und experimenteller Beitrag zur krampflosenden Wirkung der Purinderivate. Klin Wochenschr 1922; 1:615–618.
51. Mitenko PA, Ogilvie RI. Pharmacokinetics of intravenous theophylline. Clin Pharmacol Ther 1973; 14:509–513.
52. Hendeles L, Iafrate RP, Weinberger M. A clinical and pharmacokinetic basis for the selection and use of slow release theophylline products. Clin Pharmacokinet 1984; 9:95–135.
53. Simons KJ, Simons FER. Urinary excretion of dyphylline in humans. J Pharm Sci 1979; 68:1327-1328.
54. Hudson LD, Tyler ML, Petty TL. Oral aminophylline and dihydroxypropyl theophylline in reversible obstructive airway disease: a single dose, double-blind, crossover comparison. Curr Ther Res 1973; 15:367-372.
55. Selvig K. Pharmacokinetics of proxyphylline in adults after intravenous and oral administration. Eur J Clin Pharmacol 1981; 19:149–155.
56. Persson CGA. Xanthines for asthma—present status. Trends Pharmacol Sci 1982; 3:312–313.
57. Persson CGA, Kjellin G. Enprofylline, a principally new antiasthmatic medication. Arch Pharmacol Toxicol 1981; 49:313–316.
58. Hendeles L, Weinberger M. Theophylline. A "state of the art" review. Pharmacotherapy 1983; 3:2–44.
59. Sutherland EW, Robison GA, Butcher RW. Some aspects of the biological role of adenosine 3′,5′ monophosphate (cyclic AMP). Circulation 1968; 37:279–306.
60. Bergstrand H. Phosphodiesterase inhibition and theophylline. Eur J Respir Dis 1980; 61 (Suppl 109):37–44.
61. Persson CG. Development of safer xanthine drugs for treatment of obstructive airways disease. J Allergy Clin Immunol 1986; 78:817–824.
62. Grandordy B, Cuss FMC, Barnes PJ. Breakdown of phosphoinositides in airway smooth muscle: lack of influence or anti-asthmatic drugs. Life Sci 1987; 41:1661-1667.
63. Kolbech RC, Speir WA, Carrier GO, Branson ED Jr. Apparent irrelevance of

cyclic nucleotides to the relaxation of tracheal smooth muscle induced by theophylline. Lung 1976; 156:173-183.

64. Bryson SE, Rodger IW. Effects of phosphodiesterase inhibitors on normal and chemically skinned isolated guinea-pig isolated airway smooth muscle. Br J Pharmacol 1987; 92:673-681.
65. Orange RP, Kaliner MA, Laraia PJ, Austen KF. Immunological release of histamine and slow reacting substance of anaphylaxis from human lung. II. Influence of cellular levels of cyclic AMP. Fed Proc 1971; 30:1725-1729.
66. O'Neill SJ, Sitar DS, Klass DJ, Taraska VA, Kepron W, Mitenko PA. The pulmonary disposition of theophylline and its influence on human alveolar macrophage bactericidal function. Am Rev Respir Dis 1986; 134:1225-1228.
67. Nielson CP, Crowley JJ, Cusack BJ, Vestal RE. Therapeutic concentrations of theophylline and enprofylline potentiate catecholamine effects and inhibit leukocyte activation. J Allergy Clin Immunol 1986; 78:660-667.
68. Sutton PP, Pavia D, Bateman JRM, Clarke SW. The effect of oral aminophylline on lung mucocilary clearance in man. Chest 1981; 80(Suppl): 889-892.
69. Aubier M, DeTroyer A, Sampson M, Macklem PT, Roussos C. Aminophylline improves diaphragmatic contractility. N Engl J Med 1981; 130:429-433.
70. Mackay AD, Baldwin CJ, Tattersfield AE. Action of intravenously administered aminophylline on normal airways. Am Rev Respir Dis 1983; 127: 609:613.
71. Higbee MD, Kumar M, Galant SP. Stimulation of endogenous catecholamine release by theophylline: a proposed additional mechanism of action for theophylline effects. J Allergy Clin Immunol 1982; 70:377-382.
72. Whyte KF, Addis GJ, Whitesmith R, Reid JL. Failure of chronic theophylline therapy to alter circulating catecholamines. Eur J Respir Dis 1987; 70:221-228.
73. Ellis EF. Inhibition of exercise-induced asthma by theophylline. J Allergy Clin Immunol 1984; 73:690-692.
74. Cockroft DW, Killian DN, Mellow JJA, Hargreave FE. Protective effect of drugs on histamine-induced asthma. Thorax 1977; 32:429-437.
75. McWilliams BC, Menendez R, Kelly HW, Howick J. Effects of theophylline on inhaled methacholine and histamine in asthmatic children. Am Rev Respir Dis 1984; 130:193-197.
76. Cartier A, Lemire I, L'Archeveque J, Ghezzo H, Martin RR, Malo JL. Theophylline partially inhibits bronchoconstriction caused by inhaled histamine in subjects with asthma. J Allergy Clin Immunol 1986; 77:570-575.
77. Pauwels R, Van Renterghem D, Van der Straeten M, Johannesson N, Persson CG. The effect of theophylline and enprofylline on allergen-induced bronchoconstriction. J Allergy Clin Immunol 1985; 76:583-590.
78. Weinberger MM, Bronsky E. Evaluation of oral bronchodilator therapy. J Pediatr 1974; 84:421-427.

79. Ellis EF. Antiasthma xanthines and adenosine on theophylline toxicity. Excerpta 1985; 352-360.
80. Woodcock AA, Johnson MA, Geddes DM. Theophylline prescribing, serum concentrations, and toxicity. Lancet 1983; 2:610-613.
81. Wachelefsky GS, Wo J, Adelson J, Mickey MR, Spector SL, Katz RM, Siegel SC, Rohr AS. Behavior abnormalities and poor school performance due to oral theophylline use. Pediatrics 1986; 78:1133-1138.
82. Andersson KE, Johannesson N, Karlberg B, Persson CGA. Xanthine-induced increase of plasma free fatty acids and natriuresis in man may reflect adenosine antagonism. Eur J Clin Pharmacol 1985; 26:33.
83. Gandevia B. Historical review of the use of parasympathetic agents in the treatment of respiratory disorders. Postgrad Med J 1975; 51(Suppl 7): 13-20.
84. Grandordy BM, Cuss FMC, Sampson AS, Palmer JB, Barnes PJ. Phosphatidylinositol response to cholinergic agonists in airway smooth muscle: relationship to contraction and muscarinic receptor occupancy. J Pharmacol Exp Ther 1986; 238:273-279.
85. Fryer AD, Maclagan J. Muscarinic inhibitory receptors in parasympathetic nerves in the guinea pig. Br J Pharmacol 1984; 83:973-978.
86. Wahl O. Pharmacokinetics (absorption-distribution-metabolism-excretion) of C14-labelled SCH 1000 administered by inhalation, orally, and intravenously (Abstr). Postgrad Med J 1975; 51 (Suppl 7):93-94.
87. Barnes PJ. Neural control of human airways in health and disease. Am Rev Resp Dis 1986; 134:1289-1314.
88. Blaber LC, Fryer AD, Maclagan J. Neuronal muscarinic receptors attenuate vagally-induced contraction of feline bronchial smooth muscle. Br J Pharmacol 1985; 86:723-728.
89. Ingram RH, Wellman JJ, McFadden ER, Mead J. Relative contributions of large and small airways to flow limitation in normal subjects before and after atropine and isoproterenol. J Clin Invest 1977; 59:696-703.
90. Ruffin RE, Newhouse MT. Ipratropium bromide (SCH-1000) monohydrate aerosol: bronchodilator effect of three dose levels in asthmatics. Lung 1978; 155:141-146.
91. Peel ET, Anderson G. A dose response study of oxitropium bromide in chronic bronchitis. Thorax 1984; 39:453-456.
92. Gross NJ, Skorodin MS. Anticholinergic, antimuscarinic bronchodilators. Am Rev Resp Dis 1984; 129:856-870.
93. DeVries K. The protective effect of inhaled SCH-1000 MDI on bronchoconstriction induced by serotonin, histamine, acetycholine and propranolol (Abstr). Postgrad Med J 1975; 51 (Suppl 7):106.
94. Grieco MH, Pierson RN Jr. Mechanism of bronchoconstriction due to beta-adrenergic blockade. Studies with practolol, propranolol, and atrophine. J Allergy Clin Immunol 1971; 48:143-152.
95. Ruffin RE, Wolff RK, Dolovich MB, Eng P, Rossman CM, Fitzgerald JD, Newhouse MT. Aerosol therapy with SCH 1000: short-term mucociliary clearance in normal and bronchitic subjects and toxicology in normal subjects. Chest 1978; 73:501-505.

96. Molkenboer JFWM, Lardenoye JG. The effect of Atrovent in micturition function, double-blind crossover study. Scand J Respir Dis 1979; 103 (Suppl):154–158.
97. Sturgess J, Reid L. An organ culture study of the effect of drugs on the secretory activity of the human bronchial submucosal gland. Clin Sci 1972;43:533–543.
98. Blair AMJN, Woods A. The effects of isoprenaline, atropine and disodium cromoglycate on ciliary motility and mucus flow measured in vivo in cats. Br J Pharmacol 1969;35:379P–380P.
99. Iravani J, Melville GN. Ciliary movement following various concentrations of different anticholinergic and adrenergic bronchodilator solutions in animals (Abstr). Postgrad Med J 1975;51(Suppl 7):108.
100. Yeates DB, Aspin N, Levison H, Jones MT, Bryan AC. Mucociliary tracheal transport rates in man. J Appl Physiol 1975;39:487–495.
101. Pavia D, Thomson ML. Inhibition of mucociliary clearance from the human lung by hyoscine. Lancet 1971;i:449–450.
102. Pavia D, Bateman JRM, Sheahan NF, Clarke SW. Effect of ipratropium bromide on mucociliary clearance and pulmonary function in reversible airways obstruction. Thorax 1979;34:501-507.
103. Lopez-Vidriero MT, Costello J, Clark TJH, Das I, Keal EE, Reid L. Effect of atropine on sputum production. Thorax 1975;30:544–547.
104. Chapman KR, Smith DL, Rebuk AS, Leenen FHH. Hemodynamic effects of inhaled ipratropium bromide, alone and in combination with inhaled beta 2 agonist. Am Rev Resp Dis 1985;132:845-847.
105. Sackner MA, Friedman M, Silva G, Fernandez R. The pulmonary hemodynamic effects of aerosols of isoproterenol and ipratropium in normal subjects and patients with reversible airway obstruction. Am Rev Resp Dis 1977;116:1013–1022.
106. Connolly CK. Adverse reaction to ipratropium bromide. Br Med J 1982; 285:934–935.
107. Beasley CRW, Rafferty P, Holgate ST. Bronchoconstrictor properties of preservatives in ipratropium bromide (Atrovent) nebuliser solution. Br Med J 1987;294:1197–1198.
108. Cox JSG. Disodium cromoglycate (FPL 670) ('Intal'): a specific inhibitor of reaginic antibody-antigen mechanisms. Nature (London) 1967: 216: 1328–1329.
109. Altounyan REC. Inhibition of experimental asthma by a new compound disodium cromoglycate (Intal). Acta Allergol 1967;22:487.
110. Howell JBL, Altounyan REC. A double-blind trial of disodium cromoglycate in the treatment of allergic bronchial asthma. Lancet 1967;ii:539–542.
111. Morrison Smith J, Devey GF. Clinical trial of disodium cromoglycate in the treatment of asthma in children. Br Med J 1968;1:340-344.
112. Moran F, Bankier JDH, Boyd G. Disodium chromoglycate in the treatment of allergic bronchial asthma. Lancet 1968;ii:137–139.
113. Pepys J, Hargreave FE, Chan M, McCarthy DS. Inhibitory effects of

disodium cromoglycate (intal) on allergen inhalation tests. Lancet 1968; 2:134–137.
114. Davies SE. The effect of disodium cromoglycate on exercise-induced asthma. Br Med J 1968; 3:593–594.
115. Walker SR. The fate of 14-C disodium cromoglycate in man. J Pharm Pharmacol 1972; 24:525–531.
116. Richards IM, Dixon M, Jackson DM, Vendy K. Alternative modes of action of sodium cromoglycate. Agents Actions 1986; 18:294–300.
117. Church MK, Young KD. The characteristics of inhibition of histamine release from human lung fragments by sodium cromoglycate, salbutamol and chlorpromazine. Br J Pharmacol 1983; 78:671–679.
118. Capron A, Dessaint JP, Capron M, Joseph M, Ameisen JC, Tonnel AB. From parasites to allergy: a second receptor for IgE. Immunol Today 1986; 7:15–18.
119. Kay AB. The mode of action of anti-allergic drugs. Clin Allergy 1987; 17:153–164.
120. Moqbel R, Walsh GM, MacDonald AJ, Kay B. Effect of disodium cromoglycate on activation of human eosinophils and neutrophils following reversed (anti-IgE) anaphylaxis. Clin Allergy 1986; 16:73–83.
121. Skedinger MC, Augustine NH, Morris EZ, Nielson DW, Zimmerman GA, Hill HR. Effect of disodium cromoglycate on neutrophil movement and intracellular calcium mobilization. J Allergy Clin Immunol 1987; 80: 573–577.
122. Kay AB, Walsh GM, Moqbel R, MacDonald AJ, Nagakura T, Carroll MP, Richerson HB. Disodium cromoglycate inhibits activation of human inflammatory cells in vitro. J Allergy Clin Immunol 1987; 80:1–8.
123. Dixon M, Jackson DM, Richards IM. The action of sodium cromoglycate on "C" fibre endings in the dog. Br J Pharmacol 1980; 70:11–13.
124. Fuller RW, Dixon CMS, Barnes PJ. Bronchoconstrictor responses to inhaled capsaicin in humans. J Appl Physiol 1985; 58:1080–1084.
125. Collier JG, Fuller RW. Capsaicin inhalation in man and the effects of sodium cromoglycate. Br J Pharmacol 1984; 81:113–117.
126. Sheppard D, Nadel JA, Boushey HA. Inhibition of sulfur dioxide-induced bronchoconstriction by disodium cromoglycate in asthmatic subjects. Am Rev Resp Dis 1981; 124:257–259.
127. Fanta CH, McFadden ER, Ingram RH. Effects of cromolyn sodium on the response to respiratory heat loss in normal subjects. Am Rev Resp Dis 1982; 123:161–164.
128. Fuller RW, Dixon CMS, Cuss FMC, Barnes PJ. Bradykinin-induced bronchoconstriction in humans. Am Rev Resp Dis 1987; 135:176–180.
129. Allistone A, Collier JG, Davidson RN, Fuller RW, Richardson PS. The effect of intravenous sodium cromoglycate on the bronchoconstriction induced by sulphur dioxide inhalation in man. Clin Sci 1985; 68:227–232.
130. Pepys J, Hargreave FE, Chan M, McCarthy DS. Inhibitory effects of disodium cromoglycate on allergen-inhalation tests. Lancet 1968; ii:134–137.
131. Brompton Hospital, Medical Research Council Collaborative Trial. Long-

term study of disodium cromoglycate in treatment of severe extrinsic or intrinsic bronchial asthma in adults. Br Med J 1972;4:383-388.
132. Silverman M, Connelly N, Balfour-Lynn L, Godfrey S. Long-term trial of disodium cromoglycate and isoprenaline in children with asthma. Br Med J 1972;3:378-381.
133. Eady RP. The pharmacology of nedocromil sodium. Eur J Respir Dis 1986;69(Suppl 147):112-119.
134. Richards IM, Eady RP, Jackson DM, Orr TSC, Pritchard DI, Vendy K, Wells E. Ascaris-induced bronchoconstriction in primates experimentally infected with ascaris suum ova. Clin Exp Immunol 1983;54:461-468.
135. Roberts JA, Thomson NC. Attenuation of exercise-induced asthma by pretreatment with nedocromil sodium and minocromil. Clin Allergy 1985; 15:377-381.
136. Juniper EF, Kline PA, Morris MM, Hargreave FE. Airway constriction by isocapnic hyperventilation of cold, dry air: comparison of magnitude and duration of protection by nedocromil sodium and sodium cromoglycate. Clin Allergy 1987;17:523-528.
137. Dixon CMS, Fuller RW, Barnes PJ. Effect of nedocromil sodium on sulphur dioxide induced bronchoconstriction. Thorax 1987; 42:462-465.
138. Hansson L, Choudry NB, Fuller RW, Pride NB. Effect of nedocromil sodium on the airway response to inhaled capsaicin in normal subjects. Thorax 1988;43:935-936.
139. Lal S, Malhotra S, Gribben D, Hodder D. Nedocromil sodium: a new drug for the management of bronchial asthma. Thorax 1984;39:809-812.
140. Dorward AJ, Roberts JA, Thomson NC. Effect of nedocromil sodium on histamine airway responsiveness in grass-pollen sensitive asthmatics during the pollen season. Clin Allergy 1986;16:309-315.
141. Goldin JG, Bateman ED. Does nedocromil sodium have a steroid sparing effect in adult asthmatic patients requiring maintenance oral corticosteroids. Thorax 1988;43:982-986.
142. Holgate ST, Emanuel MB, Howarth PH. Astemizole and other H1-antihistaminic drug treatment of asthma. J Allergy Clin Immunol 1985; 76: 375-380.
143. Phillips MJ, Ollier S, Gould C, Davies RJ. Effect of antihistamines and antiallergic drugs on responses to allergen and histamine provocation tests in asthma. Thorax 1984;39:345-351.
144. Chung KF, Morgan B, Keyes SJ, Snashall PD. Histamine dose-response relationship in normal and asthmatic subjects. The importance of starting airway caliber. Am Rev Resp Dis 1982;126:849-854.
145. Rafferty P, Holgate ST. Terfenadine (Seldane) is a potent and selective histamine H1 receptor antagonist in asthmatic airways. Am Rev Respir Dis 1987;135:181-184.
146. Brik A, Tashkin DP, Gong H Jr, Dauphinee B, Lee E. Effect of cetirizine, a new histamine H1 antagonist, on airway dynamics and responsiveness to inhaled histamine in mild asthma. J Allergy Clin Immunol 1987; 80:51-56.

147. Church MK, Gradidge CF. Inhibition of histamine release from human lung in vitro by antihistamines and related drugs. Br J Pharmacol 1980; 69:663–668.
148. Adachi M, Kobayashi H, Aoki N, Iijima M, Kokubu F, Furuya A, Takahashi T. A comparison of the inhibitory effects of ketotifen and disodium cromoglycate on bronchial responses to house dust with special reference to the late asthmatic response. Pharmatherapeutica 1984; 4:36–42.
149. Craps L, Greenwood C, Radielovic P. Clinical investigation of agents with prophylactic anti-allergic effects in bronchial asthma. Clin Allergy 1978; 8:373–382.
150. Esau S, del Carpio J, Martin JG. A comparison of the effects of ketotifen and clemastine on cutaneous and airway reactivity to histamine and allergen in atopic asthmatic subjects. J Allergy Clin Immunol 1984; 74:270–274.
151. Tanser AR, Elmes J. A controlled trial of ketotifen in exercise-induced asthma. Br J Dis Chest 1980; 74:398–402.
152. Tan WC, Lim TK. Double-blind comparison of the protective effect of sodium cromoglycate and ketotifen on exercise-induced asthma in adults. Allergy 1987; 42:315–317.
153. Anderson SD, Seale JP, Ferris L, Schoeffel R, Lindsay DA. An evaluation of pharmacotherapy for exercise-induced asthma. J Allergy Clin Immunol 1979; 64:612–624.
154. Petheram IS, Moxham J, Bierman CW, McAllen M, Spiro S. Ketotifen in atopic asthma and exercise-induced asthma. Thorax 1981; 36:308–312.
155. Chung KF, Minette P, McCusker M, Barnes PJ. Ketotifen inhibits the cutaneous but not the airway responses to platelet-activating factor in man. J Allergy Clin Immunol 1988; 81:1192–1198.
156. Paterson JW, Yellin RH, Tarala RA. Evaluation of ketotifen (HC20-511) in bronchial asthma. Eur J Clin Pharmacol 1983; 25:187–193.
157. Lane OJ. A steroid sparing effect of ketotifen in steroid-dependent Asthmatics Clin Allergy 1980; 10:519–525.
158. Loftus BG, Price JF. Long-term, placebo-controlled trial of ketotifen in the management of preschool children with asthma. J Allergy Clin Immunol 1987; 79:350–355.
159. Groggins RC, Hiller EJ, Milner AD, Stokes GM. Ketotifen in the prophylaxis of childhood asthma. Arch Dis Childhood 1981; 56:304–305.
160. Loftus BG, Price JF, Heaton R, Costello JF. Effects of ketotifen on in vitro bronchoconstriction. Clin Allergy 1985; 15:465–471.
161. Mason HL, Myers CS, Kendall EC. The chemistry of crystalline substances isolated from the suprarenal gland. J Biol Chem 1936; 114:613–631.
162. Carryer HM, Prickman LE, Maytum CR. Effects of cortisone on bronchial asthma and hay fever occuring in subjects sensitive to ragweed pollen. Proc Mayo Clin 1950; 25:282–295.
163. Randolph TG, Rollins JP. Effect of cortisone on bronchial asthma. J Allergy 1950; 21:288–295.
164. Rose B, Pare JAP, Pump K, Stanford RL. Preliminary report on adreno-

corticotrophic hormone (ACTH) in asthma. Can Med Assoc 1950; 62: 6-9.
165. Foulds WS, Greaves DP, Herxheimer H, Kingdom LG. Hydrocortisone in treatment of allergic conjunctivitis, allergic rhinitis and bronchial asthma. Lancet 1955;i:234-235.
166. Herxheimer H, McAllen MK, Williams DA. Local treatment of bronchial asthma with hydrocortisone powder. Br Med J 1958;2:762-765.
167. Helm WH, Heyworth F. Bronchial asthma and chronic bronchitis treated with hydrocortisone acetate inhalations. Br Med J 1958;2:765-768.
168. Clark TJH. Effect of beclomethasone dipropionate delivered by aerosol in patients with asthma. Lancet 1972;i:1361-1364.
169. Brown HM, Storey G, George WHS. Beclomethasone dipropionate: a new steroid aerosol for the treatment of allergic asthma. Br Med J 1972; 1: 585-590.
170. Herzog HL, Nobile A, Tolksdorf S, Charney W, Hershberg EB, Perlman PL, Pechet MM. New anti-arthritic steroids. Science 1955; 121:176.
171. McKenzie AW. Percutaneous absorption of steroids. Arch Dermatol 1962; 86:611-614.
172. Ellul-Micallef R. The acute effects of corticosteroids in bronchial asthma. Eur J Respir Dis 1982; 63(Suppl 122):118-125.
173. Lan NC, Karin M, Nguyen T, Weisz A, Birnbaum MJ, Eberhardt NL, Baxter JD. Mechanisms of glucocorticoid hormone action. J Steroid Biochem 1984; 20:77-88.
174. Schleimer RP. The mechanisms of antiinflammatory steroid action in allergic diseases. Annu Rev Pharmacol Toxicol 1985; 25:381-412.
175. Hellewell PG, Williams TJ. An anti-inflammatory steroid inhibits tissue sensitization by IgE in vivo. Br J Pharmacol 1989; 96:5-7.
176. Schleimer RP, Schulman ES, MacGlashan DW Jr, Peters SP, Hayes EC, Adams GK III, Lichtenstein LM, Adkinson NF Jr. Effects of dexamethasone on mediator release from human lung fragments and purified human lung mast cells. J Clin Invest 1983; 71:1830-1835.
177. Altman LC, Hill JS, Hairfield WM, Mullarkey MF. Effects of steroids on eosinophilic chemotaxis and adherence. J Clin Invest 1981; 67:28-36.
178. Dale DC, Fauci AS, DePont-Guerry IV, Wolff SM. Comparison of agents producing a neutrophilic leukocytosis in man: hydrocortisone, prednisone, endotoxin and etiocholanolone. J Clin Invest 1975; 56:808-813.
179. Larson EL. Cyclosporin A and dexamethasone suppress T cell responses by selectively being at distinct sites of the triggering process. J Immunol 1980; 124:2828-2833.
180. Gerblich A, Urda G, Schuyler M. Atopic asthma: T cell response to corticosteroids. Chest 1985; 87:44-50.
181. Butler WT, Rossen RD. Effect of corticosteroids on immunity in man I. Decreased serum IgG concentration caused by 3 or 5 days of high doses of methylprednisolone. J Clin Invest 1973; 52:2629-2640.
182. Snyder DS, Unanue ER. Corticosteroids inhibit murine Ia expression and Interleukin 1 production. J Immunol 1982; 129:1803-1805.
183. Flower RJ, Blackwell GJ. Anti-inflammatory steroids induce biosyn-

thesis of phospholipase A2 inhibitor which prevents prostaglandin generation. Nature 1979; 278:456–459.
184. Wallner BP, Mattaliano RJ, Hession C, Cate RL, Tizard R, Sinclair LK, Foeller C, Chow EP, Browing JL, Ramachandran KL, et al. Cloning and expression of human lipocortin, a phospholipase A2 inhibitor with potential anti-inflammatory activity. Nature 1986; 320:77–81.
185. Marom Z, Shelhamer J, Alling D, Kaliner M. The effects of corticosteroids on mucous glycoprotein secretion from human airways in vitro. Am Rev Respir Dis 1984; 129:62–65.
186. Agnew JE, Bateman JRM, Sheahan NF, Lennard-Jones AM, Pavia D, Clarke SW. Effect of oral corticosteroids on mucus clearance by cough and mucociliary transport in stable asthma. Bull Eur Physiopathol Respir 1983; 19:37–41.
187. Dahl R, Johansson SA. Importance of duration of treatment with inhaled budesonide on the immediate and late bronchial reaction. Eur J Respir Dis 1982; 63(Suppl):167–175.
188. Hendriksen JM, Dahl R. Effects of inhaled budesonide alone and in combination with low dose terbutaline in children with exercise-induced asthma. Am Rev Resp Dis 1983; 128:993–997.
189. Jenkins CR, Woolcock AJ. Effect of prednisone and beclomethasone dipropionate on airway responsiveness in asthma: a comparative study. Thorax 1988; 43:378–384.
190. Smith MJ, Hodson ME. High-dose beclomethasone inhaler in the treatment of asthma. Lancet 1983; 1:265–269.
191. David DS, Grieco MH, Cushman P Jr. Adrenal glucocorticoids after twenty years. A review of their clinically relevant consequences. J Chron Dis 1970; 22:637–711.
192. Hoskisson C, Meades CR, Cuss FM, Palmer JBD. Inhaled beclomethasone dipropionate: systemic effects reviewed. Ed. GM Cochrane 1989;
193. Balfour-Lynn L. Growth and childhood asthma. Arch Dis Childhood 1986; 61:1049–1055.
194. Lundgren R, Soderberg M, Hostedt P, Stenling R. Morphological studies of bronchial mucosal biopsies from asthmatics before and after ten years of treatment with inhaled steroids. Eur J Respir Dis 1988; 1:883–889.
195. Williams AJ, Baghat MS, Stableforth DE, Cayton RM, Shenoi PM, Skinner C. Dysphonia caused by inhaled steroids: recognition of a characteristic abnormality. Thorax 1983; 38:813–821.
196. Nadel JA, Barnes PJ. Autonomic regulation of the airways. Ann Rev Med 1984; 35:451–467.
197. Juniper EF, Frith PA, Hargreave FE. Airway responsiveness to histamine and methacholine: relationship to minimum treatment to control symptoms of asthma. Thorax 1981; 36:575–579.
198. McFadden ER Jr. Exercise and asthma. N Engl J Med 1987; 17:502–504.
199. Anderson SD. Issues in exercise-induced asthma. J Allergy Clin Immunol 1985; 76:763–772.
200. Iikura Y, Inui H, Nagakura T, Lee TH. Factors predisposing to exercise-induced late asthmatic responses. J Allergy Clin Immunol 1985; 75:285–289.

201. Zawadski DK, Lenner KA, McFadden ER Jr. Effect of exercise on nonspecific airway reactivity in asthmatics. Clin Res 1987; 35:633A.
202. Ahrens RC, Bonham AC, Maxwell GA, Weinberger MM. A method for comparing the peak intensity and duration of action of aerosolized bronchodilators using bronchoprovocation with methacholine. Am Rev Respir Dis 1984; 129:903–906.
203. Ahrens RC, Harris JB, Milavetz G, Annis L, Ries R. Use of bronchial provocation with histamine to compare the pharmacodynamics of inhaled albuterol and metaproterenol in patients with asthma. J Allergy Clin Immunol 1987; 79:876–882.
204. Townley RJ, Hopp RJ. Inhalation methods for the study of airway responsiveness. J Allergy Clin Immunol 1987; 80:111-124.
205. Easton JG. Effect of inhaled corticosteroid on methacholine airway reactivity. J Allergy Clin Immunol 1981; 67:388–390.
206. Ryan G, Latimer KM, Juniper EF, Roberts RS, Hargreave FE. Effect of beclomethasone dipropionate on bronchial responsiveness to histamine in controlled nonsteroid-dependent asthma. J Allergy Clin Immunol 1985; 75:25–30.
207. Lowhagen O, Rak S. Modification of bronchial hyperreactivity after treatment with sodium cromoglycate during pollen season. J Allergy Clin Immunol 1985; 75:460–467.
208. Jenkins CJ, Breslin AB. Long term study of the effect of sodium cromoglycate on non-specific bronchial hyperresponsiveness. Thorax 1987; 42:664–669.
209. Butoit JI, Salome CM, Woolcock AJ. Inhaled corticosteroids reduce the severity of bronchial hyperresponsiveness in asthma but oral theophylline does not. Am Rev Respir Dis 1987; 136:1174–1178.
210. Svendsen UG, Frolund L, Madsen F, Nielsen NH, Holstein Rathlou NH, Weeks B. A comparison of the effects of sodium cromoglycate and beclomethasone dipropionate on pulmonary function and bronchial hyperreactivity in subjects with asthma. J Allergy Clin Immunol 1987; 80:68–74.
211. Kraan J, Koeter GH, v d Mark TW, Sluiter HJ, De Vries K. Changes in bronchial hyperreactivity induced by 4 weeks of treatment with antiasthmatic drugs in patients with allergic asthma: a comparison between budesonide and terbutaline. J Allergy Clin Immunol 1985; 76:628–636.
212. Kerrebijn KF, van Essen Z. andvliet EE, Neijens HJ. Effect of long-term treatment with inhaled corticosteroids and beta-agonists on the bronchial responsiveness in children with asthma. J Allergy Clin Immunol 1987; 79:653–659.
213. Vathenen AS, Knox AJ, Higgins BG, Britton JR, Tattersfield AE. Rebound increase in bronchial responsiveness after treatment with inhaled terbutaline. Lancet 1988; 1:554–558.
214. Newcomb R, Tashkin DP, Hui KK, Connolly ME, Lee ME, Dauphinee B. Rebound hyper-responsiveness to muscarinic stimulation after chronic

therapy with inhaled muscarinic agents. Am Rev Respir Dis 1985; 132: 12–15.
215. Munch EP, Taudorf E, Weeke B. Dose frequency in the treatment of asthmatics with inhaled topical steroid. Eur J Respir Dis 1982; 63(Suppl 122):143–153.
216. Booij-Noord M, De Vries K, Sluiter HJ, Orie NGM. Late bronchial obstructive reaction to experimental inhalation of house dust extract. Clin Allergy 1972; 2:43-61.
217. Cockcroft DW, Ruffin RE, Dolovich J, Hargreave FE. Allergen-induced increase in non-allergic bronchial reactivity. Clin Allergy 1977; 7:503–513.
218. De Monchy JG, Kauffman HF, Venge P, Koeter GH, Jansen HM, Sluiter HJ, De Vries K. Bronchoalveolar eosinophilia during allergen-induced late asthmatic reactions. Am Rev Respir Dis 1985; 131:373–376.
219. Burge PS, Efthimiou J, Turner-Warwick M, Nelmes PTJ. Double-blind trials of inhaled beclomethasone dipropionate and fluocortin butyl ester in allergen-induced immediate and late asthmatic reactions. Clin Allergy 1982; 12:523–531.
220. Joubert JR, Shephard E, Mouton W, Van Zyl L, Viljoen I. Non-steroid anti-inflammatory drugs in asthma: dangerous or useful therapy. Allergy 1985; 40:202–207.
221. Kirby JG, Hargreave FE, O'Byrne PM. Indomethacin inhibits allergen-induced airways hyper-responsiveness but not allergen-induced asthmatic responses (Abstr). Am Rev Respir Dis 1982; 135(Suppl):A312.
222. Sotomayor H, Badier M, Vervloet D, Orehek J. Seasonal increase of carbachol airway responsiveness in patients allergic to grass pollen. Reversal by corticosteroids. Am Rev Respir Dis 1984; 130:56–58.
223. Tinkelman DG, Webb CS, Vanderpool GE, Carroll MS, Spangler DL, Lotner GZ. The use of ketotifen in the prophylaxis of seasonal allergic asthma. Ann Allergy 1986; 56:213–217.
224. Mapp C, Boschetto P, Dal Vecchio L, Crescioli S, de Marzo N, Paleari D, Fabbri LM. Protective effect of antiasthma drugs on late asthmatic reactions and increased airway responsiveness induced by toluene diisocyanate in sensitized subjects. Am Rev Respir Dis 1987; 136:1403–1407.
225. Cuss FM, Dixon CM, Barnes PJ. Effects of inhaled platelet activating factor on pulmonary function and bronchial responsiveness in man. Lancet 1986; 2:189–192.
226. Arm JP, Spur BW, Lee TH. The effects of inhaled leukotriene E4 on the airway responsiveness to histamine in subjects with asthma and normal subjects. J Allergy Clin Immunol 1988; 82:654–660.

11

Clinical Control of Asthma

JERRY DOLOVICH

McMaster University
Hamilton, Ontario, Canada

FREDERICK E. HARGREAVE

St. Joseph's Hospital
Hamilton, Ontario, Canada

INTRODUCTION

Inflammation of the airways can elicit a number of pathophysiological abnormalities including airways hyperresponsiveness, inflammatory edema, increased secretions, and probably chronic airflow limitation. The symptoms which result from these airway abnormalities include breathlessness, wheeze, chest tightness, cough, and sputum. These symptoms are characteristic of asthma, but also present in an appreciable number of nonsmokers with no localized lung disease who, nevertheless, have not received the "asthma" label. Thus, in many populations, the recorded prevalence of asthma is 5–10%; however the number of people with recurrent or continuing symptoms of cough, wheeze, chest tightness, or breathlessness may be an additional 10–20% (1,2). People whose predominant symptom is episodic cough are commonly said to have bronchitis. Failure to use the word asthma commonly leads to failure to use an asthma-type treatment regimen which may eradicate the symptoms (3). In children, this syndrome shares many other features with characteristic asthma, including a high prevalence of allergy and blood eosinophilia and, in some cases, airways hyperresponsiveness (4,5).

The ongoing underdiagnosis and undertreatment of affected people has implications in terms of function and well-being. In a cohort of 179 seven-year-old children in the school system in Tynesdine, only 21 of the wheezing children had a designation of asthma and only one-third were on antiasthma treatment.

When affected children were placed on appropriate treatment including anti-inflammatory treatment (inhaled beclomethasone or cromoglycate) their status improved remarkably and school absenteeism was reduced tenfold (3). Experience of this type suggests that a large proportion of nonsmokers with no localized disease who experience repeated or persistent cough, wheeze, or breathlessness would benefit from a treatment regimen appropriate for asthma. More therapeutic trials of the treatment of well-documented clinical populations with various combinations of symptoms are required.

OBJECTIVES OF TREATMENT (DEFINITION OF CONTROL AND BEST STATUS)

Both the physician and the asthmatic patient require clearly expressed criteria which serve as outcome objectives. Criteria which define control of asthma can be expressed as follows: (a) no cough, wheeze, or breathlessness; (b) normal functioning of the individual; (c) no severe attacks; the requirement is for arrangements for early effective treatment of exacerbations to quickly reverse them; (d) normal pulmonary function and (e) no side effects or overdose of medication.

Control of asthma is a realistic objective for the majority of people affected by mild to moderately severe disease. In all cases, the effort should be made to reverse the underlying inflammation. In some cases, the best status achieved falls short of control as defined above. There may be complete reversal of all symptoms except, for example, the occurrence of occasional breathlessness and tightness of the chest from exertion. In a small percentage of people, there may be a need for ongoing ingested prednisone despite other treatment including high-dose inhaled steroid, and in such cases, there may be steroid side effects. In this unfortunate situation, the necessary "trade off" between complete elimination of symptoms and the occurrence of side effects requires careful individual attention, judgement, and compromise. Once the best status in the individual is determined, it should be maintained; any worsening is an indication for an appropriate increase in the level of treatment.

Pulmonary function tests provide objective quantitation of the status of the airways; the greater the severity of the asthma the greater the importance of measurements for accurate assessment. Measurements by physicians when the patient is seen should be mandatory. Daily self-administration of peak flow rate measurements to monitor the asthmatic status is an important guideline for treatment of severe asthma. Woolcock and coworkers (6) have used changes in peak expiratory flow rate (PEFR) as a basis for increased treatment. When a 10% fall in peak flow rate occurred, the treatment regimen, emphasizing an anti-inflammatory approach, was increased by doubling the dose of inhaled salbutamol and beclomethasone to regain best values. In a controlled trial, this approach was shown more likely to improve airway hyperresponsiveness than reliance upon symptoms as a basis for increasing the level of treatment.

AVOIDANCE STRATEGIES

Natural or experimental exposure to an allergen (7) or to an occupational sensitizer such as toluene diisocyanate (TDI) or plicatic acid (8) can stimulate airway mucosal inflammation and an increase in airway responsiveness to inhaled methacholine or histamine. Conversely, avoidance of offending allergen or occupational sensitizer can, over time, lead to a reversal of induced airway hyperresponsiveness and a reversal of symptoms (9,10). The importance of efforts to avoid exposure is further exemplified by the observation that the longer a symptomatic individual is exposed to an occupational sensitizer, the greater the probability of a chronic persistence of symptoms and airway hyperresponsiveness after avoidance is accomplished (11). These observations argue for efforts to minimize exposure to inhaled offending substances to the greatest extent possible. In theory, exposure to a household cat or an occupational sensitizer such as TDI can be completely prevented. Exposures to some substances such as house dust mite can be reduced but not entirely eliminated. The results of experimental efforts to eliminate exposure to house dust mite are variable, but have been sufficiently successful to warrant efforts in individual house dust mite-allergic asthmatic patients (9,12).

Beta blockers must be avoided by all asthmatics, and other substances such as food allergens, nonsteroidal anti-inflammatory agents, metabisulfite, and probably monosodium glutamate (MSG) must be avoided by people with the specific allergy or intolerance in order to prevent the occurrence of acute episodes. However, there is little to suggest that such food substances form the basis of ongoing asthma; avoiding ingestion of trace dietary quantities, for example, of salicylate or sulfites, is not likely to have therapeutic value (13,14).

METHODS OF MEDICAL TREATMENT

Choices of Medications

Bronchodilator, in the form of inhaled or ingested selective $beta_2$-agonist or ingested theophylline, alone or in combination, has typically been the initial approach or so-called "first-line" maintenance treatment of asthma. Two types of observations have led to a reconsideration of this strategy. First, $beta_2$-agonist or theophylline does not have a beneficial effect upon induced airway hyperresponsiveness (15,16), which is considered to be an indication of the underlying airway inflammation. Second, there is increasing evidence that treatment regimens which include medications which exert an anti-inflammatory effect are more effective (3,17,18).

Comparisons of ingested theophylline with inhaled cromoglycate yield a consistent message; inhaled cromoglycate efficacy is as great or greater than theophylline used under optimum conditions and cromoglycate therapy is less invasive and far less likely to elicit side effects (17,19). Moreover, clinical trials seem to confirm the short-term experimental observations that cromoglycate is beneficial for the underlying inflammatory response and the resulting airway hyperresponsiveness, whereas theophylline is not (20).

Disadvantages of using only bronchodilator therapy include:

1. Short-term benefit from bronchodilator encourages continuing exposure to adverse conditions which can aggravate asthma; the temporary improvement in symptoms without beneficial effect upon the underlying disease can lead to a false sense of security.
2. The short-term benefit delays introduction of treatment which can suppress the inflammation.
3. When control is inadequate and alternative treatment has not been an integral part of the regimen, there is a temptation to dangerously overuse the bronchodilator.

Inhaled beta$_2$-agonist is much more effective than the corresponding ingested beta$_2$-agonist or theophylline in reversing established bronchoconstriction or preventing bronchoconstriction by stimuli such as exercise (21). One situation in which long-acting theophylline preparations can be uniquely beneficial and can be employed to advantage is before sleep to prevent early morning waking due to airway symptoms when this cannot be prevented by anti-inflammatory treatment. Long-acting ingested beta$_2$-agonist such as long-acting salbutamol may also accomplish this purpose. It is important to remember in such cases that greater efforts at improving the basic status of the asthma, such as by an increased dose of inhaled steroid, can often eliminate the nocturnal symptoms which are a reflection of the underlying airways hyperresponsiveness (22).

First-line use of inhaled steroid or inhaled cromoglycate or both in maintenance treatment of asthma is finding increasing acceptance. It permits control of the asthma in many cases, or, short of that, the achievement of the best status for the individual. Unlike bronchodilator, inhaled steroids can prevent airway hyperresponsiveness induced by allergen or a chemical sensitizer and probably by respiratory virus infection.

Long-term use of conventional doses of inhaled cromoglycate or inhaled steroid such as beclomethasone, budesonide, flunisolide, or triamcinolone has proven effective and safe. Inhaled steroid, particularly in high doses, can lead to oropharyngeal side effects including pharyngitis, dysphonia, or oropharyngeal candidiasis (23). With usual doses, clinical systemic side effects do not occur although there may be a reduction in the early morning blood cortisol level and in the 24-h urine cortisol excretion and also in blood eosinophil counts (24,25).

The practical significance of the former systemic changes is not known but seems to be negligible.

Side-by-side comparison of cromoglycate with inhaled beclomethasone diproprionate in treatment of asthma in children suggests that the latter is more potent. For example, two sprays of beclomethasone diproprionate taken four times a day yielded more wheeze-free days in children than Intal taken four times a day (26). Inhaled steroid but not inhaled cromoglycate has been shown to prevent the airway hyperresponsiveness induced by inhalation challenge with TDI (27). Thus a rational first-line treatment could consist of inhaled steroid or perhaps inhaled cromoglycate or both taken in the minimum dose needed to maintain the best control of symptoms and airway function.

A treatment regimen consisting of inhaled steroid and inhaled $beta_2$-agonist taken in amounts needed to achieve specified objectives has good rationale. In this approach, inhaled steroid is used in a dose sufficient to achieve and maintain control or the best status possible. Bronchoconstriction is an indication of a failure to completely eliminate airway hyperresponsiveness but, to the extent that it occurs, inhaled beta agonist is needed on a demand basis. Advantages of the use of steroid together with the beta agonist include:

1. Both immediate and long-term efficacy
2. Both anti-inflammatory and bronchodilatation effect
3. If there is bronchoconstriction at the time of use of the inhalers, bronchodilatation produced by the preliminary use of $beta_2$-agonist permits a more effective peripheral delivery of the subsequently used inhaled steroid

Allergen injection treatment in asthma remains controversial. It has the hypothetical advantage of reducing host responsiveness to inhaled allergen, thereby reducing symptoms and the requirement for medications. The observation that allergen injection treatment seems to selectively eliminate the late phase asthmatic response to inhaled allergen seemed encouraging insofar as there is a close association between the late response and the occurrence of allergen-induced airway hyperresponsiveness. However, the beneficial effects of allergen injection treatment on methacholine or histamine airway hyperresponsiveness remains to be convincingly demonstrated. Major practical disadvantages are that allergen injection treatment remains cumbersome and unpredictable in contrast with currently available medications which are rapid and reasonably predictable and have a favorable profile in terms of suppression of the underlying disease processes while controlling the symptoms.

Ketotifen is a medication for asthma, taken by ingestion, presently available in many countries. The onset of action is slow; in controlled trials, improvement in symptoms and reduction in dosage of supplemental inhaled $beta_2$-agonist or theophylline has been observed only after a treatment period of 2 or 3 months (28,29). However, beneficial effects can persist up to a month after the medication is discontinued, suggesting a suppression of basic disease mechanisms. Its place in treatment, in relation to alternative medications, has not been established.

Medication by the Inhalant Route

Use of the metered dose inhaler by proper technique is surprisingly difficult and subject to error. For optimal results, the following technique should be followed (30,31). Shake the inhaler while exhaling. The device is then held about 2 inches outside the wide open mouth with the canister pointed upward and the device pointed toward the throat. Following the onset of a slow inhalation, the canister is actuated and the inhalation is continued slowly without interruption until complete. Then breath holding commences, lasting for 10 seconds, followed by exhalation. In repeated studies, steps in the procedure shown to be important in delivery of medication to the lungs include the proper timing of actuation, the slow rate of inhalation, and the breath holding. With optimal use, there is about 10% delivery of the aerosol medication to the intrapulmonary airways and about 70% oropharyngeal deposition (32,33).

The oropharyngeal deposition of inhaled steroid can lead to local side effects including pharyngitis, dysphonia, and oropharyngeal candidiases. Techniques which probably reduce the likelihood of these local complications include:

1. Actuation of the canister outside the mouth.
2. Rinsing the throat by gargling after use of the inhaler.
3. Use of the inhaler before meals whereby eating can then wash away locally deposited steroid.
4. Use of a holding chamber (spacer). With a holding chamber there is no reduction in intrapulmonary deposition but pharyngeal deposition is reduced from about 70% to about 10% of the aerosolized medication. This generally serves to reduce or eliminate local adverse effects of inhaled steroid. It is reasonable to prescribe a holding chamber routinely in the adult if more than 800 μg per day of beclomethasone is needed to reduce the risk of oropharyngeal side effects. Since much of the locally deposited medication is ultimately swallowed, there is also possible reduction in systemic adverse effects of inhaled $beta_2$-agonist.

Infancy and childhood present special problems in the use of inhaled medication. The effectiveness of the combination of $beta_2$-agonist combined with steroid has been shown even in infants under 12 months of age; thus, there is good rationale for efforts to achieve a successful use of metered dose inhalers in the young. In practice, various failings of technique, including poor synchronization are probably more prevalent in children than adults. Nevertheless, children down to the age of 4 or 5 can use the metered dose inhaler. One technical problem which seems largely limited to childhood and has been observed in as many as 40% of children is the so-called "cold freon effect" (35). When the spray reaches the back of the throat, inhalation stops, and there is a resulting poor delivery to the lungs. These problems are largely eliminated by the use of a holding chamber; as such, the holding chamber has a unique and important place in the use of metered dose inhalers in children and probably should be used by the majority of children who require metered dose inhaler therapy.

The delivery of aerosol by compressors has the advantage of requiring no synchronization of delivery with inhalation. The high flow rate achieved by intermittent positive pressure machines is such that the delivery of aerosolized medication to intrapulmonary airways is less efficient than by a conventional compressor. Accordingly, there is no place for intermittent positive pressure delivery of aerosolized medication unless there is a separate requirement for the intermittent positive pressure for the treatment of respiratory insufficiency. With compressor/nebulizer-driven aerosol treatment, about 3% of the total dose is delivered to the intrapulmonary airways (36). This accounts, at least in part, for the higher dose of beta$_2$-agonist placed in the nebulizer for a course of treatment. Nevertheless, with the nebulized doses usually used, the effective lung dose is still higher than with a few puffs from a metered dose inhaler. With the higher dose and with the reliability of delivery, the "mask treatment" has become the standard for acute asthmatic episodes. It could be argued that the metered dose inhaler combined with a holding chamber can accomplish the same results, and indeed this has been demonstrated (37). The latter represents a reasonable option for emergency treatment such as in an ambulance where a compressor and nebulizer may not be available.

In infants, the compressor-driven nebulizer is a reliable method of provision of inhalation treatment. Cromoglycate, delivered via a nebulizer, has proved highly successful inhalational treatment in infants and young children (19) and is commonly used effectively in the same nebulizer as a beta$_2$-agonist such as salbutamol. If an additional agent, such as ipratropium bromide is to be added, the compatibility should be ascertained. It may, for example, be incompatible with cromoglycate solution. Steroid for nebulizer use is receiving clinical trial and seems to provide the expected beneficial effects in young children (38). The Aerochamber with mask, a pediatric version of a holding chamber, is now available commercially and is appropriate for the delivery of steroid or beta$_2$-agonist from a metered dose inhaler in young children.

Treatment (Medication) Regimens

In the person with a stable long-standing history of only brief episodes of breathlessness elicited by circumstances such as exercise or cold air exposure, inhaled

$beta_2$-agonist to prevent or reverse the symptoms is probably sufficient treatment.

If a person has only cough with no other chest symptoms, it is likely that bronchoconstriction is not a clinically relevant problem and many such people have normal methacholine airway responsiveness (5,39). As such, there would seem to be little rationale to the use of bronchodilator; inhaled steroid or cromoglycate would seem more appropriate although definitive controlled clinical trials have not yet been done.

If there is cough, wheeze, and breathlessness, the requirement is to try to reverse the underlying inflammation with inhaled steroid or cromoglycate. The drugs need to be used in sufficient dose and duration to reverse the episode. Optimum regimes still need to be investigated. However, if the patient is not on corticosteroid, we use beclomethasone diproprionate in a dose of 200 μg, two or four times daily, until symptoms and lung function are improved to the previous best result for several days. The drug is then discontinued or reduced to the minimum required to maintain this best result for at least months at a time. If the patient is already on beclomethasone, the dose is doubled at least until the exacerbation is reversed. Additional bronchodilator, usually in the form of inhaled $beta_2$-agonist is used on demand to the extent needed. When the best result is achieved the bronchodilator requirement should be minimal.

When the best status is not achieved or maintained by the above treatment regimen or if the exacerbation is more severe, it is necessary to add prednisone. We usually use prednisone in doses of 30-50 mg immediately and then 30 mg in single or divided doses daily for 5 days or until control or the patient's best status is achieved; then the total daily dose can be taken after breakfast and rapidly reduced by 5 mg daily to zero or to the minimum required to prevent deterioration. A maintenance dose may be required for months at a time. Often the dose can then be reduced slowly, for example, by 5 mg off the daily dose each week. In this situation, when an exacerbation begins, the high dose is resumed until the patient's best status is again achieved and then the dose is rapidly reduced to 5 mg above the one on which the previous exacerbation began. Theophylline or ipratropium are not usually required. However, if they have been used, an attempt should be made to discontinue them once best status has been restored.

Severe Exacerbations of Asthma

A detailed consideration of the assessment and treatment of a severe attack of asthma is reviewed in Chapter 12. Some principles will be briefly considered. Exacerbations of asthma generally develop over many hours and days; there is time for intervention to prevent the episode from becoming severe. The key is early intervention. With an exacerbation, if the patient has not been on inhaled steroid and the tempo of worsening is slow, the introduction of inhaled steroid with $beta_2$-agonist may be sufficient to reverse the episode. In the usual case where steroid and $beta_2$-agonist are already in use, the addition of ingested prednisone is generally required. In instances where, (1) there has been a failure to intervene early, (2) early intervention has not been effective, or (3) the tempo of development has been unusually rapid, assessment and treatment in an emergency unit or even an intensive care unit may be required.

Emergency treatment of an asthmatic episode requires monitoring the FEV_1 and PEFR and, if the episode is clearly severe or not responding well to initial treatment, monitoring of blood gases. Treatment is initiated with an augmented oxygen mixture and with inhaled $beta_2$-agonist. Use of intravenous aminophylline in the person already well-treated with $beta_2$-agonist is controversial and evidence of any added benefit is inconclusive. It is clear that the addition of intravenous theophylline does add to the risk of side effects. In the adult, initial and regular corticosteroid is required in a dose of 40-100 mg of ingested prednisone or an equivalent quantity of intravenous hydrocortisone repeated perhaps in 6 hours and then daily until full recovery. Once there is definite clinical and pulmonary function improvement, it is usual, so long as treatment is maintained, for the improvement process to continue. Once it is possible to comfortably take food and drink by mouth, any intravenous line can be discontinued.

It is important to determine whether the severe exacerbation could have been prevented and how such exacerbations could be prevented in the future. The patient should understand that severe exacerbations are commonly the result of inappropriate exposure to an aggravating factor or inappropriate delay in treatment with adequate doses of steroid. Methods to achieve and maintain the best status and provide for future early intervention should be reviewed.

PATIENT EDUCATION

Asthma is a condition where treatment choices and methods of administration of treatment have a major impact upon the well-being of the affected person. As such, the patient can benefit greatly from being well-instructed and well-indoctrinated. Instructions that work, that is, instructions that improve well-being are those which pertain to decisions the patient is obliged to make concerning treatment. Part of the treatment is the avoidance of offending substances. Probably no one with moderate to severe asthma should use ASA or any comparable nonsteroidal anti-inflammatory drug unless under careful monitoring and for special reasons. If there is intolerance to a substance such as metabisulfite or monosodium glutamate, a list of potential sources should be provided. If the asthma is induced by exposure to an occupational sensitizer such as TDI or plicatic acid, it is likely that an alternative job to avoid this exposure will be required. If there is allergy to pollen or mold spore which originates outdoors,

TABLE 1 Patient Education: What the Patient Needs to Know

1. How to avoid causal factors
2. Correct techniques of use of inhalant medication
3. Proper doses and times to use the medications prescribed
4. The early indications that control or best result of the individual has been lost
5. How to treat exacerbations
6. When and how to get help in treatment

closed windows and the use of an air conditioner, with the vent closed if it is a window-type, can be recommended since indoor counts can be reduced to near zero. Avoidance of other allergens such as pets in the home or house dust mite might also be relevant.

To assure successful use of inhalers, patients should be asked repeatedly to demonstrate the technique with their inhalers or a placebo inhaler. Assurances, without demonstration, that the technique of inhaler use is excellent should not be accepted. When a compressor is available in the home, a brochure containing instructions on how to keep it clean, how to use it safely, and the exact dosages of medications should be provided. There should be a demonstration of the ability to accurately measure out the correct dose of medications.

Successful adherence to a treatment regimen and proper choices in changing doses of medications at home require some understanding of the mode of action and the purpose of prescribed medication. For example, it is useful for the patient to know that an inhaled $beta_2$-agonist is rapid acting and useful in reversing or preventing episodes of breathlessness, but has no long-term effect insofar as it does not beneficially affect the underlying inflammatory process. In contrast, inhaled steroid does not have an immediate effect and would not be helpful to quickly relieve or prevent acute breathlessness. The requirement for steroid is not easily understood unless the timing and mechanism of action on the underlying processes is explained. The relative merits and the appropriate time of use of the different types of medication can then be understood. For example, the patient troubled by cough with no wheeze, tight chest, or breathlessness could understand that there may be no requirement for bronchodilator at that time but regular use of inhaled steroid is indicated. The importance of effective delivery to the periphery of the lung should be understood; usually inhaled $beta_2$-agonist can be followed immediately by inhaled steroid. However, when airflow limitation is present, inhaled $beta_2$-agonist 5 minutes prior to inhaled steroid can improve the delivery and thereby the efficacy of the latter (41).

Rules should be established for appropriate increase or decrease of the dosage of medications. Typically, the correct dosage is the minimum amount of medication needed to maintain control or the best result which has been established for the individual. Patients should learn that it is reasonable to increase medications suddenly up to the specified upper limit of dosage if symptoms are not controlled, and to decrease medication dosage only when baseline status has been achieved. Decrease in dosage is accomplished over days or weeks. There should be a well-defined plan to obtain additional treatment advice by telephone, an immediate office visit or visit to an emergency unit when there is failure to reverse any exacerbation. Criteria for an increase in the level of treatment are as follows:

1. The appearance of cough, wheeze, or breathlessness not previously present or requirement for an increased dose of inhaled bronchodilator is reason to increase the level of treatment, usually in the form of inhaled or ingested steroid.
2. Excessive inhaled $beta_2$-agonist such as a regular requirement more than 4 times daily or requirement at any time more than 6 times daily is generally an urgent indication for a major increase in the level of treatment, usually in the form of inhaled or ingested steroid.
3. Persistent fall of postbronchodilator peak flow rate of 20% or more.
4. If all treatment modalities available have been used and there is, one hour later, any evidence of the acquisition of airflow limitation such as wheeze, breathlessness, tight chest, or reduction in measured airflow rates, there should be an immediate major increase in the level of treatment, usually in the form of ingested steroid.

Patients who are subject to severe episodes of asthma with little warning or who sometimes find themselves in remote areas, need provision for self-administration of augmented treatment. Prednisone can be made available and used when control cannot otherwise be readily restored. If the patient displays poor perception of the onset of worsening, it is particularly important to use daily peak flow meter measurements as a basis of the decision to increase the level of treatment.

Asthma generally is a chronic condition that requires continuing attention to details. It is generally necessary to make provision for a regular review of aspects of treatment including methods of avoidance of offending substances, choices of medications, methods of use of medications, criteria which indicate the need for increased treatment, and methods to obtain such treatment.

REFERENCES

1. Peat JK, Britton WJ, Salome CM, Woolcock AJ. Bronchial hyperresponsiveness in two populations of Australian schoolchildren. II Relative importance of associated factors. Clin Allergy 1987; 17:283-290.

2. Kerigan AT, Pengelly LD, Goldsmith CH, Garside BK. *The Effect of Environmental Factors on the Respiratory Health of Schoolchildren in Hamilton*. Health & Welfare Canada Project 6606-1752-53; Ontario Ministry of the Environment Air Research Branch Project 20: Final Report. June 30.
3. Speight ANP, Lee DA, Hey EN. Underdiagnosis and undertreatment of asthma in childhood. Br Med J 1983; 286:1253–1258.
4. McNicol KN, Williams HE. Spectrum of asthma in children—I clinical and physiological components. Br Med J 1973; 4:7–11.
5. Salome CM, Peat JK, Britton WJ, Woolcock AJ. Bronchial hyperresponsiveness in two populations of Australian children. I Relation to respiratory symptoms and diagnosed asthma. Clin Allergy 1987; 17:271–281.
6. Woolcock AJ, Yan K, Salome CM. Effect of therapy on bronchial hyperresponsiveness in the long-term management of asthma. Clin Allergy 1988; 18:165–176.
7. Cockcroft DW, Ruffin RE, Dolovich J, Hargreave FE. Allergen-induced increase in non-allergic bronchial reactivity. Clin Allergy 1977; 7:503–513.
8. Chan-Yeung M, Lam S. Occupational asthma. Am Rev Respir Dis 1986; 133:686–703.
9. Platts-Mills TAE, Heymann PW, Chapman MD, Moszoro H, Nock P, Wilkins SR. Reduction of bronchial hyperreactivity during prolonged allergen avoidance. Lancet 1982; ii:675–677.
10. Mapp CE, Corona PC, de Marzo N, Fabbri L. Persistent asthma due to isocyanates. A follow-up study of subjects with occupational asthma due to toluene diisocyanate (TDI). Am Rev Respir Dis 1988; 137:1326–1329.
11. Chan-Yeung M, MacLean L, Paggiaro PL. Follow-up study of 232 patients with occupational asthma caused by western red cedar (Thuja plicata). J Allergy Clin Immunol 1987; 79:792–6.
15. Dutoit JI, Salome CM, Woolcock AJ. Inhaled corticosteroids reduce the severity of bronchial hyperresponsiveness in asthma but oral theophylline does not. Am Rev Respir Dis 1987; 136:1174–1178.
16. Cockcroft DW, Murdock KY. Comparative effects of inhaled salbutamol, sodium cromoglycate, and beclomethasone dipropionate on allergen-induced early asthmatic responses, late asthmatic responses, and increased bronchial responsiveness to histamine. J Allergy Clin Immunol 1987; 79:734–740.
17. Furukawa CT, Shapiro GG, Bierman W, Kraemer MJ, Ward DJ, Pierson WE. A double-blind study comparing the effectiveness of cromolyn sodium and sustained-release theophylline in childhood asthma. Pediatrics 1984; 74: 453–459.
18. Broder I, Tarlo SM, Davies GM, Thomas P, Leznoff A, Sturgess J, Baumal R, Mintz S, Corey PN. Safety and efficacy of long-term treatment with inhaled beclomethasone dipropionate in steroid-dependent asthma. CMAJ 1987; 136:129–134.
19. Newth CJL, Newth CV, Turner JAP. Comparison of nebulised sodium cromoglycate and oral theophylline in controlling symptoms of chronic asthma in pre-school children: A double blind study. Aust NZJ Med 1982; 12:232–238.

20. Lowhagen O, Rak S. Modification of bronchial hyperreactivity after treatment with sodium cromoglycate during pollen season. J Allergy Clin Immunol 1985;75:460-467.
21. Shim C, Williams MH Jr. Bronchial response to oral versus aerosol metaproterenol in asthma. Ann Intern Med 1980;93:428-431.
22. Horn CR, Clark TJH, Cochrane GM. Inhaled therapy reduces morning dips in asthma. Lancet 1984;May:1143-1145.
23. Salzman GA, Pyszczynski DR. Oropharyngeal candidiasis in patients treated with beclomethasone dipropionate delivered by metered-dose inhaler alone and with Aerochamber. J Allergy Clin Immunol 1988; 81: 424-428.
24. Messerli C, Studes H, Scherrer M. Systemic side effects of beclomethasone dipropionate aerosols (becotide, aldecine, sanasthmyl) in otherwise nonsteroid treated asthmatic patients. Pneumonology 1975;153:29-42.
25. Wyatt R, Waschek J, Weinbergen M, Sherman B. Effects of inhaled beclomethasone dipropionate and alternate day prednisone on pituitary-adrenal function in children with chronic asthma. N Engl J Med 1978;299:1387-1392.
26. Francis RS, McEnery G. Disodium cromoglycate compared with beclomethasone dipropionate in juvenile asthma. Clin Allergy 1984; 14:537-540.
27. Mapp C, Boschetto P, Vecchio LD, Crescioli S, de Marzo N, Paleari D, Fabbri LM. Protective effect of antiasthma drugs on late asthmatic reactions and increased airway responsiveness induced by toluene diisocyanate in sensitized subjects. Am Rev Respir Dis 1987;136:1403-1407.
28. Tinkelman DG, Moss BA, Bukantz SC, Shaffer AL et al. A multicenter trial of the prophylactic effect of ketotifen, theophylline, and placebo in atopic asthma. J Allergy Clin Immunol 1985;76:487-497.
29. Neijens HJ, Knol K. Oral prophylactic treatment. Immunol Allergy Practice 1988;10:17-23.
30. Dolovich M, Ruffin RE, Roberts R. Optimal delivery of aerosols from metered dose inhalers. Chest 1981;80S:911S-915S.
31. Newman SP, Pavia D, Clarke SW. Bronchodilator response after administration of pressurized aerosols at different lung volumes in patients with airways obstruction. Clin Sci 1980;56:10P-11P.
32. Dolovich M, Ruffin R, Corr D, Newhouse MT. Clinical evaluation of a simple demand inhalation MDI aerosol delivery device. Chest 1983; 84: 36-41.
33. Newman SP, Moren F, Pavia D, Little F, Clarke SW. Deposition of pressurized suspension aerosols inhaled through extension devices. Am Rev Respir Dis 1981;124:317-320.
34. Corr D, Dolovich M, McCormack D, Ruffin R, Obminski G, Newhouse M. Design and characteristics of a portable breath actuated, particle size selective medical aerosol inhaler. J Aerosol Sci 1982;13:1-7.
35. Crompton GK. Problems patients have using pressurized aerosol inhalers. Eur J Respir Dis 1982;63(suppl 119):101-104.

36. Berenberg MJ, Cupples LA, Baigelman W, Pearce L. Comparison of metered-dose inhaler attached to an Aerochamber with an updraft nebulizer for the administration of metaproterenol in hospitalized patients. J Asthma 1985;22(2):87-92.
37. Fuglsang G, Pedersen S. Comparison of nebulizer and nebulizer treatment of acute severe asthma in children. Eur J Respir Dis 1986;69:109-113.
38. Godfrey S, Avital A, Rosler A, Mandelberg A, Vwyyed K. Nebulized budesonide in severe infantile asthma. Lancet 1987;ii:851-852.
39. Cockcroft DW, Killian DN, Mellon JJA, Hargreave FE. Bronchial reactivity to inhaled histamine: a method and clinical survey. Clin Allergy 1977; 7:235-243.

12

Management of Acute Life-Threatening Asthma

J. MARK FITZGERALD

University of British Columbia
Vancouver, British Columbia, Canada

FREDERICK E. HARGREAVE

St. Joseph's Hospital
Hamilton, Ontario, Canada

Asthma is a common medical emergency. Unfortunately its assessment and management are frequently not appropriate to its potentially fatal outcome. The potential for asthma to be fatal, and the cause for this, have recently been reviewed in detail (1,2). The significant factors contributing to avoidable deaths include failure by the physician and the patient to appreciate the severity of the attack and to delay implementing the adequate use of corticosteroids. The importance of this problem is shown in a British survey (3) of emergency room deaths from medical conditions. A significant minority of patients dying in the emergency room did so from asthma. In addition, the majority of these patients were young.

HISTORY OF SYMPTOMS

In acute life-threatening asthma the patient may find it difficult to speak. When the attack is less severe, a number of details need to be obtained. The duration of the attack and any exacerbating factors need to be elicited. The time frame over which the symptoms develop, particularly if they have occurred over a prolonged period, will give an indication of the development of significant airway inflammation. The historical features which need to be elicited at this time which will indicate the need for greater caution are listed in Figure 1. In particu-

1. Recent emergency room visit. *2*. Current requirement for corticosteroids. *3*. A previous history of hospitalization. *4*. Previous mechanical ventilation. *5*. A history of rapid deterioration in symptoms.

FIGURE 1 Features indicating increased caution in assessing patients with asthma.

lar, a previously documented history of rapid deterioration, recurrent hospitalization, and especially a history of mechanical ventilation and current use of corticosteroids should lead to a heightened level of caution and increased awareness of the potential need for hospitalization. This not only gives an indication of the severity of the current attack but also highlights features of the patient's management that need attention during the convalescent period.

The intensity of the symptoms can be gauged from their interruption of sleep, presence on waking, and restriction of normal activities, as well as the increased requirement for $beta_2$-agonists for symptomatic relief. Sometimes a prodromal upper respiratory tract infection will precipitate an attack. Alternatively, exposure to an allergen or an agent to which the patient is intolerant (e.g., acetylsalicyclic acit) will be elicited.

A prospective evaluation of 261 consecutive episodes of acute asthma suggested that 46% occurred within 24 hours of presentation and 13% occurred in less than 1 hour (4). In our experience this rapid deterioration is not usual. The problem in this analysis (4) may well relate to the fact that it defined the onset of an acute attack as when the patient 'perceived that wheezing was worse than usual.' In our experience, patients are usually unable to define this period accurately and close questioning will elicit a more protracted onset of symptoms than this study would suggest.

Another feature which should be noted at this time is whether the patient and family physician responded appropriately to an acute deterioration, for example, was beclomethasone increased or was prednisolone instituted or increased, and were these carried out early enough and in adequate doses. The appropriate attention to these matters at this time should prevent the future development of acute life-threatening episodes.

Asthmatic patients often have a better appreciation of the degree of airflow limitation than their physician (5), but considerable airflow limitation can be present when they are symptom free. This poor perception of the presence of airflow limitation has been shown both in patients recovering from severe asthma in hospital where patients may be asymptomatic and still have an FEV_1 of 50% of predicted (6), and in experimental conditions where airflow obstruction has been induced by methacholine or histamine (7,8). These points stress that, while the history obtained is important, the use of objective measurements of airflow limitation by spirometer or a peak flow meter is more important. Unfortunately, most patients are still treated in the emergency room without these measurements being made (9-11).

CLINICAL EXAMINATION

Although objective data are always required to document the severity of an asthmatic attack, the presence of certain clinical signs may be considered markers for a life-threatening attack (6). The physical signs normally associated with severe airflow limitation are tachycardia, tachypnea, hyperinflation, wheeze, accessory muscle use, pulsus paradoxous, and diaphoresis. It should be stressed that the absence of these signs should not be taken as indicative that the episode in question is not life threatening. The use of accessory muscles, pulsus paradoxicus, and diaphoresis are considered the most significant in terms of grading the severity of an attack. There is an added problem in the ability of the physician to detect the presence of an abnormality (12,13), and the high rate of inter- and intraobserver error in evaluating clinical signs, again indicating the need for objective measurements.

Various attempts have been made to formulate a scoring index to assess the severity of an acute attack and the need for hospitalization. Fischl et al. (14), in 1981, reported one such index. An index score was formed using a combination of factors including pulse rate >120/min, respiratory rate >30/min, pulsus paradoxus ⩾18 mmHg, peak expiratory flow rate ⩽120 l/min, moderate to severe dyspnea, use of accessory muscles, and wheezing. Each of these signs was scored with one point. The authors calculated that a score ⩾4 was 95% accurate in predicting relapse and 96% accurate in predicting the need for hospitalization. Unfortunately the clinical usefulness of the index was not borne out in two subsequent studies (15,16), which failed to show such a useful predictive value. In fact these studies indicated that decisions made on the basis of chance were just as likely to be correct.

INVESTIGATIONS

Spirometry

The primary investigation in assessing patients with acute life-threatening asthma involves measurement of their airflow rates. This can be achieved with a peak flow meter such as a Wright minipeak flow meter or optimally with a spirometer. The difficulties in evaluating patients clinically and, in particular, their response to therapy makes one of these investigations mandatory in the assessment of all asthmatics. These values are particularly helpful if one has, for comparison, the patient's previous best spirometry or peak flow meter readings.

Arterial Blood Gas

Measurement of arterial blood gases (ABG) can be important in the assessment of an acute asthmatic attack, particularly in regards to estimation of alveolar ventilation. Initially the $PaCO_2$ may be low; a "normal" $PaCO_2$ may indicate impending respiratory muscle fatigue; values above 40 mmHg indicate a need for careful subsequent monitoring and possible mechanical ventilation. The difficulty of assessing hypoxaemia clinically is well documented. Raffin (17) has recently reviewed the use of ABG in clinical practice and noted the poor correlation of arterial blood gas tension with the severity of asthma, as measured by ventilatory function. A recent prospective study (18) showed that every patient with an FEV_1 >1 liter or a peak expiratory flow rate >200 l/min had a PaO_2 >60 mmHg and a $PaCO_2$ <42 mmHg. They therefore suggested that ABGs were not warranted when flow rates were above these values, especially when the patient was responding appropriately to therapy. In contrast to the data outlined above for adult patients, a recent report in a pediatric population found oximetry useful (19). Of 13 children sent home with an initial saturation >91%, only one presented again. In contrast, 10 of the 11 children with an initial saturation of 91% or less, all but one child had a relapse and required hospitalization subsequent to their initial presentation. Oximetry may therefore have specific indications in a paediatric population, particularly where children (as in the quoted study) may be too young to perform spirometry. Obviously when a patient has an elevated $PaCO_2$ and is deteriorating objectively and clinically, close monitoring of ABG is indicated because mechanical ventilation may be required. However, the optimum frequency of arterial blood gas assessment is poorly defined (20) and awaits appropriate prospective study.

Chest X-ray

A chest x-ray is often performed in the assessment of the acute asthmatic patient. The reason for this has been to examine for evidence of infection or the complications of hyperinflation (i.e., pneumothorax or pneumomediastinum) however, there is no objective data to support their routine use. Findley and Sahn (21), in 1981, reviewed 90 consecutive chest x-rays in patients presenting with acute asthma; the results of this prospective study were that 55 (55%) films were reported as normal, 33 (37%) showed hyperinflation, and 6 (7%) showed minimal interstitial abnormalities unchanged from previous films. In a further study (22), 371 consecutive children older than one year presenting with an initial episode of wheeze were reviewed. Three hundred and fifty children (94.3%) had negative films. Twenty-one (5.7%) had positive findings. These authors found that 20 of these 21 children could be identified before treatment on the basis of a combination of tachypnea, tachycardia, fever, and localized rales or decreased breath sounds. Although these data would support the policy of not routinely performing chest x-rays in the assessment of acute asthma, x-rays should be considered in certain situations. For example, Rebuck and Read (23) found two instances of unsuspected pneumothorax and one of pneumomediastinum in 58 patients during 80 hospital admissions. This suggests that a chest x-ray is indicated in patients with attacks of such severity requiring hospital admission or where the patient is not responding appropriately to therapy.

Electrocardiogram

Rebuck and Read (23) have also described the electrocardiographic changes, apart from sinus tachycardia, found in his patients. These abnormalities were present in 40% (35/88) of patients. The most common changes were those of right axis deviation (12.5%), clockwise rotation of the heart (10%) and, more rarely, evidence of right ventricular hypertrophy. These changes usually reverse completely within a few hours of the patient's response to initial therapy. These data suggest that electrocardiograms are not routinely indicated in the assessment of patients with acute life-threatening asthma.

Miscellaneous

The sputum must be examined for color, yellow or green suggesting infection or eosinophilia. A gram stain, culture and sensitivity, are only required if there is lung consolidation or if the purulence does not respond to initial therapy. Other hematological and biochemical investigations are not usually required with regard to decision making in the management of the acute asthmatic attack. The biochemical investigations which may have some importance in terms of monitoring patients during the acute phase are serum potassium (beta$_2$ agonists may cause hypokalemia) and serum glucose (corticosteroids may cause hyperglycemia).

CRITERIA FOR HOSPITAL ADMISSION

Criteria for hospital admission with severe asthma have recently been reviewed (24,25). Verbeek and Chapman (24) have used an FEV_1 of 2.0 liters or less as a criteria for hospital admission. In addition, these authors quote a number of features indicating the need for extra caution as outlined in Figure 1. It is difficult to support a recommendation of using an absolute value for the FEV_1, but rather a percent of predicted FEV_1 is more useful. In their more comprehensive review of the currently available literature, Core and Rothstein support this approach. MacFadden and Lyons (26) have used a value of >51% of predicted FEV_1 as indicative of a mild attack. More recently, Nowak et al. (18) used 60% as a cutoff point while also mentioning an absolute value of 2 liters.

However, the same author has previously used a value of $\leqslant 1.6$ liters (27). Kelsen et al. (28) looked at improvement after treatment and found that where there was an increase in the FEV_1 $\leqslant 400$ ml, these patients had a 67% relapse rate while those with an improvement >400 ml had a relapse rate of only 29%.

Certain historical features obtained from the patient are indications for a more cautious approach, but even in the absence of these, an FEV_1 of at least 60% of predicted has been suggested as the cutoff point between discharge or admission. Although, this value seems high, there is no objective prospective data to support a lower value, although anecdotally with close supervision we have been able to manage patients with lower levels as outpatients.

THERAPY

While the above process of assessment is being carried out, therapy will have been initiated. Therapy should consist of aggressive use of bronchodilators, supplemental oxygen, and, most importantly, corticosteroids.

$Beta_2$ Agonists

Studies have shown that $beta_2$ sympathomimetic agents such as salbutamol are effective bronchodilators in severe asthma (29). Traditionally these agents have been given in the form of nebulized solutions in normal saline. However, delivery of therapy using a metered dose inhaler (MDI) alone, has been successfully reported (30-35). Indeed, bronchodilator therapy can be administered successfully in this way even with the most severe asthmatics requiring hospital admission. The advantages of this system include cost, speed at which therapy can be commenced and equipotent bronchodilatation. In addition, this mode of delivery avoids the problems of paradoxical bronchoconstriction which has been noted with nebulized ipratropium bromide (36). Our method is to routinely administer four puffs of salbutamol followed by further inhalations to a total of 12 puffs (or less if the patient is limited by tremor). This dose may be repeated at hourly intervals until subjective and objective improvement as measured by spirometry occurs, at which time dose requirements may be reduced to more orthodox levels. Aggressive MDI therapy eliminates the need for intravenous forms of $beta_2$ agonists. The latter route adds considerably to systemic toxicity without appreciable gain in efficacy.

A recent study (37) noting greater efficacy with intravenous salbutamol versus nebulized salbutamol, also cautioned the presence of unacceptable cardiovascular side effects. An important feature of this study was the failure to use any anticholinergic therapy, in particular ipratropium bromide which could have added significantly to the efficacy of the intervention and avoid the side effects of intravenous salbutamol therapy.

Another feature of the emergency room management of acute asthma is that many patients have pretreated themselves with beta$_2$ sympathomimetic agents prior to arrival in the emergency room and therefore physicians assume they may not be responsive to further therapy. Rossing et al. (38) compared two groups of asthmatics presenting with acute exacerbations who were similar in all respects except that one group had sympathomimetic therapy in the 6 hours prior to admission and the other had received no such therapy. When data from both groups were analyzed there was no significant difference in baseline FEV_1 nor in response to beta$_2$ sympathomimetic therapy in the emergency room.

Anticholinergic Agents

A recent study (39) has indicated that the combination of an anticholinergic agent, ipratropium bromide, to fenoterol (another beta$_2$ agonist) is more effective than either agent alone. This additive effect is not surprising as the anticholinergic agents differ in their mode of action from beta$_2$ agonists. Rebuck and coworkers studied patients with asthma as well as a group with chronic airflow limitation who were treated in a randomized double-blind control study with either fenoterol, ipratropium bromide, or a combination of both administered in nebulized solutions. The greatest improvement followed treatment with the ipratropium-fenoterol combination (0.53 ± 0.40 liters at 45 minutes; 0.57 ± 0.51 liters at 90 minutes) and was significantly greater than following either ipratropium alone ($p<0.001$) or fenoterol alone in asthmatics but not patients with chronic airflow limitation ($p<0.05$). In contrast to Rafferty et al. (40), no paradoxical bronchoconstriction was reported in this study.

Corticosteroids

Corticosteroids must be considered the most essential part of the management of acute life-threatening asthma (41). The rationale for their use is based on the fact that most attacks of this severity are associated with airway inflammation which will not be influenced by bronchodilator therapy alone (42–44). Unfortunately, in the emergency room setting, patients may be discharged without corticosteroid treatment, when they respond symptomatically to bronchodilator therapy. In all reviews of asthma mortality, failure to appreciate the severity of the attack by the physician or patient and failure to treat the condition with steroids have been important contributing factors (1). Corticosteroids are believed to act in a number of ways to speed the resolution of an acute asthmatic attack (45). These mechanisms include an anti-inflammatory effect by decreasing leukocyte accumulation, potentiation of beta$_2$ agonists, lysosomal membrane stabilization, reduction of capillary permeability, and inhibition of histamine release.

Although the role of steroids in the acute asthmatic attack is not in doubt, there is some question as to the optimum dose, frequency and route of administration as well as type of preparation used. Harrison et al. (46) reported a randomized control study in which 52 severely ill asthmatic patients, requiring hospitalization, were treated by conventional means with one group receiving intravenous hydrocortisone (3 mg/kg bolus and then six hourly as an infusion) or ingested prednisolone (45 mg orally followed by 15 mg q8h po). At the end of 24 hours there was no difference in outcome between the two groups. A more recent study (47) confirms these findings. This prospective study in a group of 70 patients showed that methylprednisolone, 160 mg ingested daily, was as effective as 320 mg ingested, to 500 mg or 1,000 mg intravenously. Two methodological criticisms of this study are that it was not blinded and that 21 of the patients in the oral group versus 11 in the intravenous group were receiving oral prednisone at the time of presentation. These data are not surprising given that prednisolone is rapidly absorbed from the gut and peak plasma levels are obtained within 15 minutes of oral administration (48).

Despite the above data, intravenous therapy continues to be used in current clinical practice. Haskell et al. (49), in another randomized double-blind study, compared three dosing schedules, 15 mg, 40 mg, and 125 mg methylprednisolone q6h i.v. for three days. The best response was with the high-dose group who improved significantly within the first 24 hours; the medium dose improved in the middle of the second day, while the low dose group failed to improve significantly over the three-day study period. There were no significant side effects at the different doses and the authors concluded that the 125 mg dose regimen was the most appropriate. In view of Harrison and Ratto's data a logical compromise would seem to be to use the intravenous form for up to 24 hours and, if the patient is responding, substitute oral therapy.

Although intravenous steroids are routinely used in the hospitalized patient, there are fewer data available on patients discharged from the emergency room. The only well controlled study addressing this issue was published by Littenberg and Gluck (50). In this study 97 acutely ill patients with bronchial asthma were enrolled in a double-blind, placebo-controlled trial of intravenous methylprednisolone (125 mg) given on presentation in the emergency room, in addition to standard emergency treatment for asthma. Subjective and objective assessment of airflow limitation was similar in both groups at baseline. Subsequently, only 9 of 48 patients (19%) treated with intravenous corticosteroids required hospital admission compared with 23 of 49 patients (47%) in the control group ($p<0.003$). When the decision was made to admit or discharge, all the admitted patients started i.v. steroids while the discharge group were placed on oral prednisolone. There were only three patients among the discharge patients who relapsed, one from the i.v. methylprednisolone group and two from the placebo group. This relapse rate is much lower than the reported rate in the literature which ranges as high as 26%. The low relapse rate is most likely related to the routine use of oral steroids in the discharge group. It is our policy to treat with prednisolone 30 to 40 mg daily for approximately five days at least or until symptoms are under control. Once control has been achieved with the oral dose of prednisolone, the dose is rapidly discontinued or reduced to the minimum needed to maintain control (42). The benefits of this approach are well documented in the literature (51). An alternative method of delivery of corticosteroids, particularly where compliance is a problem, is the one of a depot preparation. There have been a number of reports using this method with success (52,53).

In conclusion, corticosteroids are effective in the treatment of acute severe asthma. The oral route has been shown to be as effective as the i.v. route, although there are some methodological concerns with regards to at least one of the studies showing this efficacy. It is, therefore, our policy to use intravenous corticosteroids initially followed by continued i.v. therapy in admitted patients for the first 24 hour period and oral therapy in the discharged patients tapered as outlined above.

Aminophylline

Traditionally aminophylline has been given for acute life-threatening episodes of asthma. However, Rossing et al. (29) have shown that the use of aminophylline confers no additional benefit to the use of $beta_2$-agonists alone. A more recent study (54) confirms these findings. A recent meta analysis of 13 adequately designed studies in patients with severe, acute asthma decided the evidence for its use was inconclusive (55). Not only does aminophylline have a low therapeutic ration, it also has a marked potential for toxicity in the hypoxemic patient. In addition, obtaining a therapeutic dose is further hampered by the large number of variables affecting its metabolism (i.e., age, coincidental congestive cardiac failure, and concomitent therapy with such agents as erythromycin, cimetidine, and also a history of smoking). An additional concern mitigating against its use is the concern that its combined use with $beta_2$ agonists may lead to increased toxicity, in particular cardiac toxicity. In animals, an increased risk of tachyarrhythmias when these drugs are combined has been documented. This has led to a warning from the FDA cautioning their combined use and suggesting that further studies should be carried out (56). Therefore, if optimal doses of $beta_2$-agonists are being given, there appears to be no advantage and several disadvantages in using aminophylline.

Adrenaline

Adrenaline has been used in the management of acute life-threatening asthma since 1951 (57,58). However, adrenaline is not needed when the other therapeutic modalities as outlined here are used to their optimal doses.

A recent study (59) compared the subcutaneous administration of terbutaline and adrenaline in the treatment of acute severe asthma. In this study there was no significant difference between the use of both these measures in patients who were otherwise treated the same. This therapy was given as initial treatment and followed by more orthodox therapy with nebulized salbutamol, hydrocortisone, and aminophylline. The authors comment on the fact that previous studies have reported significant side effects with adrenaline but they relate this to inappropriate high dosage and also intravenous use, particularly in elderly patients.

In summary, despite this recent study, most authors agree that adrenaline is not required in the management of acute life-threatening asthma. However, it is reassuring in that this study indicates that adrenaline in a dose of 0.5 mg subcutaneously is well tolerated in this patient population without significant side effects and, therefore, can be considered if the other manoeuvers outlined are ineffective.

Mechanical Ventilation

Occasionally, despite the above measures or before they can be implemented, the patient will progress to respiratory failure. In this instance, endotracheal intubation is a life-saving intervention. The approach to ventilating the asthmatic patient has undergone a change in recent years. The main problem with ventilation in these patients is the high peak airway pressures (PAP) and associated risk of barotrauma (60). A novel approach to overcome this problem has now been successfully reported by two groups of investigators (61,62). In these studies, a reduction in tidal volume, peak flow ventilatory rate, and paralysis with pancuronium bromide resulted in hypoventilation. Prolonged hypercapnia was successfully tolerated, once the $PaCO_2$ remained below 90 mmHg. In contrast to other studies, where ventilated patients have a reported mortality from 9 to 35% related to pneumothorax (60), no patient died in these two series.

Extraordinary Measures

Other approaches which have been reported anecdotally in the literature, in patients resistant to orthodox therapy, have included general anesthesia (63–65). Problems encountered with this approach include hypotension and arrhythmias, presumably exacerbated by the hypoxemia experienced by these patients. Other dramatic interventions reported have included selective whole lung lavage to relieve inspissated secretions (66). The use of extracorporeal membrane oxygenator support has also been described (67). There is no control data to support the use of these interventions, but their use may be required if the measures outlined previously fail to improve the patient.

Oxygen Therapy

Acute life-threatening asthma fulfills accepted criteria for the empiric use of oxygen therapy (20,68). It should be instituted on an empiric basis while the patient is being evaluated and receiving drug therapy. Ongoing use should be based on objective evaluation. The use of a face mask with an inspired oxygen concentration of 31% is usually sufficient to maintain an adequate oxygenation and poses no potential difficulties in the presence of hypercarbia. A recent pediatric study (19) showed significant levels of hypoxemia as judged by pulse oximetry at the time of presentation. With the documented occurrence of hypoxemia induced by beta-$_2$ agonist therapy (69) even in the presence of adequate oxygenation at presentation, therapy with supplemental oxygen is indicated in the initial period of stabilization.

Antibiotics

As noted above, there are a host of noninfectious precipitating causes for acute life-threatening asthma. In the absence of obvious markers for bacterial infection (i.e., presence of purulent sputum, fever, leukocytosis, and infiltrates on chest x-ray), antibiotics are not routinely indicated. Two controlled studies (70,71) have shown no benefit in their routine use.

Intravenous Fluids

Historically it has been assumed that patients with acute asthma often have tenacious mucous plugs and rapid hydration should form part of the therapy for such attacks (72). In contrast to this therapy, at least one study has shown no effect on sputum production with hydration in chronic bronchitis (73). In addition there has been further concern expressed regarding the risk of overhydration and the development of increased lung water (74). It would therefore seem prudent not to give excessive intravenous fluids unless there is objective evidence of volume depletion (i.e., postural hypotension).

Access to Medical Care

Delay in referral and access to medical care has been identified as factors contributing to asthma mortality (75). More direct access to emergency services has been shown to improve the outcome in the management of acute asthma (76–78). We conclude that patients with the historical features outlined in Figure 1 should have immediate self-referral access to acute medical care. In our clinic, patients have direct access to a respiratory physician 24 hours per day. It is our contention that this form of access optimizes patient management during episodes of life-threatening asthma. Medical care used appropriately in the early stages of an acute episode may contribute to the prevention of a more acute episode.

Prevention of Future Life-Threatening Exacerbations

As outlined above (4), approximately 50% of emergency visits, hospital admissions, and life-threatening exacerbations develop over days and there is time to increase treatment to reverse them before they become severe. The other attacks usually develop over a 24-hour period and there is a significant minority (13%) that has a sudden onset often associated with the accidental ingestion of food, nonsteroidal anti-inflammatory drug, sulfite preservatives, or monosodium glutamate to which the patient is sensitive or intolerant. Occasionally, also a severe attack can develop after overexposure to an allergen or occupational chemical sensitizer (e.g., isocyanate) to which the patient is hypersensitive. These sudden attacks are best prevented by the patient initiating avoidance strategy plus the use of drugs prophylactically (42).

Asthma should usually be maintained under the best control, which means that symptoms should be reduced to a minimum and FEV_1 or FEFR after bronchodilator should be normal or at a maximum for that patient (42,43). Exacerbations of asthma are due to airway inflammation triggered by respiratory infections, allergens, or occupational chemical sensitizers or inadequate maintenance treatment with anti-inflammatory drugs (79). Any exacerbation should be treated at the earliest indication by the addition of or an increase in anti-inflammatory treatment, of which corticosteroids are the most effective. The patient needs an individualized plan to treat exacerbations.

The life-threatening exacerbation must be taken as an opportunity to identify why the exacerbation was allowed to become so severe and to discuss future management to prevent a recurrence. Did the patient know when to increase treatment? Did the patient know how to increase treatment? Did the patient know that they should have phoned early for advice if they did not know how to treat the exacerbation or if the increased treatment was not successful? Was there an exacerbating factor which could be avoided in future?

Occasionally, the history will not identify how the exacerbation could have been prevented. In this instance, especially, the possibility of poor perception of airflow limitation should be considered (6,7). This is identified by an absence of symptoms when the PEFR or FEV_1 are reduced. Such patients will not detect symptoms, or will not be bothered by them, until the FEV_1 is severely reduced when there may be little or no time to prevent a severe exacerbation. These patients, in particular, must own a peak flow meter to measure their PEFR before and after an inhaled bronchodilator at least once daily until the best values are determined, minimum medication requirements are established, and it is determined whether regular measurements are required to detect an exacerbation. The use of a peak flow meter should also be considered by other adults and children to help detect the severity of exacerbations and to start appropriate treatment early.

CONCLUSION

Acute life-threatening asthma is a common medical emergency. It requires careful assessment with an appropriate history focusing on current symptoms, requirement for $beta_2$-agonist therapy, previous or concurrent history of steroid use, as well as a history of previous hospitalization, in particular requirements for mechanical ventilation. Appropriate physical examination assessing respiratory rate, pulse rate, the presence of pulsus paradoxus, as well as signs of fatigue and the level of consciousness of the patient are indicated. The most valuable form of assessment is the measurement of airflow limitation, ideally with spirometer but, at the very least, with a peak flow meter. These measurements allow comparison with the patient's previous best status, as well as objectively establishing the severity of the current attack. In addition, they can be used subsequently to monitor the patient's response to therapy. The majority of patients requiring assessment in the emergency room, whether admitted or discharged, will require steroid therapy for control of airway inflammation. In addition, therapy for the acute attack should proceed with optimum bronchodilator therapy using a combination of $beta_2$ sympathomimetic agents as well as atropine derivatives (i.e., ipratropium bromide). If the patient is discharged, he or she must be reviewed by their family physician or referred to an appropriate specialist. Life-threatening asthma is usually preventable and the opportunity must be taken to determine why the severe exacerbation occurred so that the patient can be given an individualized plan to prevent a recurrence in future.

ACKNOWLEDGMENT

We thank Mrs. Ellen Hatlevik for typing the manuscript.

REFERENCES

1. Benatar SR. Fatal asthma. N Engl J Med 1986; 314:423–429.
2. Robin ED. Death from bronchial asthma. Chest 1988; 93:614–620.
3. Shalley MJ, Cross AB. Which patients are likely to die in an accident and emergency department. Br Med J 1984; 289:419–421.
4. Arnold AG, Lane DJ, Zapata E. The speed of onset and severity of acute severe asthma. Br J Dis Chest 1982; 76:157–163.
5. Shim CS, Williams MH. Evaluation of the severity of asthma: patients versus physicians. Am J Med 180; 68:11–13.

6. McFadden ER. Clinical physiologic correlates in asthma. J Allergy Clin Immunol 1986;77:1-5.
7. Rubinfield AR, Pain MC. Perception of asthma. Lancet 1976; 7932:882-884.
8. Burdon JG, Juniper EF, Killian KJ. The perception of breathlessness in asthma. Am Rev Respir Dis 1982;126:825-828.
9. Reed S, Diggle S, Cushley MJ, et al. Assessment and management of asthma in an accident and emergency department. Thorax 1985;40:897-902.
10. Westerman DE, Benatar SR, Potgieter PD. Identification of the high-risk asthmatic patient. Am J Med 1979;66:565-572.
11. Ebden P, Carey OJ, Quinton D, Cookson JB. A study of acute asthma in the accident and emergency department. Br J Dis Chest 1988; 82:162-167.
12. Godfrey S, Edwards RHT, Campbell EJM. Repeatability of physical signs in airway obstruction. Thorax 1969;24:4-9.
13. Campbell EJM. Physical signs of diffuse airway obstruction and lung distension. Thorax 1969;24:1-4.
14. Fischl MA, Pitchenik A, Gardner LB. An index predicting relapse and need for hospitalization in patients with acute bronchial asthma. N Engl J Med 1981;305:783-789.
15. Rose CC, Murphy JG, Schwartz JS. Performance of an index predicting the response of patients with acute bronchial asthma to intensive emergency department treatment. N Engl J Med 1984;310:573-576.
16. Centor RM, Yarbrough B, Wood JQ. Inability to predict relapse in acute asthma. N Engl J Med 1984;310:577-580.
17. Raffin TA. Indications for arterial blood gas analysis. Ann Intern Med 1986;105:390-398.
18. Nowak RM, Tomlanovich, Sarker DD, et al. Arterial blood gases and pulmonary function testing in acute bronchial asthma: predicting patient outcomes. JAMA 1983;249:2043.
19. Geelhoed GC, Landau LI, Lesouef PN. Predictive value of oxygen saturation in emergency evaluation of asthmatic children. Br Med J 1988; 297: 395-396.
20. Fitzgerald JM, Baynham R, Powles ACP. Oxygen utilization among patients outside critical care areas in a university hospital. Lancet 1988; 8592:981-982.
21. Findley LJ, Sahn S. The value of chest roentogenograms in acute asthma in adults. Chest 1981;80:535-536.
22. Gershel JC, Goldman HS, Stein RE, Steven T, Shelov MD, Ziprokowski M. The usefulness of chest radiographs in first asthma attacks. N Engl J Med 1983;309:336-339.
23. Rebuck AS, Read J. Assessment and management of severe asthma. Am J Med 1971;51:788-798.
24. Verbeek PR, Chapman KR. Asthma: who to send home, when to hospitalize. J Respir Dis 1986;7(12):15-31.
25. Core CA, Rothstein RJ. Assessing severity of adult asthma and need for hospitalization. Ann Emerg Med 1985;14:103-110.

26. MacFadden ER Jr, Lyons HA. Arterial blood gas tension in asthma. N Engl J Med 1968; 278:1027-1032.
27. Nowak RN, Gordon KR, Wroblewski DA, et al. Spirometric evaluation of acute bronchial asthma. JACEP 1979; 8:9-12.
28. Kelsen SG, Kelsen DP, Fleegler BF, et al. Emergency room assessment and treatment of patients with acute asthma. Adequacy of the conventional approach. Am J Med 1978; 64:622-628.
29. Rossing TH, Fanta CH, Goldstein DH, et al. Emergency therapy of asthma: comparison of the acute effects of parenteral and inhaled sympathomimetics and infused aminophylline. Am Rev Respir Dis 1980; 122:365-371.
30. Shim CS, Williams HM. Effect of bronchodilator therapy administered by cannister versus jet nebulizer. J Allergy Clin Immunol 1984; 387-390.
31. Turner JR, Corkery KJ, Eckman D, Gelb A, et al. Equivalence of continuous flow nebulizer and metered dose inhaler with reservoir bag for treatment of acute airflow obstruction. Chest 1988; 93:476-481.
32. Morgan MDL, Singh BV, Frame MH, Williams SJ. Terbutaline aerosol given through pear spacer in acute severe asthma. Br Med J 1982; 285:849-850.
33. Madsen EB, Bundgaard A, Hidinger KG. Cumulative dose-response study comparing terbutaline pressurized aerosol administered via a pear shaped spacer and terbutaline in a nebulized solution. Eur J Clin Pharm 1982; 23:27-30.
34. Morley TF, Marozsan E, Zappason SJ, Griesback R, Giudice JC. Comparison of beta-adrenergic agents delivered by nebulizer versus metered dose inhaler in hospitalized asthmatic patients. Chest 1988; 94:1:51S.
35. Hodder RV, Calcutt LE, Leech JA. Metered dose inhaler with spacer is superior to wet nebulization for emergency room treatment of acute, severe asthma. Chest 1988; 94:1:52S.
36. Nebulizers and paradoxical bronchoconstriction. Lancet (Editorial) 1988; 8604:202.
37. Cheong B, Reynolds SR, Rajan G, Ward MJ. Intravenous B-agonist in severe acute asthma. Br Med J 1988; 297:448-449.
38. Rossing TH, Fanta CH, McFadden ER. Effect of outpatient treatment of asthma with beta agonists on the response to sympathomimetics in an emergency room. Am J Med 1983; 75:781-784.
39. Rebuck AS, Chapman KR, Abboud P. Nebulized anticholinergic and sympathomimetic treatment of asthma and chronic airways disease in the emergency room. Am J Med 1987; 82:59-64.
40. Rafferty P, Beasley R, Holgate ST. Comparison of the efficacy of preservative free ipratropium bromide and atrovent nebulizer solution. Thorax 1988; 446-450.
41. Fanta CH, Rossing TH, McFadden ER. Glucocorticoids in acute asthma: a critical controlled trial. Am J Med 1983; 74:845-851.
42. Hargreave FE. The drug treatment of asthma: How can it be better applied? Q J Med (in press).

43. Woolcock AJ. Therapies to control airway inflammation of asthma. Eur J Respir Dis 1986; 69(suppl 147):166–174.
44. Bond TJ. The changing face of asthma. Q J Med 1987; 63:359-365.
45. Morris HG. Mechanisms of action and therapeutic role of corticosteroids in asthma. J Allergy Clin Immunol 1985; 75:1-13.
46. Harrison BD, Stokes TC, Hart GJ, et al. Need for intravenous hydrocortisone in addition to oral prednisolone in patients admitted to hospital with severe asthma without ventilatory failure. Lancet 1986; 8474:181-184.
47. Ratto D, Alfaro C, Sipsey J, Glovsky MM, Sharma OP. Are intravenous corticosteroids required in status asthmaticus? JAMA 1988; 260:527–529.
48. Morrison PJ, Bradbrook ID, Rogers HJ. Plasma prednisolone levels from enteric and nonenteric coated tablets estimated by an original technique. Br J Clin Pharmacol 1977; 4:597–603.
49. Haskell RJ, Wong BM, Hansen JE. A double blind randomized clinical trial of methylprednisolone in status asthmaticus. Arch Intern Med 1983; 143: 1324–1327.
50. Littenberg B, Gluck E. A controlled trial of methylprednisolone in the emergency department of acute asthma. N Engl J Med 1986; 314(3):150–152.
51. Fiel SB, Swartz MA, Glans K, Francis ME. Efficacy of short-term corticosteroid therapy in outpatient treatment of acute bronchial asthma. Am J Med 1983; 75:259–262.
52. Patterson R, Greenberger PA, Grammer LC. Some indications for depot methylprednisolone for asthma or other severe allergic disease. J Allergy Clin Immun 1986; 77:686–689.
53. McLeod DT, Capewell SJ, Law J, McLaren W, Seaton A. Intramuscular triamcinolone acetonide in chronic severe asthma. Thorax 1985; 40:840–845.
54. Ruffin R, Bryant D, Burdon J, Marlin G, Mitchell C, O'Hehir R, Wilson J, Woolcock A, Webb S. Comparison of the effect of nebulized terbutaline versus intravenous enprofylline in patients with acute asthma. Chest 1988; 3:510–514.
55. Littenberg B. Aminophylline treatment in severe, acute asthma. JAMA 1988; 259:1670–1684.
56. Nicklas RA, Whitehurst VE, Donahue RF. Combined use of beta adrenergic agonists and methylxanthines. N Engl J Med 1982; 307:557–558.
57. Freedman BJ. Adrenalin in status asthmaticus. Lancet 1955; ii:575.
58. Broom B. Adrenaline in status asthmaticus. Lancet 1961; ii:1174.
59. Spiteri MA, Millar AB, Pavia D, Clarke SW. Subcutaneous adrenaline versus terbutaline in the treatment of acute severe asthma. Thorax 1988; 43:19–23.
60. Haake R, Schlictig R, Ulstad D, Henschen RR. Barotrauma. Pathophysiology, risk factors and prevention. Chest 1987; 91(4):608–613.
61. Darioli E, Perret C. Mechanical controlled hypoventilation in status asthmaticus. Am Rev Respir Dis 1984; 129:385–387.

62. Menitoue SM, Goldring RM. Combined ventilator and bicarbonate strategy in the management of status asthmaticus. Am J Med 1983; 94:898–901.
63. Robertson CE, Steedman D, Sinclair CJ, Brown D, Malcolm-Smith N. Use of ether for life-threatening acute severe asthma. Lancet 1985; 8422:187–188.
64. O'Rourke PO, Crane RK. Halothane in status asthmaticus. Crit Care Med 1982; 10:341.
65. Schwartz SH. Treatment of status asthmaticus with Halothane. JAMA 1984; 257:2688–2689.
66. Ramirez-R J, Obenour WH Jr. Bronchopulmonary lavage in asthma and chronic bronchitis: Clinical and physiologic observations. Chest 1971; 59: 146–152.
67. MacDonnell KS. Extracorporeal membrane oxygenator support in a case of severe status asthmaticus. Ann Thorac Surg 1981; 31:171–175.
68. Fulmer JD, Snider GL. Conference on oxygen therapy. American College of Chest Physicians/National Heart Lung, and Blood Institute, National Conference on Oxygen Therapy. Chest 1984; 86:234–247.
69. Harris L. Comparison of the effect on blood gases, ventilation and perfusion of isoproterenol-phenylephrine and salbutomol aerosols in chronic bronchitis and asthma. J Allergy Clin Immun 1972; 49:63–71.
70. Shapiro GG, Egeston PA, Pierson WE, Rau CG, Bierman CW. Double blind study of the effectiveness of a broad spectrum antibiotic in status asthmaticus. Pediatrics 1974; 53:867–872.
71. Graham VA, Knowles GK, Milton AF, Davies RJ. Routine antibiotics in hospital management of acute asthma. Lancet 1982; 8269:418–421.
72. Clark TJH. Acute severe asthma. *Asthma*, 2nd Ed. Clark TJH, Godfrey S (Eds.). Chapman and Hall, London, 1983.
73. Shim CS, King M, Williams MH. Lack of effect of hydration on sputum production in chronic bronchitis. Am Rev Resp Dis 1986; 133:A98.
74. Marchette LC, Marchette BE, Abraham WM, Wanner A. The effect of systemic hydration on normal and impair mucociliary function. Pediatr Pulmonol 1985; 1:107.
75. British Thoracic Association. Death from asthma in two regions. Br Med J 1982; 285:1251–1255.
76. Crompton GK, Grant IWB, Bloomfield P. Edinburgh Emergency Asthma Admission Service. Br Med J 1975; 4:680–682.
77. Cromptom GK, Grant IWB, Bloomfield P. Edinburgh Emergency Asthma Admission Service: Report on 10 years experience. Br Med J 1980; 281: 1191–1194.
78. Barriot P, Riou B. Prevention of fatal asthma. Chest 1987; 92:460–466.
79. Hargreave EE, Ramsdale EH, Kirby JG, O'Byrne PM. Asthma and the role of inflammation. Eur J Respir Dis 1986; 69(Suppl 147):16–21.

13

Prophylactic Anti-inflammatory Treatment of Asthma: Variations Throughout the World

MICHAEL DUDDRIDGE and E. HAYDN WALTERS

Newcastle General Hospital
University of Newcastle Upon Tyne
Newcastle Upon Tyne, England

INTRODUCTION

Asthma—An Inflammatory Disease of the Airways

Asthma has been recognized as a respiratory disease from the time of the ancient Chinese and Greek civilizations. In more modern times, following Floyer's description in 1698 (1), asthma has been principally considered as an intermittent, paroxysmal bronchospastic disorder which could be relieved with sympathomimetic agents. However, Aretaeus (81-131 AD) was probably one of the first to observe that asthma also affected the individual between episodes of bronchospasm, when he stated: "During remissions, though they walk erect, they bear the traces of the affection" (2). Only within the last decade has the basis for this been explained by the emerging and increasingly accepted view that clinical asthma is a manifestation of an inflammatory disease of the airways (3-7). Detailed evidence for this has been extensively reviewed and discussed in earlier chapters of this monograph.

The importance of this new understanding of asthma, and its implications for the prophylactic treatment of asthma, has only recently started to be appreciated. This is reflected in the varied current use, and perhaps underuse, of treatments with anti-inflammatory properties in asthma in different cultural and geographic regions of the world. The aim of this chapter is to discuss these differences in therapeutic practice in relation to our current understanding of the actions of the different pharmaceutical agents in common use. However, we must stress that as our understanding of asthma as an inflammatory disease of the airways is still incomplete, our understanding of the pharmacology of the drugs with which we treat asthma prophylactically is even more inadequate.

We need to consider the manifestations of airway inflammation in asthma by which we are going to judge whether the pharmaceutical agents used in its treatment have anti-inflammatory actions. The methods by which inflammatory activity has been assessed are listed in Table 1.

Bronchial Biopsies and Bronchoalveolar Lavage

Infiltration of the bronchial epithelium by inflammatory cells in asthma, and in animal models of asthma, has been well described (8–13), and increased numbers of these cells have been found in bronchoalveolar lavage (BAL) fluid from asthmatics. Although the total cell count may be in the normal range (14,15), or elevated (16), eosinophilia (14-16) has been reported consistently and in some studies related to the degree of nonspecific airway responsiveness (15,17). Neutrophilia has not been a feature of bronchoalveolar lavage fluid from stable asthmatic subjects, although the percentage neutrophil count has been positively correlated with the degree of airway responsiveness (14), as has the percentage of mast cells (15,17,18). A lymphocytosis has also been recognized (14,19) but negatively correlated to airway responsiveness (14) (i.e., more lymphocytes were present in the least responsive subjects), with the CD8 ("suppressor") lymphocyte phenotype principally responsible for this relationship (20). Bronchoalveolar lavage neutrophil metabolic activity has been shown to be increased in asthma, although not related to the degree of airway responsiveness (14), whereas the extent of pulmonary macrophage activation was positively correlated with the degree of airways responsiveness (14), (i.e., the most metabolically active macrophages were present in the most responsive subjects).

Airway Responsiveness and Late Asthmatic Reactions

The role of inflammation and inflammatory cells in the induction of airways hyperresponsiveness have been extensively reviewed recently (4,6,21). The late asthmatic reaction to allergen or chemical challenge, which is associated with

TABLE 1 Methods Which May be Used to Assess Inflammatory Activity Within Asthmatic Airways

Airway biopsies
Bronchoalveolar lavage
Nonspecific airway responsiveness
Late asthmatic reactions to allergen challenge
Cellular inflammatory mediator release

an increase in airways hyperresponsiveness, has been characterized by infiltration of the airways by inflammatory cells, including eosinophils (22-24), neutrophils (23,25), and lymphocytes (23), without similar changes accompanying the early asthmatic response. These studies have also been recently reviewed (26).

Proinflammatory Mediators

Phospholipid-derived proinflammatory mediators, such as platelet-activating factor, the leukotrienes, and prostaglandins, have been proposed as promoting airway inflammation in asthma and as being responsible in part for the induction of the late asthmatic response and the associated increase in airways responsiveness (4-6,21). Such mediators may be released from a variety of inflammatory cells within the airways, including mast cells, macrophages, polymorphonuclear neutrophils and eosinophils, and platelets. Pulmonary macrophages from asthmatics have been shown to produce greater quantities of such mediators when compared to those from nonasthmatics in response to in vitro stimulation (27-29), which would further support this unifying concept.

Asthma–the Recognition of the Need for Prophylactic Treatment

The persistence of airway inflammation (8,9) and variable airflow obstruction (30,31) in asymptomatic asthmatics underlies Aretaeus' observation. It is well known that an individual's perception of the severity of their asthma is notoriously unreliable (31), yet, despite the extensive chronic inflammatory changes in their airways (13), the majority of patients with mild asthma (with the general consensus of the medical profession) (32,33) are solely treated with bronchodilators taken as necessary for symptomatic relief. If symptoms are the tip of the iceberg, then the inflammation present in the asthmatic's airways is probably best represented by the submerged majority of that same iceberg, and it is the appreciation of this by both the asthmatic patient and the physician that is necessary in the assessment of the requirements for regular prophylactic treatment.

The Chinese were probably the first to use prophylactic treatment in asthma, with two popular herbal remedies prepared from the leaves of the ***Ginkgo biloba*** tree and the herb haifenteng. Increased interest has recently been shown in these, as extracts have been demonstrated to be potent antagonists of platelet-activating factor, a proinflammatory mediator which may have an important role in the induction of persistent airways hyperresponsiveness (34).

Recently, the need for an increased use of prophylactic treatment in asthma has been highlighted (35-39) as a consequence of the increasing morbidity and mortality from the disease as is reviewed in Chapter 3. At the same time, caution has been advised in the reliance on the chronic use of solely bronchodilator agents (39), notably methylxanthines and β_2-agonists.

This increase in morbidity and mortality has occurred despite increased sales of asthma treatments (40,41). In the United States sales have risen fourfold in the last ten years (37), although the principal increase has been in the use of bronchodilators, with inhaled steroids and cromoglycate accounting for less than 10% and 1% of the sales, respectively. In France, the use of inhaled steroids has, in fact, fallen in recent years (42). This situation exists despite the recommendations made in earlier reports (35,36) where underuse of these latter two treatments was identified as a possible factor associated with increased mortality.

Prophylactic Treatment–Anti-inflammatory Treatment?

An effective prophylactic treatment is one that diminishes the degree of airway inflammation, which is an important, or even fundamental, feature of asthma. It is therefore surprising to find that although we now accept the need for prophylactic treatment in the management of chronic asthma, there is a great lack of consensus among physicians worldwide on the "correct" approach to the use of the available treatments. The principal divergence is between those using methylxanthines and β_2-agonists as the mainstay of their "prophylactic" regimen and those prefering the early use of inhaled steroids and cromoglycate.

In this chapter we first examine the geographical differences around the world in the prophylaxis of asthma and in physicians' opinions on treatment. We then consider the evidence as to whether the pharmacological agents commonly used have anti-inflammatory actions, and how appropriate they actually are for a prophylactic role in asthma as we are now coming to understand it.

WORLDWIDE VARIATION IN PROPHYLACTIC TREATMENT

Estimation from Sales Figures

When considering the worldwide geographical patterns of treatment, differing cultural influences have to be borne in mind. For example, in the United Kingdom and Ireland, the Scandinavian countries and Australasia, topical inhaled therapy is almost universally accepted as the prime method of treating asthma. However, this is far from the case in Japan, where predominantly for cultural reasons inhaled treatment, in general, is not widely accepted and there is a reliance on oral medication for the treatment of asthma. In Arabic cultures there is again a reluctance to accept the inhaled route of treatment as it has the widely perceived connotation of terminal illness. We must therefore bear these and similar factors in mind as we consider the information presented in this section. In general, however, the use of inhaled treatment in asthma is becoming increasingly accepted (33).

Further important factors to consider are compliance with the treatment regimen and the severity of asthma. It is estimated that only 50% of patients accept their physicians' advice concerning the need for long-term prophylactic treatment of their asthma. However, no information is available on worldwide variation in compliance with prophylactic treatment regimens, which is also potentially influenced by cultural factors, and estimates derived from drug sales may therefore be an underestimate of the prevalence of attempted prophylactic management on the part of physicians.

When we consider the question of asthma severity, it is widely presumed that mild asthmatics, those with symptomatic bronchospasm less frequently than once daily, only require treatment with a short-acting β_2-agonist or methylxanthine as necessary for the relief of bronchospasm, or its prevention if exercise related (33). Therefore, as the majority of asthmatic individuals have only mild asthma they are not taking regular treatment. Thus, the overall use of inhaled and short-acting oral preparations of β_2-agonists and nonsustained release preparations of methylxanthines needs to be interpreted accordingly. Much therapy with these agents is not "prophylactic" in the strict sense of the word.

Despite these difficulties in making wholly meaningful comparisons, trends in the patterns of treatment use in different geographical regions of the world are illustrated in Table 2. This shows estimated data for 1987 based on the total days of treatment "sold" in different countries; the figures for Scandinavia are a mean estimate for Norway, Sweden, Finland, and Denmark, and the figures for Australasia are for Australia and New Zealand combined. The figures for Europe refer to the mean of estimates for the countries of continental Europe, excluding the United Kingdom and Ireland, and the Scandinavian countries. Ireland is similar in its practice to that of the United Kingdom and is therefore not listed separately. Generally speaking, within continental Europe, prescribing habits are similar, although within both The Netherlands and Italy the use of inhaled steroids approximates to that of the United Kingdom, Australasia, and Canada. In Holland and Italy there is also less emphasis on treatment with the methylxanthine derivatives compared with France and West Germany, but still more than in the United Kingdom. On the other hand, the West Germans use almost twice as much cromoglycate as the rest of Europe, but their combined use of inhaled steroids and inhaled cromoglycate is still lower than the use of these prophylactic treatments in the United Kingdom, Scandinavia, Australasia, and Canada. The total estimates of drug use shown in Table 2 do not sum to 100%; the deficit comprises the use of sympathomimetic treatment other than the more conventional and specific β_2-agonists.

The current tendency, therefore, is for a predominant use of inhaled β_2-agonists and inhaled steroids in the United Kingdom, Scandinavia, and Australasia, with a lower use of prophylactic inhaled steroids in the United States,

TABLE 2 Geographical Variations in the Pattern of Asthma Treatment (Expressed as Percentage of Total Days Treatment for 1987)

	United Kingdom	Scandinavia	Australasia	Canada	United States	Europe	Japan
Inhaled β_2-agonist	51	50	60	31	30	40	2
Inhaled steroids	18	11	16	18	6	6	2
Inhaled cromolyn	5	2	4	3	2	4	3
Ketotifen	<1	–	1	–	–	4	9
Methylxanthines	12	18	12	37	43	28	34
Oral β_2-agonist	6	10	2	3	8	7	22
Others	6	5	4	5	2	9	15

continental Europe, and Japan. Canada occupies an intermediate position with the higher use of inhaled steroids of the former grouping, but the lower use of inhaled β_2-agonists of the latter grouping. The use of inhaled cromoglycate appears to be more uniform, although its use is generally not as great as that of inhaled steroids. Ketotifen is very region specific in its pattern of use, being almost exclusively used in some countries of continental Europe and Japan.

Methylxanthines are used both in the immediate treatment of bronchospasm and as prophylactic treatment depending upon the formulation of the medication. Table 3 shows the balance between the use of these different preparations in the geographical regions already described. In all areas the long-acting formulations used for prophylactic treatment comprise the majority of use, with an inverse relationship between the use of methylxanthines and the use of inhaled steroids. The partial exception to this generalization is Japan where the use of ketotifen, and similar locally available products, hold a middle ground as putative "antiallergic" treatments. Treatments such as antihistamines and leukotriene inhibitors are also now commercially available for the treatment of asthma in Japan, which accounts for the larger proportion within the "other" treatment category compared with the remainder of the world.

Analysis of treatment use patterns from estimates of the proportional daily use of the various treatments, as quoted herein, is preferred to the alternative analysis using the percentage of total monetary sales in U.S. dollars (37,45). The latter does not account for the discrepancy in cost between the cheaper inhaled β_2-agonists and the more expensive inhaled steroids for example, and does not allow for local changes in price. This is clearly illustrated for the use of inhaled steroids in Japan (45), where, as a proportion of dollar sales of all asthma treatment, inhaled steroids accounted for 7% of the total in 1984, but only approximately 2% of the volume of treatment, by days of use, even by 1987, although the actual use of inhaled steroids had almost certainly continued to rise, as it had before 1984. This apparent paradox is explained by the high cost of the inhaled steroid therapy.

Physicians Opinions on the Choice of Prophylactic Treatment

An alternative approach to addressing geographical regional differences in the prophylactic treatment of asthma, avoiding some of the interpretive difficulties mentioned above (including those caused by difficulties in differentiating between truly prophylactic use of therapy and "as needed" use of therapy), is to consider the opinion of physicians as to their preferences for prophylactic therapies. Unfortunately, there is relatively little such information available, with only single studies in Europe and North America, and no published studies at all on the attitudes of Japanese or Australasian physicians. In 1984, the

TABLE 3 Proportion of the Methylxanthine Preparations Used in Asthma (Expressed as a Percentage of the Total Methylxanthine Use)

	United Kingdom	Scandinavia	Australasia	Canada	United States	Europe	Japan
Long-acting	95	89	89	84	81	80	62
Rapid-acting	5	11	11	16	19	20	38

European Audit on the Diagnosis and Treatment of Asthma sampled the attitudes of physicians in 16 countries across Europe (46–48), and the following year a similar survey was carried out, using the same questionnaire, in the United States (49).

The orders of preference for the prophylactic treatment of chronic asthma found by both studies are shown in Tables 4 and 5, for adults and children, respectively. A disadvantage in considering Europe as a whole rather than as continental Europe, Scandinavia, and the United Kingdom, as in the previous section, is the wide divergence of opinion on the preferred first choice, and subsequent order of choice, of prophylactic treatment between different regions. This is illustrated by the provision of the preferences expressed by the physicians of the United Kingdom and France, in addition to the orders for Europe as a whole and the United States.

The general tendency in these studies was again to illustrate that physicians in the United Kingdom and Scandinavia favored the use of inhaled β_2-agonists and inhaled steroids, often at higher doses compared to those used throughout continental Europe and the United States, with the Scandinavian countries rating cromoglycate lower than the United Kingdom as previously seen. In France and the rest of continental Europe, the trend was toward the use of oral theophylline as first-line treatment, although in West Germany this was relegated into second place by inhaled β_2-agonists. Overall, France (a representative of the continental European approach) and the United States show great similarities, although oral β_2-agonists were still rated more highly in the United States than either inhaled cromoglycate or inhaled steroids.

In children the pattern was even more complicated, with inhaled cromoglycate enjoying a high rating as first-line prophylactic treatment in Europe, although relegated to second place by inhaled β_2-agonists in the United Kingdom. It fared relatively poorly in the United States behind theophylline and both inhaled and oral β_2-agonists. The United Kingdom and Scandinavia considered treatment with inhaled steroids in children at a far earlier stage than any other country, although it was still only the third preference behind inhaled cromoglycate. This contrasted with the opinions for the treatment of adults. It seems that worries about the possibility that inhaled steroids may affect the child's growth and development, although now generally overcome in those countries where they are widely used, still prevail in many countries.

The overall verdict from these surveys was that physicians in the United States tended to be more conservative in their attitude to the use of inhaled β_2-agonists and inhaled steroids as prophylactic treatment of asthma compared with their European counterparts, and even more so compared with the British and Scandinavians. However, the American chest specialists surveyed were more likely than "generalists" to use inhaled β_2-agonists as their first-line treatment. No such subtrends were analyzed in the European study, although general prac-

TABLE 4 Physicians' Stated Preferences (in Order of Choice) for the Prophylactic Treatment of Adults

United Kingdom	Europe[a]	France	United States
Inhaled β_2-agonists	Inhaled β_2-agonists	Theophylline	Theophylline
Inhaled steroids	Theophylline	Inhaled β_2-agonists	Inhaled β_2-agonists
Inhaled cromolyn	Inhaled steroids	Inhaled cromolyn	Oral β_2-agonists
Theophylline	Inhaled cromolyn	Inhaled steroids	Inhaled steroids
Oral β_2-agonists	Oral β_2-agonists	Ketotifen	Inhaled cromolyn
Oral steroids	Oral steroids	Oral β_2-agonists	Oral steroids
Ketotifen	Ketotifen	Oral steroids	—

[a]Europe here refers to the whole of Western Europe.

TABLE 5 Physicians' Stated Preferences (in Order of Choice) for the Prophylactic Treatment of Children

United Kingdom	Europe[a]	France	United States
Inhaled β_2-agonists	Inhaled cromolyn	Inhaled cromolyn	Theophylline
Inhaled cromolyn	Inhaled β_2-agonists	Theophylline	Inhaled β_2-agonists
Inhaled steroids	Theophylline	Ketotifen	Oral β_2-agonists
Oral β_2-agonists	Oral β_2-agonists	Inhaled β_2-agonists	Inhaled cromolyn
Theophylline	Ketotifen	Oral β_2-agonists	Inhaled steroids
Oral steroids	Inhaled steroids	Inhaled steroids	—

[a]Europe here refers to the whole of Western Europe.

titioners, general physicians, and chest specialists were all included within the survey.

It is interesting to note one of the conclusions from the European survey regarding the apparently greater acceptance of recent clinical pharmacological developments in the United Kingdom and Scandinavia, where physicians were more likely to follow the conclusion of studies recommending the practice of prophylactic treatment with inhaled β_2-agonists and inhaled steroids. It seems as though this message is still not generally accepted in continental Europe nor the United States, as the treatment statistics for 1987 have shown, despite the American study also concluding that the therapeutic interventions in practice in other countries for years prior to their consideration in America could benefit their own asthmatic patients. However, this advice is probably now starting to have an impact, to the extent that the use of inhaled cromoglycate has apparently increased within the last year.

Although both surveys included attitudes toward allergen desensitization, this together with allergen avoidance are not considered in detail in this chapter. However, suffice it to say that although it is generally recognized that simple allergen avoidance measures are effective and important, there is no consensus as to the role of allergen desensitization (50,51).

Summary

Whether prophylactic treatment trends are assessed by physicians' subjective attitudes or objectively by drug sales, there is considerable agreement about the variations described throughout geographical areas of the world, with several broad groupings into which countries or regions can be placed. The United Kingdom, Scandinavia, Australasia, and Canada (to some extent) tend to use inhaled steroids more than the methylxanthine derivatives which are favored by continental Europe and the United States. Japan, on the other hand, falls into its own distinct niche using a relatively high proportion of oral β_2-agonists and methylxanthines with ketotifen, and the newer antihistamines and leukotriene antagonists which are only currently being evaluated elsewhere.

In the following section we consider which of these prophylactic treatments are appropriate as prophylactic agents in terms of their anti-inflammatory properties in asthma.

THE ANTI-INFLAMMATORY PROPERTIES OF PROPHYLACTIC TREATMENTS

Beta$_2$-agonists

Airway Inflammation

Unfortunately, there is no information available on the effects of physiological doses of β_2-agonists on airway inflammation in asthma, whether assessed by bronchial biopsies or bronchoalveolar lavage findings. In isolated tissue from experimental animals, β_2-agonists have reduced vascular permeability and edema formation in models of inflammation (52-54), although, worryingly, a deterioration has been shown in the lungs of rats treated with β_2-agonists and subjected to in vivo injury (55). Airway secretion of mucus has been stimulated by β_2-agonists (56), and particularly viscous mucus with a high protein content (57), which may not be desirable in asthmatic patients.

We have recently found that salbutamol, at physiological concentrations, had no effect on the metabolic activity (the respiratory burst) of either bronchoalveolar lavage neutrophils or pulmonary macrophages in vitro (unpublished observations), and it is unlikely to affect the increased metabolic activity that has been described in bronchoalveolar macrophages and neutrophils in asthma (14). Similarly, the production of thromboxane and leukotriene B_4 by pulmonary macrophages in vitro was not inhibited by β_2-agonists (58).

Airway Responsiveness

β_2-agonists have been shown to be potent acute inhibitors of airway responsiveness during the bronchodilator phase of their action (59-61), with up to a fourfold doubling dose reduction in responsiveness. However, the long-term use of β_2-agonists (over 1 to 6 months) has not, in general, been associated with any improvement in baseline airway responsiveness once the treatment is stopped (62-65), although one study showed an exception to this (66). A small increase in responsiveness was observed in two of these studies (63,64), and more recently was also found following cessation of two weeks treatment with regular terbutaline, but not following a single day's treatment (67).

Late Asthmatic Reaction

In parallel with the absence of a long-term beneficial effect on airway responsiveness, β_2-agonists have had no demonstrable effect on the late asthmatic response to allergen challenge (65,68), nor did they prevent the induction of airway hyperresponsiveness associated with the late response (65). Furthermore, β_2-agonists given during the late response following allergen challenge do not fully reverse the decrement in pulmonary function observed (26), presumably as the mucosal inflammation associated with the late asthmatic response accounts for a significant proportion of this flow limitation.

Proinflammatory Mediators

β_2-agonists have been shown to be potent inhibitors of mast cell histamine release in vitro (69) and in vivo (70), with inhibition of the early asthmatic response (65,68). The question has been asked as to why β_2-agonists are not, therefore, effective as prophylactic agents in reducing airway inflammation and airway responsiveness after allergen challenge. The most likely explanation is that mast cells are not as important as previously thought in the genesis of the late response and the airway inflammation of asthma, despite their importance in the immediate bronchoconstriction following allergen or osmotic challenge (69).

Anticholinergics

Although anticholinergics were not listed in our review of asthma treatment on a world-wide basis, they have been considered by some as an alternative bronchodilator to the β_2-agonists. In an acute dosing study, ipratropium was found to be equipotent as a bronchodilator when compared to salbutamol, although it produced significantly less acute reduction in airway responsiveness (61). There are no reports, however, of their effect on long-term baseline airway responsiveness. They have been shown to have no effect on the late asthmatic response (71) nor on histamine release in vivo (70). Other parameters of airway inflammation (Table 1) have not been addressed.

Methylxanthines–Theophylline and Aminophylline

Airway Inflammation

Although there are no reports of the effect of methylxanthines on airway inflammation in chronic asthma, in a sensitized guinea pig model of the late asthmatic response, theophylline has been demonstrated to reduce the bronchoalveolar neutrophilia of the late response, but only when administered during the early response and not when given immediately prior to provocation (72). Theophylline has also inhibited allergen- or mediator-induced inflammatory plasma exudation into the airways of guinea pigs (73,74), although these observations have not been extended to asthma. The metabolic activity of peripheral blood neutrophils (75) and pulmonary macrophages (76) in vitro has been inhibited by in vivo treatment of healthy volunteers with theophylline at therapeutic levels, but this has not been repeated in subjects with asthma. T lymphocytes from the peripheral blood of asthmatic subjects have been examined before and after one month's treatment with theophylline (77), and although the total number of T lymphocytes was no different from the non-asthmatic control population, there was a significantly lower "suppressor" T-lymphocyte count in the asthmatics before treatment, which rose to normal levels following treatment. An increased number of "suppressor T lymphocytes has also been found in asthmatics on long-term treatment with theophylline (78), although there have been no studies looking directly at an effect of treatment in the airways.

Airway Responsiveness

Theophylline treatment for three months has been shown to have no effect on baseline airway responsiveness (79,80), and in one study (80) the improvement gained during an initial three months treatment with inhaled steroids was significantly reduced following cross-over to treatment with theophylline.

Late Asthmatic Reaction

Methylxanthines have been shown to inhibit the late asthmatic response to allergen challenge (81,82), although it has recently been demonstrated that the reduction in its magnitude is only of a small degree (83). Partial inhibition of the late response following toluene diisocyanate challenge in sensitized workers by theophylline has also been observed (84). However, in neither circumstance did theophylline pretreatment inhibit the increase in airway hyperresponsiveness associated with the late response (82,84).

Proinflammatory Mediators

Mast cell mediator release in vivo has been inhibited during the early asthmatic response by pretreatment with theophylline (85), although mediator release during the late response has not been investigated. Inhibition of the production of leukotriene B_4 by peripheral blood neutrophils in vitro has also been demonstrated following in vivo treatment (75).

Inhaled Steroids

Airway Inflammation

Bronchial biopsies have been assessed following inhaled steroid treatment to exclude deleterious effects, but only two studies have reported the effect of steroid treatment on the airway damage in asthma (86,87), and they have shown epithelial repair, in particular ciliogenesis, without commenting on the inflammatory cell infiltrate. The neutrophilia and increased albumin levels found in bronchoalveolar lavage during the late asthmatic response to toluene diisocyanate challenge have been inhibited by treatment with oral prednisolone concomitantly with inhibition of the late response (88), but the effect of treatment with inhaled steroids on the lavage findings in chronic asthma have not been reported.

Glucocorticosteroids have been shown to reduce the increased permeability and microvascular leakage produced in animal models of inflammation (54,89), and to inhibit proteinaceous mucus secretion in animal airways in vitro (90). In stable asthma mucus formation has been reduced and its clearance accelerated following treatment (91).

A wide range of in vitro cell activities associated with the inflammatory process have been inhibited or suppressed by corticosteroids, following both in vitro incubation of cells with steroids and in vivo exposure of peripheral blood leukocytes to steroids, as recently reviewed (92). Treatment of chronic asthma with oral prednisolone has also resulted in a downregulation of peripheral blood leukocyte activity (93), but the effect of topical treatment on the function of airway cells has not been addressed.

Airway Responsiveness

Both oral and inhaled corticosteroids have been shown to improve the airway hyperresponsiveness of chronic asthma over durations of 3 weeks to 30 months (63,64,80,94-97), with a comparable dose of inhaled beclomethasone dipropionate proving more efficacious than oral prednisolone (97). An early study using a low dose of inhaled steroid reported no effect (98), but more recently the improvement in responsiveness has been shown to be dependent on both the dose and duration of therapy used (99). Oral steroids have also been demonstrated to prevent the airway hyperresponsiveness associated with the grass pollen season in sensitized subjects (100). A recent comparative crossover study showed inhaled steroids to improve airway responsiveness whereas no benefit was found from inhaled cromoglycate (101).

Late Asthmatic Reaction

The late asthmatic response, and the subsequent increase in airway responsiveness, induced by both allergen and chemical challenge in sensitized subjects and animals has been shown to be inhibited by both oral and inhaled steroids (65, 84,88,102-104), even after as little as a single low dose of inhaled therapy immediately prechallenge (65,103).

Proinflammatory Mediators

Human and rat pulmonary macrophage production of thromboxane and leukotriene B_4 have been inhibited by preincubation of the cells with corticosteroids for both 1 and 16 hours (105,106), and human peripheral blood granulocytes have shown a reduced production of leukotriene C_4 following the treatment of chronic asthma with oral prednisolone for one week (93). Corticosteroids have also been shown to inhibit the in vitro release of leukotrienes, prostaglandins, and thromboxane from stimulated human (107) and guinea pig (108) lung strips, and rat lungs (109), and more recently to reduce the level of mediators in nasal washings after allergen challenge (110).

Inhaled Cromoglycate and Nedocromil

Airway Inflammation

In the only study to directly examine the effect of asthma treatment on the inflammatory cell profile in the airways, Diaz et al. showed that four weeks treatment with cromoglycate reduced the bronchoalveolar lavage eosinophilia and the IgA/albumin ratio, but had no effect on other cell populations (111). The effect of treatment on the activity or function of the inflammatory cells obtained was not examined. In vitro incubation of pulmonary macrophages from asthmatics with nedocromil has been found to reduce their production of leukotriene B_4 (112), but not thromboxane (113).

In sensitized guinea pigs, nedocromil given prior to allergen challenge inhibited the bronchoalveolar neutrophilia of the late asthmatic response, without influencing the eosinophilia, whereas when given after the challenge the eosinophilia, but not the neutrophilia, was inhibited. A greater inhibition of the late response was shown when treatment was given following the challenge, i.e., in association with inhibition of the eosinophila influx (114). In other models nedocromil has been found to inhibit the increased permeability of anaphylactic injury (115).

Airway Responsiveness

There are conflicting reports of the efficacy of cromoglycate treatment on baseline airway hyperresponsiveness in asthma. Studies of one to twelve months in duration have demonstrated no improvement (101,116,117), although Lowhagen and Rak found an improvement in more than half their group (116), while one three-month study did report that cromoglycate was effective in reducing hyperresponsiveness (79). During the grass pollen season, both cromoglycate and nedocromil were effective in preventing the increase in hyperresponsiveness that usually occurs in sensitized patients (118,119), although the effect of nedocromil was not marked.

Late Asthmatic Reaction

Both cromoglycate and nedocromil inhibited the late asthmatic response to allergen challenge (65,103,120) in acute dosing studies, although in children the late response was only delayed in onset, with no effect on the magnitude of the response (121). Cromoglycate has also been reported to inhibit the increase in airway responsiveness seen after allergen challenge (65,121). Following one week of treatment with cromoglycate, the late response to toluene diisocyanate was not found to be affected in sensitized subjects (84), nor was there inhibition of the associated increase in airway hyperresponsiveness. Inhibition of both the late contractile response and the rise in airway responsiveness occurred in a sensitized sheep model following therapy with cromoglycate and nedocromil (122,123).

Proinflammatory Mediators

The activation of pulmonary macrophages was inhibited in vitro by nedocromil, with a reduction of the respiratory burst and lysosomal enzyme release (124), and inhibition of leukotriene production (112). However, neither cromoglycate nor nedocromil inhibited the production of thromboxane by pulmonary macrophages in vitro (113,125). Peripheral blood neutrophil and eosinophil activation have been inhibited in vitro by both cromoglycate and nedocromil (126–128), although both agents were less potent inhibitors of mast cell histamine release in vitro (128,129). Platelet activation was inhibited in vivo by cromoglycate during exercise-induced asthma (130), although salbutamol also had a similar effect.

Ketotifen

Airway Inflammation

In a baboon model, ketotifen was found to prevent the development of a bronchoalveolar eosinophilia following challenge with platelet activating factor (131), but no studies have been performed following allergen challenge. In humans, three weeks of treatment with ketotifen has been shown to decrease the number of neutrophils, eosinophils and bronchial epithelial cells in sputum (132), although more direct studies of bronchoalveolar lavage or airway biopsies have not been performed.

Airway Responsiveness

Two studies of three months duration reached opposite conclusions regarding the effect of ketotifen on airway hyperresponsiveness: in children no effect of ketotifen was found (133), but in adults a significant improvement was demonstrated (134), albeit with an unusual method of acetylcholine challenge. Platelet activating factor-induced increases in airway responsiveness have been inhibited by ketotifen in guinea pigs (135), but not in humans (136).

Late Asthmatic Reactions

A similar impasse is also found concerning possible effects on the late response. Both European and Australasian studies have shown no inhibition of the late response (137,138), whereas a Japanese study reported ketotifen to be as effective as cromoglycate in inhibiting late responses to allergen challenge (139).

Proinflammatory Mediators

The metabolic activity of human pulmonary macrophages has been inhibited by ketotifen in vitro (140), and a reduction in leukotriene, thromboxane and prostaglandin E_2 production by rat pulmonary macrophages has also been reported (141). Leukotriene release from human granulocytes has also been inhibited (142), although no such inhibition was observed following antigen challenge of sensitized rat lungs (109). A similar paradox has also been described for histamine release, with inhibition of histamine release from isolated basophils but no inhibition from chopped lung preparations (143).

Others

Alternative therapies, such as gold salts, antihistamines (H_1), and leukotriene receptor antagonists, are now available for the treatment of asthma in Japan, although they are still undergoing evaluation elsewhere. Little information is

TABLE 6 Efficacy of "Prophylactic" Treatments Used Worldwide as Assessed by Their Effect on Manifestations of Airway Inflammation

	Biopsies	BAL	AHR	LAR	Mediators
β_2-agonists	?	0	0/–	0	0
Anticholinergics	?	?	?	0	?
Methylxanthines	?	[+]	0	(+)/0	+
Inhaled steroids	+	[+]	+	+	+
Cromolyn/nedocromil	?	+	+/0	+/0	+/0
Ketotifen	?	[+]	+/0	+/0	+/0
Others	?	?	(+)	?	?

Key: + improvement; – deterioration; 0 no effect; ? no data.
Abbreviations: BAL, bronchoalveolar lavage; [ ] for changes with LAR; AHR, airway hyperresponsiveness; LAR, late asthmatic response to allergen challenge (including increased responsiveness); Mediators, phospholipid-derived proinflammatory mediators.

available regarding their effects on the manifestations of inflammation in asthma as listed in Table 1. However, a significant reduction in airway hyperresponsiveness was reported in half the patients treated with oral gold in an open study (144).

Summary

The effects on airway inflammation of the treatments commonly used throughout the world in the prophylaxis of asthma are summarized in Table 6. From this inhaled steroids can be judged to be the most efficacious prophylactic therapy for asthma, given our current knowledge and assuming an inflammatory pathophysiological basis for the disease.

RATIONAL CHOICE OF THE PROPHYLACTIC TREATMENT OF ASTHMA

If airway inflammation is a fundamental characteristic of asthma, then we should logically choose as prophylaxis a therapy which has been shown to reduce it. Table 6 provides a summary of the anti-inflammatory profiles of the "prophylactic" therapies in common use worldwide. In Table 7 treatments have been listed in order of their proven anti-inflammatory efficacy, with inhaled corticosteroids clearly at the head of the list. This should therefore provide us with a rational order of choice for the prophylactic treatment of asthma.

However, there are obviously great discrepancies between the order listed in Table 7 and the order of both treatment sales outlined in Table 2 and the order of choice expressed by physicians in Europe and the United States, as listed in

TABLE 7 Rational Order of Choice of the Prophylactic Therapy of Asthma Based Upon Proven Anti-inflammatory Effects

1. Inhaled steroids
2. Inhaled cromoglycate/nedocromil
3. Ketotifen[a]
4. Methylxanthines[a]
5. β_2-agonists[b]

[a]Some evidence for anti-inflammatory effects.
[b]Little evidence for anti-inflammatory effects.

Tables 4 and 5 for adults and children. The most notable contrast is provided by the high placing of regularly taken β_2-agonists in the "prophylaxis" of asthma throughout the world and the virtual lack of evidence as to their exerting an anti-inflammatory influence in asthma. Methylxanthines are commonly used in continental Europe, the United States, and Japan, yet their apparent efficacy as anti-inflammatory agents is low in comparison with that of inhaled steroids, whose use is low in these countries. Even in the United Kingdom, Scandinavia, and Australasia, where inhaled steroids are most frequently used, they are still a second choice to the use of regular inhaled β_2-agonists. The closest that practice approaches the rational choice of prophylaxis is in the treatment of children in Europe, where inhaled cromoglycate is rated as the first choice therapy, and this should be commended, although it could be argued that inhaled steroids would be even more effective.

Cultural factors may influence our prescribing practice, and a lack of patient compliance may reduce the prevalence of effective prophylactic practice, but if the current morbidity and mortality of our patients is to be improved, then surely we should follow the advice of earlier studies (35,36,39,49) and make greater efforts to promote the acceptance of efficaceous anti-inflammatory therapies delivered topically to the airways, especially inhaled corticosteroids in adult asthmatics, but also possibly cromoglycate and nedocromil, and reduce dependence on combinations of bronchodilators. We should also educate our patients more on the need for prophylactic treatment by increasing their understanding of asthma as an inflammatory disease of the airways: the bulk of the iceberg below the waterline, compared with the visible peak representing bronchospasm. Unfortunately, the results of one such attempt in general practice in the United Kingdom has not proved promising (145), although with a growing social awareness of health issues this situation may change both in the United Kingdom and worldwide.

REFERENCES

1. Floyer J. *A Treatise of the Asthma*. London, R. Wilkin, 1726.
2. Aretaeus (translated by Adams F). *The Extant Works of Aretaeus, the Cappadocian*. London, Syndenham Society, 1856, pp. 255-258.
3. Nadel JA. Inflammation and asthma. J Allergy Clin Immunol 1984; 73: 651-653.
4. Chung KF. Role of inflammation in the hyperreactivity of the airways in asthma. Thorax 1986;41:657-661.
5. Barnes PJ. The changing face of asthma. Q J Med 1987; 63:359-365.
6. Holgate ST, Finnerty JP. Recent advances in understanding the pathogenesis of asthma and its clinical implications. Q J Med 1988; 66:5-19.
7. Reed CE. Basic mechanisms of asthma. Role of inflammation. Chest 1988; 94:175-177.
8. Dunnill M. *Pulmonary Pathology*. Edinburgh, Churchill Livingston, 1987; pp. 61-79.
9. Cutz E, Levison H, Cooper DM. Ultrastructure in airways in children with asthma. Histopathology 1978;2:407-411.
10. Holtzman MJ, Fabbri LM, O'Byrne PM, Gold BD, Aizawa H, Walters EH, Alpert SE, Nadel JA. Importance of airway inflammation for hyperresponsiveness induced by ozone. Am Rev Respir Dis 1983; 127:686-690.
11. Hutson PA, Church MK, Clay TP, Miller P, Holgate ST. Early and late-phase bronchoconstriction after allergen challenge of nonanaesthetized guinea pigs. The association of disordered airway physiology to leukocyte infiltration. Am Rev REspir Dis 1988; 137:548-557.
12. Bacci E, Paggiaro PL, Paoletti P, Bernard P, Dente FL, Talini D, Marchetti G, Menconi G, Guintini C. Morphological findings in toluene-diisocyanate asthmatic patients. Am Rev Respir Dis 1988; 137:A296.
13. Beasley RC, Roberts JA, Roche WM, Holgate ST. Bronchial lavage and biopsy findings before and after allergen challenge in mild atopic asthma. Thorax 1988;43:812P.
14. Kelly CA, Ward C, Stenton SC, Bird G, Hendrick DJ, Walters EH. Number and activity of inflammatory cells in bronchoalveolar lavage fluid in asthma and their relation to airway responsiveness. Thorax 1988; 43:684-692.
15. Wardlaw AJ, Dunnette S, Gleich GJ, Collins JV, Kay AB. Eosinophils and mast cells in bronchoalveolar lavage in subjects with mild asthma. Relationship to bronchial hyperreactivity. Am Rev Respir Dis 1988; 137:62-69.
16. Chan-Yeung M, LeRiche J, Maclean L, Lam S. Comparison of cellular and protein changes in bronchial lavage fluid of symptomatic and asymptomatic patients with red cedar asthma on follow-up examination. Clin Allergy 1988; 18:359-365.
17. Kirby JG, Hargreave FB, Gleich G, O'Byrne PM. Bronchoalveolar lavage cell profiles of asthmatic and non-asthmatic subjects. Am Rev Respir Dis 1987; 136:379-383.

18. Flint KC, Leung KBP, Hudspith BN, Brostoff J, Pearce FL, Johnson NM. Bronchoalveolar mast cells in extrinsic asthma: a mechanism for the initiation of antigen specific bronchoconstriction. Br Med J 1985; 291:923-926.
19. Godard P, Aubas P, Calvayrac P, Taib J, Michel FB. Endoscopie et lavage bronchoalveolaire chez l'asthmatique allergique. Nouv Presse Med 1981; 10:3141-3148.
20. Kelly CA, Stenton SC, Ward C, Bird G, Hendrick DJ, Walters EH. Lymphocyte subsets in bronchoalveolar lavage fluid obtained from stable asthmatics, and their correlations with bronchial responsiveness. Clinical Experimental Allergy 1989; 19:169-175.
21. Holgate ST, Beasley R, Twentyman OP. The pathogenesis and significance of bronchial hyperresponsiveness in airways disease. Clin Science 1987; 73:561-572.
22. De Monchy JGR, Kauffman HF, Venge P, Koeter GH, Jansen HM, Sluiter HJ, de Vries K. Bronchoalveolar eosinophilia during allergen-induced late asthmatic reaction. Am Rev Respir Dis 1985; 131:373-376.
23. Metzger WJ, Zavala D, Richerson HB, Moseley P, Iwamota P, Monick M, Sjoerdsma K, Hunninghake GW. Local allergen challenge and bronchoalveolar lavage of allergic asthmatic lungs. Description of the model and local airway inflammation. Am Rev Respir Dis 1987; 135:433-440.
24. Lam S, LeRiche J, Phillips D, Chan H, Chan-Yeung M. Cellular and protein changes in bronchial lavage fluid following late asthmatic reaction in patients with red cedar asthma. J Allergy Clin Immunol 1987; 80:44-50.
25. Fabbri LM, Boschetto P, Zocca E, Milani G, Pivirotto F, Plebani M, Burlina A, Licata B, Mapp CE. Bronchoalveolar neutrophilia during late asthmatic reactions induced by toluene diisocyanate. Am Rev Respir Dis 1987; 136: 36-42.
26. O'Byrne PM, Dolovich J, Hargreave FE. Late asthmatic responses. Am Rev Respir Dis 1987; 136:740-751.
27. Godard P, Bousquet J, Lebel B, Michel FB. Le lavage bronchoalveolaire chez l'asthmatic. Bull Eur Physiopathol Respir 1987; 23:73-83.
28. Arnoux B, Joseph M, Simoes MH, Tonnel AB, Duroux P, Capron A, Benveniste J. Antigenic release of PAF-acether and β-glucuronidase from alveolar macrophages of asthmatics. Bull Eur Physiopathol Respir 1987; 23:119-124.
29. MacDermot J, Fuller RW. Macrophages. In: *Asthma: Basic Mechanisms and Clinical Management*. Barnes PJ, Rodger IW, Thomson NC, eds. London, Academic Press, 1988; pp 97-113.
30. Ferguson AC. Persisting airway obstruction in asymptomatic children with asthma with normal peak expiratory flow rates. J Allergy Clin Immunol 1988; 82:19-22.
31. Canny GJ, Levison H. Pulmonary function abnormalities during apparent clinical remission in childhood asthma. J Allergy Clin Immunol 1988; 82:1-4.
32. Canny GJ, Levison H. Management of asthma. A Canadian perspective. Chest 1986; 90:46S-52S.

33. Newhouse MT, Dolovich MB. Control of asthma by aerosols. N Engl J Med 1986;315:870-874.
34. Barnes PJ, Chung KF, Page CP. Platelet activating factor as a mediator of allergic disease. J Allergy Clin Immunol 1988;81:919-934.
35. British Thoracic Association. Death from asthma in two regions of England. Br Med J 1982;285:1251-1255.
36. Stableforth D. Death from asthma. Thorax 1983;38:801-805.
37. Reed CE. New therapeutic approaches in asthma. J Allergy Clin Immunol 1986;77:537-543.
38. Buist AS. Is asthma mortality increasing? Chest 1988;93:449-450.
39. Robin ED. Death from bronchial asthma. Chest 1988;93:614-618.
40. Keating G, Mitchell EA, Jackson R, Beaglehole R, Rea H. Trends in sales of drugs for asthma in New Zealand, Australia, and the United Kingdom, 1975-81. Br Med J 1984;289:348-351.
41. Bosco LA, Knapp DE, Gerstman B, Graham CF. Asthma drug therapy trends in the United States, 1972 to 1985. J Allergy Clin Immunol 1987; 80:398-402.
42. Marsac J. French audit of asthma therapy. Chest 1986;90:78S-80S.
43. Haynes RL, Ingram RH, McFadden ER. An assessment of the pulmonary response to exercise in asthma and an analysis of the factors influencing it. Am Rev Respir Dis 1976;116:739-752.
44. Jenkins PF, Benfield GFA, Smith AP. Predicting recovery from acute severe asthma. Thorax 1981;36:835-841.
45. Miyamoto T. Treatment of bronchial asthma in Japan. Chest 1986; 90: 71S-73S.
46. Vermeire PA. *A European Audit of Asthma Diagnosis and Treatment*. London, Castle Press, 1985.
47. Vermeire P. A European audit of asthma diagnosis and treatment based on the ESP asthma questionnaire. In: *Asthma and Bronchial Hyperreactivity*. Progress in respiratory research. Vol 19. Herzof H, Perruchoud AP, eds. Basel, Karger, 1985; pp 476-480.
48. Vermeire PA, Wittesaele WM, Janssens E, de Backer WA. European audit of asthma therapy. Chest 1986;90:58S-61S.
49. Hodgkin JE. United States audit of asthma therapy. Chest 1986; 90:62S-66S.
50. Grant IWB, Mosbech H, Weeke B. Does immunotherapy have a role in the treatment of asthma? Clin Allergy 1986;16:7-16.
51. Bousquet J, Michel FB. Allergen avoidance and immunotherapy. In: *Asthma: Basic Mechanisms and Clinical Management*. Barnes PJ, Rodger IW, Thomson NC, eds. London, Academic Press, 1988; pp 551-562.
52. Persson CGA, Ekman M, Erjefalt I. Terbutaline preventing permeability effects of histamine in the lung. Acta Pharmacol Toxicol 1978; 42:395-397.
53. Mizus I, Summer W, Farrukh I, Michael JR, Gurtner GH. Isoproterenol or aminophylline attenuate pulmonary edema after acid lung injury. Am Rev Respir Dis 1985;131:256-259.

54. Persson NH, Erlansson M, Bergqvist D, Takolander R, Svensjo E. Terbutaline and budesonide as inhibitors of postischaemic permeability increase. Acta Physiol Scand 1987; 129:517-524.
55. Braude S, Royston D. Infused salbutamol accentuates acid-induced lung injury in the rat. Clin Sci 1986; 71:205-209.
56. Phipps RJ, Williams IP, Richardson PS, Pell J, Pack RJ, Wright N. Sympathomimetic drugs stimulate the output of secretory glycoproteins from human bronchi *in vitro*. Clin Sci 1982; 63:23-28.
57. Borson B, Nadel J. Neurophysiological control of airway secretions in experimental animals. Am Rev Respir Dis 1986; 134:614-617.
58. Fuller RW, O'Malley G, Baker AJ, MacDermot J. β-adrenoceptor stimulation does not inhibit activation of human alveolar macrophages. Am Rev Respir Dis 1987; 135:A206.
59. Cockcroft DW, Killian DN, Mellon JJA, Hargreave FE. Protective effect of drugs on histamine-induced asthma. Thorax 1977; 32:429-437.
60. Salome CM, Schoeffel RE, Yan K, Woolcock AJ. Effect of aerosol fenoterol on the severity of bronchial hyperreactivity in patients with asthma. Thorax 1983; 38:854-858.
61. Britton J, Hanley SP, Garrett HV, Hadfield JW, Tattersfield AE. Dose related effects of salbutamol and ipratropium bromide on airway reactivity in subjects with asthma. Thorax 1988; 43:300-305.
62. Peel ET, Gibson GJ. Effects of long-term inhaled therapy on the provocation of asthma by histamine. Am Rev Respir Dis 1980; 121:973-978.
63. Kraan J, Koeter GH, Mark TW, Sluiter HJ, de Vries K. Changes in bronchial hyperreactivity induced by 4 weeks of treatment with anti-asthmatic drugs in patients with allergic asthma: A comparison between budesonide and terbutaline. J Allergy Clin Immunol 1985; 76:628-636.
64. Kerrebijn KF, van Essen-Zandvliet EEM, Neijens HJ. Effect of long-term treatment with inhaled corticosteroids and beta-agonists on the bronchial responsiveness in children with asthma. J Allergy Clin Immunol 1987; 79:653-659.
65. Cockcroft DW, Murdock KY. Comparative effects of inhaled salbutamol, sodium cromoglycate, and beclomethasone dipropioate on allergen-induced early asthmatic responses, late asthmatic responses, and increased bronchial responsiveness to histamine. J Allergy Clin Immunol 1987; 79:734-740.
66. Walters EH, Bevan M, Davies BH. Interactions between response to inhaled prostaglandin E_2 in human airways and chronic β-adrenergic agonist therapy with inhaled salbutamol. Thorax 1982; 37:430-437.
67. Vathenen AS, Knox AJ, Higgins BG, Britton JR, Tattersfield AE. Rebound increase in bronchial responsiveness after treatment with inhaled terbutaline. Lancet 1988; i:554-558.
68. Hegardt B, Pauwels R, Van der Straten M. Inhibitory effect of KWC2131, terbutaline and DSCG on the immediate and late allergen-induced bronchoconstriction. Allergy 1981; 36:115-122.
69. Kay AB. The mode of action of anti-allergic drugs. Clin Allergy 1987; 17:153-164.

70. Howarth PH, Durham SR, Lee TH, Kay AB, Church MK, Holgate ST. Influence of albuterol, cromolyn sodium and ipratropium bromide on the airway and circulating mediator responses to allergen bronchial provocation in asthma. Am Rev Respir Dis 1985; 132:986-992.
71. Cockcroft DW, Ruffin RE, Hargreave FE. Effect of Sch 1000 in allergen-induced asthma. Clin Allergy 1978; 8:361-372.
72. Andersson P, Brange C, Sonmark B, Stahre G, Erjefalt I, Wieslander E, Persson CGA. Anti-anaphylactic and anti-inflammatory effects of xanthines in the lung. In: *Anti-asthma Xanthines and Adenosine*. Andersson KE, Persson CGA, eds. Amsterdam, Excerpta Medica, 1985; pp 187-191.
73. Persson CGA, Erjefalt I, Andersson P. Leakage of macromolecules from the guinea pig tracheobronchial microcirculation: effects of allergen, leukotrienes, tachykinins and antiasthma drugs. Acta Physiol Scand 1986; 127: 95-105.
74. Erjefalt I, Persson CGA. Antiasthma drugs attenuate inflammatory leakage of plasma into airway lumen. Acta Physiol Scand 1986; 128:653-654.
75. Nielson CP, Crowley JJ, Morgan ME, Vestal RE. Polymorphonuclear leukocyte inhibition by therapeutic concentrations of theophylline is mediated by cyclic-3′,5′-adenosine monophosphate. Am Rev Respir Dis 1988; 137:25-30.
76. O'Neill SJ, Sitar DS, Klass DJ, Taraska VA, Kepron W, Mitenko PA. The pulmonary disposition of theophylline and its influence on human alveolar macrophage bactericidal function. Am Rev Respir Dis 1986; 134:1225-1228.
77. Shohat B, Volovitz B, Varsano I. Induction of suppressor T cells in asthmatic children by theophylline treatment. Clin Allergy 1983; 13:487-493.
78. Fink G, Mittelman M, Shohat B, Spitzer SA. Theophylline-induced alterations in cellular immunity in asthmatic patients. Clin Allergy 1987; 17: 313-316.
79. Furukawa CT, Shapiro GG, Bierman CW, Kraemer MJ, Ward DJ, Pierson WE. A double-blind study comparing the effectiveness of cromolyn sodium and sustained-release theophylline in childhood asthma. Pediatrics 1984; 74:453-459.
80. Dutoit JI, Salome CM, Woolcock AJ. Inhaled corticosteroids reduce the severity of bronchial responsiveness in asthma but oral theophylline does not. Am Rev Respir Dis 1987; 136:1174-1178.
81. Pauwels R, van Renterghem D, van der Straeten M, Johannesson N, Persson CGA. The effect of theophylline and enprofylline on allergen-induced bronchoconstriction. J Allergy Clin Immunol 1985; 76:583-590.
82. Crescioli S, Spinazzi A, Paleari D, Pozzan M, Mapp CE, Fabbri LM. Theophylline inhibits early and late asthmatic reactions induced by allergens in atopic subjects with asthma. Am Rev Respir Dis 1988; 137:A35.
83. Cockcroft DW, Murdock KY, Gore BP, O'Byrne PM, Manning PJ. Theophylline does not inhibit allergen-induced increases in airway response to methacholine. J Allergy Clin Immunol 1989; 83:913-920.
84. Mapp C, Boschetto P, dal Vecchio L, Crescioli S, de Marzo N, Paleari D,

Fabbri LM. Protective effect of antiasthma drugs on late asthmatic reactions and increased airway responsiveness induced by toluene diisocyanate in sensitized subjects. Am Rev Respir Dis 1987; 136:1403-1407.
85. Martin GL, Atkins PC, Dunsky EH, Zweiman B. Effects of theophylline, terbutaline, and prednisone on antigen-induced bronchospasm and mediator release. J Allergy Clin Immunol 1980; 66:204-212.
86. Lundgren R. Scanning electron microscopic studies of bronchial mucosa before and during treatment with beclomethasone dipropionate inhalations. Scand J Resp Dis 1977; (Suppl.) 101:179-187.
87. Heino M, Karjalainen J, Ylikoski J, Laitinen A, Laitinen LA. Bronchial ciliogenesis and oral steroid treatment in patients with asthma. Br J Dis Chest 1988; 82:175-178.
88. Boschetto P, Fabbri LM, Zocca E, Milani G, Pivirotto F, dal Vecchio A, Plebani M, Mapp CE. Prednisone inhibits late asthmatic reactions and airway inflammation induced by toluene diisocyanate in sensitized subjects. J Allergy Clin Immunol 1987; 80:261-267.
89. Svensjo E, Roempke K. Time dependent inhibition of bradykinin and histamine induced increase in microvascular permeability by local glucocorticosteroid treatment. In: *Glucocorticosteroids, Inflammation and Bronchial Hyperreactivity*. Hogg JC, Ellul-Micallef R, Brattsand R, eds. Amsterdam, Excerpta Medica, 1984; pp 136-153.
90. Lundgren JD, Hirata F, Marom Z, Logun C, Steel L, Kaliner M, Shelhamer J. Dexamethasone inhibits respiratory glycoconjugate secretion from feline airways in vitro by the induction of lipocortin (lipomodulin) synthesis. Am Rev Respir Dis 1988; 137:353-357.
91. Agnew JE, Bateman JRM, Pavia D, Clarke SW. Peripheral airways mucus clearance in stable asthma is improved by oral corticosteroid therapy. Bull Eur Physiopathol Respir 1984; 20:295-301.
92. Ellul-Micallef R. Glucocorticosteroids–the pharmacological basis of their therapeutic use in bronchial asthma. In: *Asthma: Basic Mechanisms and Clinical Management*. Barnes PJ, Rodger IW, Thomson NC, eds. London, Academic Press, 1988; pp 653-691.
93. Gin W, Shaw RJ, Kay AB. Airways reversibility after prednisolone therapy in chronic asthma is associated with alterations in leukocyte function. Am Rev Respir Dis 1985; 132:1199-1203.
94. Juniper EF, Frith PA, Hargreave FE. Long-term stability of bronchial responsiveness to histamine. Thorax 1982; 37:288-291.
95. Ryan G, Latimer KM, Juniper EF, Roberts RS, Hargreave FE. Effect of beclomethasone dipropionate on bronchial responsiveness to histamine in controlled nonsteroid-dependent asthma. J Allergy Clin Immunol 1985; 75:25-30.
96. Bhagat RG, Grunstein MM. Effect of corticosteroids on bronchial responsiveness to methacholine in asthmatic children. Am Rev Respir Dis 1985; 131:902-906.
97. Jenkins CR, Woolcock AJ. Effect of prednisolone and beclomethasone dipropionate on airway responsiveness in asthma: a comparative study. Thorax 1988; 43:378-384.

98. Easton JG. Effect of an inhaled corticosteroid on methacholine airway reactivity. J Allergy Clin Immunol 1981; 67:388–390.
99. Kraan J, Koeter GH, Van der Mark ThW, Boorsma M, Kukler J, Sluiter HJ, de Vries K. Dosage and time effects of inhaled budesonide on bronchial hyperreactivity. Am Rev Respir Dis 1988; 137:44–48.
100. Sotomayor H, Badier M, Vervloet D, Orehek J. Seasonal increase of carbachol airway responsiveness in patients allergic to grass pollen. Reversal by corticosteroids. Am Rev Respir Dis 1984; 130:56–58.
101. Svendsen UG, Frolund L, Madsen F, Nielson NH, Holstein-Rathlou NH, Weeke B. A comparison of the effects of sodium cromoglycate and beclomethasone dipropionate on pulmonary function and bronchial hyperreactivity in subjects with asthma. J Allergy Clin Immunol 1987; 80:68–74.
102. Fabbri LM, Chiesura-Corona P, dal Vecchio L, di Giacomo GR, Zocca E, de Marzo N, Maestrelli P, Mapp CE. Prednisone inhibits late asthmatic reactions and the associated increase in airway responsiveness induced by toluene diisocyanate in sensitized subjects. Am Rev Respir Dis 1985; 132:1010–1014.
103. Pelikan Z, Pelikan-Filipek M, Remeijer L. Effects of disodium cromoglycate and beclomethasone dipropionate on the asthmatic response to allergen challenge. II. Late response. Ann Allergy 1988; 60:217–225.
104. Abraham WM, Lanes S, Stevenson JS, Yerger LD. Effect of an inhaled glucocorticosteroid (budesonide) on post-allergen induced increases in airway responsiveness. Bull Eur Physiopathol Respir 1986; 22:387–392.
105. Fuller RW, Kelsey CR, Cole PJ, Dollery CT, MacDermot J. Dexamethasone inhibits the production of thromboxane B_2 and leukotriene B_4 by human alveolar and peritoneal macrophages in culture. Clin Sci 1984; 67:653–656.
106. Peters-Golden M, Thebert P. Inhibition by methylprednisolone of zymosan-induced leukotriene synthesis in alveolar macrophages. Am Rev Respir Dis 1987; 135:1020–1026.
107. Schleimer RP, Schulman ES, MacGashan DW, Peter SP, Hayes EC, Adams GK, Lichtenstein LM, Adkinson NF. Effect of dexamethasone on mediator release from human lung fragments and purified human lung mast cells. J Clin Invest 1983; 71:1830–1835.
108. Schleimer RP, Undem BJ, Meeker S, Bollinger ME, Adkinson NF, Lichtenstein LM, Adams GK. Dexamethasone inhibits the antigen-induced contractile activity and release of inflammatory mediators in isolated guinea pig lung tissue. Am Rev Respir Dis 1987; 135:562–566.
109. Ottenhof M, Ufkes JGR, van Rooij HH. The effect of prednisolone and ketotifen on the antigen-induced bronchoconstriction and mediator release in rat isolated lungs. Br J Pharmacol 1985; 86:627–636.
110. Pipkorn U, Proud D, Lichtenstein LM, Kagey-Sobotka A, Norman PS, Naclerio RM. Inhibition of mediator release in allergic rhinitis by pretreatment with topical glucocorticosteroids. N Engl J Med 1987; 316: 1506–1510.
111. Diaz P, Galleguillos FR, Gonzalez MC, Pantin CFA, Kay AB. Broncho-

alveolar lavage in asthma: the effect of disodium cromoglycate (cromolyn) on leukocyte counts, immunoglobulins, and complement. J Allergy Clin Immunol 1984; 74:41–48.

112. Godard P, Chavis C, Daures JP, Crastes de Paulet A, Michel FB, Damon M. Leukotriene B_4 and 5-HETE release by alveolar macrophages in asthmatic patients: inhibition by nedocromil sodium. Am Rev Respir Dis 1987; 135:A318.

113. Damon M, Chavis C, Crastes de Paulet A, Michel FB, Godard P. Effect of nedocromil sodium on TXB_2, LTB_4 and LTD_4 synthesis by alveolar macrophages from asthmatic patients. Eur J Respir Dis 1986; 69(Suppl 147):206–209.

114. Hutson PA, Holgate ST, Church MK. Inhibition by nedocromil sodium of early and late phase bronchoconstriction and airway cellular infiltration provoked by ovalbumin inhalation in conscious sensitized guinea-pigs. Br J Pharmacol 1988; 94:6–8.

115. Evans TW, Rogers DF, Roberts NM, Chung KF, Barnes PJ. Mediators of increased vascular permeability during anaphylaxis in sensitized guinea-pigs. Thorax 1987; 42:221P.

116. Lowhagen O, Rak S. Bronchial hyperreactivity after treatment with sodium cromoglycate in atopic asthmatic patients not exposed to relevant allergens. J Allergy Clin Immunol 1985; 75:343–347.

117. Jenkins CJ, Breslin ABX. Long term study of the effect of sodium cromoglycate on non-specific bronchial hyperresponsiveness. Thorax 1987; 42:664–669.

118. Lowhagen O, Rak S. Modification of bronchial hyperreactivity after treatment with sodium cromoglycate during pollen season. J Allergy Clin Immunol 1985; 75:460–467.

119. Dorward AJ, Roberts JA, Thomson NC. Effect of nedocromil sodium on histamine airway responsiveness in grass-pollen sensitive asthmatics during the pollen season. Clin Allergy 1986; 16:309–315.

120. Shaw RJ, Youngchaiyud P, Orr TSC, Wells E, Greenwood B, Lee TB, Kay AB. Nedocromil, a mucosal and connective tissue mast cell stabilizer, inhibits allergen and exercise induced asthma. Br J Dis Chest 1985; 79: 385–389.

121. Mattoli S, Foresi A, Corbo GM, Valente S, Ciappi G. Effects of two doses of cromolyn on allergen-induced late asthmatic response and increased responsiveness. J Allergy Clin Immunol 1987; 79:747–754.

122. Abraham WM, Stevenson JS, Chapman GA, Tallent MW, Jackowski J. The effect of nedocromil sodium and cromolyn sodium on antigen-induced responses in allergic sheep in vivo and in vitro. Chest 1987; 92: 913–917.

123. Abraham WM, Stevenson JS, Tallent M. Effect of nedocromil sodium on antigen-induced airways responsiveness in allergic sheep. Am Rev Respir Dis 1987; 135:A318.

124. Thorel T, Joseph M, Tonnel AB, Capron A. Inhibition by nedocromil

sodium of IgE-mediated activation of human mononuclear phagocytes and platelets in allergy. Int Arch Allergy Appl Immunol 1988; 85:232–237.

125. Fuller RW, MacDermot J. Stimulation of IgE sensitized human alveolar macrophages by anti-IgE is unaffected by sodium cromoglycate. Clin Allergy 1986; 16:523–526.
126. Moqbel R, Walsh GM, MacDonald AJ, Kay AB. Effect of disodium cromoglycate on activation of human eosinophils and neutrophils following reversed (anti-IgE) anaphylaxis. Clin Allergy 1986; 16:73–83.
127. Kay AB, Walsh GM, Moqbel R, MacDonald AJ, Nagakura T, Carroll MP, Richerson HB. Disodium cromoglycate inhibits activation of human inflammatory cells in vitro. J Allergy Clin Immunol 1987; 80:1–8.
128. Moqbel R, Cromwell O, Walsh GM, Wardlaw AJ, Kurlak L, Kay AB. Effects of nedocromil sodium (Tilade) on the activation of human eosinophils and neutrophils and the release of histamine from mast cells. Allergy 1988; 43:268–276.
129. Flint KC, Leung KBP, Pearce FL, Hudspith BN, Brostoff J, Johnson NM. Human mast cells recovered by bronchoalveolar lavage: their morphology, histamine release and the effects of sodium cromoglycate. Clin Sci 1985; 68:427–432.
130. Johnson CE, Belfield PW, Davis S, Cooke NJ, Spencer A, Davies JA. Platelet activation during exercise induced asthma: effect of prophylaxis with cromoglycate and salbutamol. Thorax 1986; 41:290–294.
131. Arnoux B, Denjean A, Page CP, Nolibe D, Morley J, Benveniste J. Accumulation of platelets and eosinophils in baboon lung after PAF-acether challenge. Inhibition by ketotifen. Am Rev Respir Dis 1988; 137:855–860.
132. Radielovic P, Steiner A. Short-term effects of ketotifen in chronic bronchial asthma. Am Rev Respir Dis 1980; 121:A85.
133. Graff-Lonnevig V, Hedlin G. The effect of ketotifen on bronchial hyperreactivity in childhood asthma. J Allergy Clin Immunol 1985; 76:59–63.
134. Girard JP. Ketotifen and bronchial hyperreactivity in asthmatic patients. Clin Allergy 1981; 11:449–452.
135. Mazzoni L, Morley J, Page CP, Sanjar S. Prophylactic anti-asthma drugs impair the airway hyper-reactivity that follows exposure to platelet activating factor. Br J Pharmacol 1985; 86:571P.
136. Chung KF, Minette P, McCusker M, Barnes PJ. Ketotifen inhibits the cutaneous but not the airway responses to platelet-activating factor in man. J Allergy Clin Immunol 1988; 81:1192–1198.
137. Pelikan Z, Pelikan M. Early and late asthmatic response to allergen challenge and their pharmacological modulation. Ann Allergy 1985; 55:318.
138. Wells A, Taylor B. A placebo-controlled trial of ketotifen (HC 20-511, Sandoz) in allergen induced asthma and comparison with disodium cromoglycate. Clin Allergy 1979; 9:237–240.
139. Adachi M, Kobayashi H, Aoki N, Iijima M, Kokubu F, Furuya A, Takahashi T. A comparison of the inhibitory effects of ketotifen and disodium

cromoglycate on bronchial responses to house hust, with special reference to the late asthmatic response. Pharmatherapeutica 1984; 4:36–42.
140. Kakuta Y, Kato T, Sasaki H, Takishima T. Effect of ketotifen on human alveolar macrophages. J Allergy Clin Immunol 1988; 81:469–474.
141. Wilhelms OH. Inhibition profiles of picumast and ketotifen on the in vitro release of prostanoids, slow-reacting substance of anaphylaxis, histamine and enzyme from human leukocytes and rat alveolar macrophages. Int Arch Allergy Appl Immunol 1987; 82:547–549.
142. Wang SSM, Wang SR, Shieh WS. The inhibitory effects of ketotifen on SRS activity and SRS production from human leukocytes. J Allergy Clin Immunol 1984; 73:193.
143. Moodley I, Davies RJ. Inhibition and stimulation of mediator release from human leucocytes and chopped human lung by ketotifen. Clin Sci 1982; 62:13P–14P.
144. Bernstein DI, Bernstein IL, Bodenheimer SS, Pietrusko RG. An open study of Auranofin in the treatment of steroid-dependent asthma. J Allergy Clin Immunol 1988; 81:6–16.
145. Modell M, Harding JM, Horder EJ, Williams PR. Improving the care of asthmatic patients in general practice. Br Med J 1983; 286:2027–2030.

Index

About the Editor

Paul M. O'Byrne is Associate Professor in the Department of Medicine, McMaster University, Hamilton, Ontario, Canada. The author or coauthor of many book chapters, abstracts, and articles in peer-reviewed journals, Dr. O'Byrne is Associate Editor of ***Pulmonary Pharmacology***, and serves as a peer reviewer for numerous medical publications. He is a Fellow of the Royal College of Physicians of Canada and Royal College of Physicians of Ireland, member of the American Thoracic Society, American College of Physicians, and Canadian Medical Association, and elected member of the American Physiological Society and Canadian Society for Clinical Investigation. Dr. O'Byrne received the M.B. and B.Ch. degrees (1975) from University College, Dublin, Ireland.